Methods in Molecular Biology

For further volumes:
http://www.springer.com/series/7651

For over 35 years, biological scientists have come to rely on the research protocols and methodologies in the critically acclaimed *Methods in Molecular Biology* series. The series was the first to introduce the step-by-step protocols approach that has become the standard in all biomedical protocol publishing. Each protocol is provided in readily-reproducible step-by-step fashion, opening with an introductory overview, a list of the materials and reagents needed to complete the experiment, and followed by a detailed procedure that is supported with a helpful notes section offering tips and tricks of the trade as well as troubleshooting advice. These hallmark features were introduced by series editor Dr. John Walker and constitute the key ingredient in each and every volume of the *Methods in Molecular Biology* series. Tested and trusted, comprehensive and reliable, all protocols from the series are indexed in PubMed.

Trinucleotide Repeats

Methods and Protocols

Edited by

Guy-Franck Richard

Department Genomes & Genetics, Institut Pasteur, Paris, France

Humana Press

Editor
Guy-Franck Richard
Department Genomes & Genetics
Institut Pasteur
Paris, France

ISSN 1064-3745 ISSN 1940-6029 (electronic)
Methods in Molecular Biology
ISBN 978-1-4939-9783-1 ISBN 978-1-4939-9784-8 (eBook)
https://doi.org/10.1007/978-1-4939-9784-8

Cover illustration: "Trinucleotide repeat secondary structures: an artist view". Original painting by Emily Richard.

This Humana imprint is published by the registered company Springer Science+Business Media, LLC, part of Springer Nature.
The registered company address is: 233 Spring Street, New York, NY 10013, U.S.A.

Preface

Since the discovery of the first human disorder linked to trinucleotide repeat expansions, almost three decades ago, researchers in the field have been fascinated by the unusual properties of these peculiar microsatellites. In order to understand the complex dynamics of trinucleotide repeats, experimental designs were conceived in model systems such as bacteria, yeast, flies, human cells, and transgenic mouse. One aspect of the problem's complexity is reflected by the technical challenges raised by secondary structure-forming repeats and their propensity to contract and expand over time. These will be dealt with in Chapters 1 to 4. Genetic screens in *Saccharomyces cerevisiae* will be described in Chapters 5 to 7, whereas experimental systems to study trinucleotide repeat instability in human cells will be detailed in Chapters 8 to 11. Another aspect of the trinucleotide repeat complexity is displayed by the large collection of tissues and cell types affected by these different pathologies. For instance, in myotonic dystrophy type 1 (Steinert disease), the skeletal muscles, the heart, and the central nervous system are defective, whereas in Friedreich ataxia, neurons of the dorsal root ganglia are the primary affected cells. This variety of tissues led scientists to develop dedicated experimental systems in appropriate cell types. Some of them will be described in Chapters 10, 14, and 15. Finally, tentative gene therapy approaches using the CRISPR-Cas family of endonucleases will be presented in the last two chapters.

We hope that this series of methods and protocols will be valuable to confirmed researchers in the field, as well as to newcomers to the fascinating and ever-expanding world of trinucleotide repeats.

Paris, France *Guy-Franck Richard*

Contents

Contributors

LUDOVIC ARANDEL • *Centre de Recherche en Myologie, Sorbonne Univeristé, Paris, France; Centre de Recherche en Myologie, Inserm, Paris, France; Association Institut de Myologie, Paris, France*
LATA BALAKRISHNAN • *Department of Biology, Indiana University Purdue University Indianapolis, Indianapolis, IN, USA*
JOANNA BARTHELEMY • *Department of Biochemistry and Molecular Biology, Boonshoft School of Medicine, Wright State University, Dayton, OH, USA*
SANDRA O. BRAZ • *Laboratory CTGDM, Inserm UMR1163, Paris, France; Institut Imagine, Université Paris Descartes—Sorbonne Paris Cité, Paris, France*
CINZIA CINESI • *Center for Integrative Genomics, University of Lausanne, Lausanne, Switzerland*
MAGDALENA DABROWSKA • *Department of Genome Engineering, Institute of Bioorganic Chemistry, Polish Academy of Sciences, Poznan, Poland*
PRADEEP K. DAGUR • *Flow Cytometry Core, National Heart, Lung and Blood Institute, National Institutes of Health, Bethesda, MD, USA*
DIANA M. DINCA • *Laboratory CTGDM, Inserm UMR1163, Paris, France; Institut Imagine, Université Paris Descartes—Sorbonne Paris Cité, Paris, France*
VINCENT DION • *Dementia Research Institute, Cardiff University, Cardiff, UK*
BRUNO DUMAS • *Biologics Research, Sanofi R&D, Vitry sur Seine, France*
THOMAS EBERSOLE • *Department of Biology, Tufts University, Medford, MA, USA*
CATHERINE H. FREUDENREICH • *Department of Biology, Tufts University, Medford, MA, USA*
DENIS FURLING • *Centre de Recherche en Myologie, Sorbonne Univeristé, Paris, France; Centre de Recherche en Myologie, Inserm, Paris, France; Association Institut de Myologie, Paris, France*
RUJUTA YASHODHAN GADGIL • *Department of Biochemistry and Molecular Biology, Boonshoft School of Medicine, Wright State University, Dayton, OH, USA*
MÁRIO GOMES-PEREIRA • *Laboratory CTGDM, Inserm UMR1163, Paris, France; Institut Imagine, Université Paris Descartes—Sorbonne Paris Cité, Paris, France; Centre de Recherche en Myologie (CRM), Inserm UMRS974, Association Institut de Myologie, Sorbonne Université, Paris, France*
GENEVIÈVE GOURDON • *Laboratory CTGDM, Inserm UMR1163, Paris, France; Institut Imagine, Université Paris-Descartes–Sorbonne Paris-Cité, Paris, France; Centre de Recherche en Myologie (CRM) INSERM UMRS 974, Association Institut de Myologie, Sorbonne Université, Paris, France*
OLIVIER GRISO • *Institut de Génétique et de Biologie Moléculaire et Cellulaire (IGBMC), Illkirch, France; INSERM, U1258, Illkirch, France; CNRS, UMR7104, Illkirch, France; Université de Strasbourg, Strasbourg, France*

Wenying Guo • *Institute for Bioengineering and Bioscience, School of Biological Sciences, Georgia Institute of Technology, Atlanta, GA, USA*
Arnaud F. Klein • *Centre de Recherche en Myologie, Sorbonne Univeristé, Paris, France; Centre de Recherche en Myologie, Inserm, Paris, France; Association Institut de Myologie, Paris, France*
Artem V. Kononenko • *Department of Biology, Tufts University, Medford, MA, USA*
Robert S. Lahue • *Centre for Chromosome Biology, National University of Ireland, Galway, Galway, Ireland; Galway Neuroscience Centre, National University of Ireland, Galway, Galway, Ireland*
Michael Leffak • *Department of Biochemistry and Molecular Biology, Boonshoft School of Medicine, Wright State University, Dayton, OH, USA*
Todd Lewis • *Department of Biochemistry and Molecular Biology, Boonshoft School of Medicine, Wright State University, Dayton, OH, USA*
Kirill S. Lobachev • *Institute for Bioengineering and Bioscience, School of Biological Sciences, Georgia Institute of Technology, Atlanta, GA, USA*
Huiyan Lu • *Laboratory Animal Sciences Section, National Institute of Diabetes, Digestive and Kidney Diseases, National Institutes of Health, Bethesda, MD, USA*
Joelle Marie • *Centre de Recherche en Myologie, Sorbonne Univeristé, Paris, France; Centre de Recherche en Myologie, Inserm, Paris, France; Association Institut de Myologie, Paris, France*
Sergei M. Mirkin • *Department of Biology, Tufts University, Medford, MA, USA*
Marta Olejniczak • *Department of Genome Engineering, Institute of Bioorganic Chemistry, Polish Academy of Sciences, Poznan, Poland*
Athena K. Petrides • *Department of Pathology, Harvard Medical School, Boston, MA, USA*
Lucie Poggi • *Institut Pasteur, CNRS, UMR3525, Paris, France; Collège Doctoral, Sorbonne Université, Paris, France; Biologics Research, Sanofi R&D, Vitry sur Seine, France*
Erica J. Polleys • *Department of Biology, Tufts University, Medford, MA, USA*
Hélène Puccio • *Institut de Génétique et de Biologie Moléculaire et Cellulaire (IGBMC), Illkirch, France; INSERM, U1258, Illkirch, France; CNRS, UMR7104, Illkirch, France; Université de Strasbourg, Strasbourg, France*
Guy-Franck Richard • *Department Genomes & Genetics, Institut Pasteur, CNRS UMR3525, Paris, France*
S. Dean Rider Jr. • *Department of Biochemistry and Molecular Biology, Boonshoft School of Medicine, Wright State University, Dayton, OH, USA*
Jennifer A. Surtees • *Department of Biochemistry, Jacobs School of Medicine and Biomedical Sciences, State University of New York at Buffalo, Buffalo, NY, USA; Genetics, Genomics and Bioinformatics Program, Jacobs School of Medicine and Biomedical Sciences, State University of New York at Buffalo, Buffalo, NY, USA*
Stéphanie Tomé • *Laboratory CTGDM, Inserm UMR1163, Paris, France; Institut Imagine, Université Paris-Descartes-Sorbonne Paris-Cité, Paris, France; Centre de Recherche en Myologie, CRM, Association Institut de Myologie, INSERM UMRS 974, Sorbonne Université, Paris, France*

KAREN USDIN • *Section on Gene Structure and Disease, Laboratory of Cell and Molecular Biology, National Institute of Diabetes, Digestive and Kidney Diseases, National Institutes of Health, Bethesda, MD, USA*
REMCO T. P. VAN CRUCHTEN • *Department of Cell Biology, Radboud Institute for Molecular Life Sciences, Radboud University Medical Center, Nijmegen, The Netherlands*
DAVID VITERBO • *Institut Pasteur, CNRS, UMR3525, Paris, France*
DERICK G. WANSINK • *Department of Cell Biology, Radboud Institute for Molecular Life Sciences, Radboud University Medical Center, Nijmegen, The Netherlands*
GREGORY M. WILLIAMS • *Department of Biochemistry, Jacobs School of Medicine and Biomedical Sciences, State University of New York at Buffalo, Buffalo, NY, USA; Center for Chromosome Biology and Galway Neuroscience Centre, School of Natural Sciences, National University of Ireland, Galway, Ireland*
BIN YANG • *Center for Integrative Genomics, University of Lausanne, Lausanne, Switzerland*
XIAONAN ZHAO • *Section on Gene Structure and Disease, Laboratory of Cell and Molecular Biology, National Institute of Diabetes, Digestive and Kidney Diseases, National Institutes of Health, Bethesda, MD, USA*

Chapter 1

Experimenting with Trinucleotide Repeats: Facts and Technical Issues

Guy-Franck Richard

Abstract

Trinucleotide repeats are a peculiar class of microsatellites involved in many neurological as well as developmental disorders. Their propensity to generate very large expansions over time is supposedly due to their capacity to form specific secondary structures, such as imperfect hairpins, triple helices, or G-quadruplexes. These unusual structures were proposed to trigger expansions in vivo. Here, I review known technical issues linked to these structures, such as slippage during polymerase chain reaction and aberrant migration of long trinucleotide repeats during agarose gel electrophoresis. Our current understanding of interactions between trinucleotide repeat secondary structures and the mismatch-repair machinery is also quickly reviewed, and critical questions relevant to these interactions are addressed.

Key words Trinucleotide repeat, Secondary structure, PCR, Agarose gel electrophoresis, Mismatch repair

1 Introduction

Trinucleotide repeats are a peculiar class of microsatellites, extremely frequent in all eukaryotic genomes sequenced so far (reviewed in [1]). They became more famous almost 30 years ago when it was demonstrated that the large expansion of trinucleotide repeat tracts was linked to some neurological human pathologies [2–4]. At the present time, trinucleotide repeat expansions are involved in more than two dozen human neurological disorders, including Huntington disease, Steinert disease (myotonic dystrophy type 1), fragile X syndrome, and Friedreich's ataxia. These disorders are monogenic, one single locus is responsible for the disease in association studies, although *cis*- and *trans*-acting genetic factors are known to modulate trinucleotide repeat instability in human cells as well as in model systems (reviewed in [1, 5–9]). Therefore, each disease is associated to the expansion of one single trinucleotide repeat tract at one single genomic location; for example, CTG triplets are expanded in Steinert disease, GAA in Friedreich's ataxia,

Guy-Franck Richard (ed.), *Trinucleotide Repeats: Methods and Protocols*, Methods in Molecular Biology, vol. 2056,
https://doi.org/10.1007/978-1-4939-9784-8_1,

CGG in fragile X syndrome, etc. (Fig. 1). Interestingly, other microsatellites besides trinucleotide repeats were also found to be responsible for several disorders: CCTG tetranucleotide repeats in myotonic dystrophy type 2, ATTCT and TGGAA pentanucleotides or GGCCTG hexanucleotides in spinocerebellar ataxias type 10, 31, and 36, respectively, and GGGGCC hexanucleotide repeat in amyotrophic lateral sclerosis (ALS) (Fig. 1). Note also that the expansion of a 12-bp GC-rich minisatellite is associated to progressive myoclonic epilepsy, a rare epileptic syndrome including seizures together with progressive neurological decline.

The molecular mechanism responsible for these large expansions is not totally understood, but past experiments in model systems (bacteria, yeast, mouse, and human cells) showed that de novo repeat-templated DNA synthesis was prone to generate contractions and expansions of the repeat tract: S-phase replication, double-strand break repair, nucleotide excision repair, and base excision repair all induce trinucleotide repeat instability in various experimental systems. It is not the purpose of the present chapter

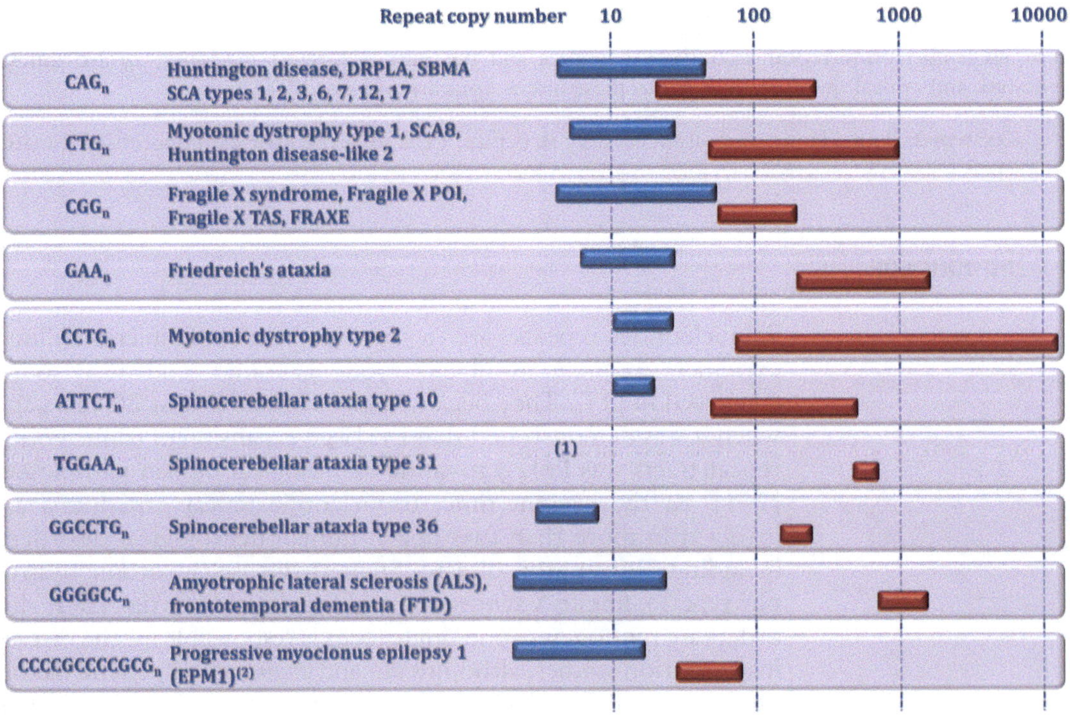

Fig. 1 Microsatellite expansion disorders. For each microsatellite, the corresponding disease(s) are indicated, as well as normal (in blue) and pathological allele lengths (in red), on a logarithmic scale. Abbreviations used: *DRPLA* dentatorubral-pallidoluysian atrophy, *SBMA* spinal and bulbar muscular atrophy, *SCA* spinocerebellar ataxia, *Fragile X POI* Fragile X-associated primary ovarian insufficiency, *Fragile X TAS* Fragile X-tremor/ataxia syndrome, *FRAXE* Fragile X mental retardation syndrome. (1) The TGGAA pentanucleotide repeat is inserted within a low complexity (TAGAA)n (TAAAATAGAA)n repeat. (2) The expanded sequence in EPM1 is not a microsatellite but is technically considered to be a minisatellite (base motif >10 bp)

to describe molecular mechanisms involved in trinucleotide repeat instability; those have been thoughtfully reviewed in many places [1, 5–8]. I will rather try to focus on the peculiar properties of such sequences and on the technical issues raised by their study.

2 Trinucleotide Repeats Form Secondary Structures In Vitro

In a seminal article by the McMurray laboratory, it was early demonstrated that CAG, CTG, and CGG DNA repeats prone to expansions exhibited the property to form stable imperfect hairpins in vitro [10] (Fig. 2a, b). This work was rapidly followed by others studying hairpin properties of single-stranded CTG [11], CAG and GAC [12], GTC [13], and CGG [14] trinucleotide repeats. It must be noted that RNA molecules containing CAG, CCG, CGG, or CUG triplet repeats also fold into stable hairpins in

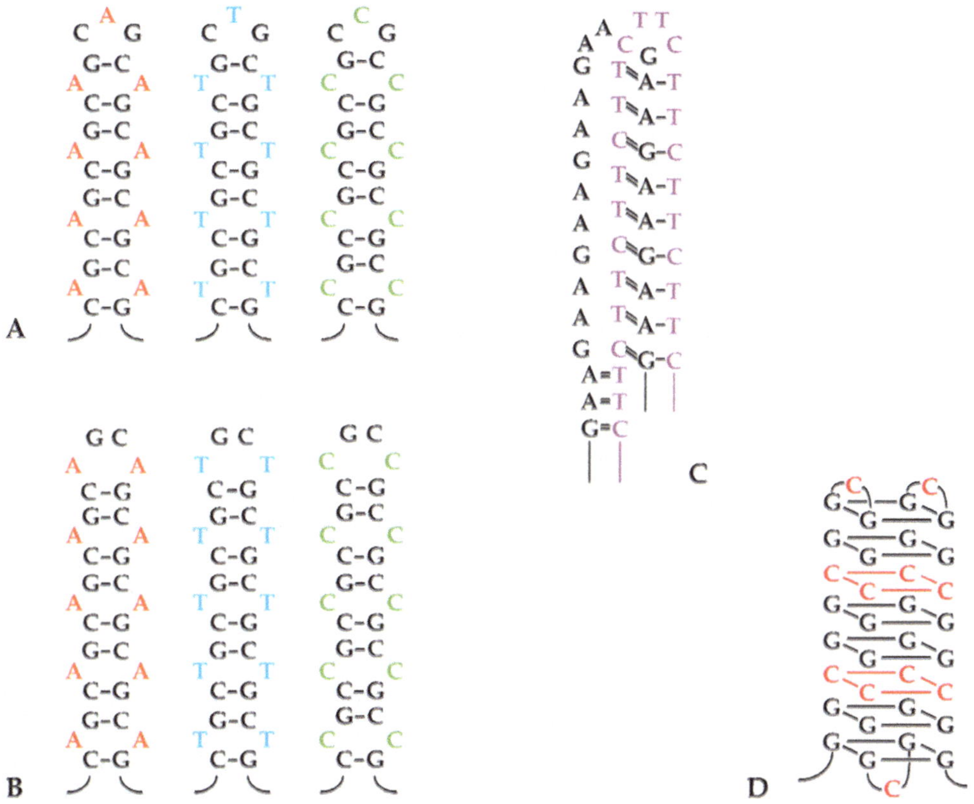

Fig. 2 Secondary structures formed by different trinucleotide repeats. (**a**) CAG, CTG, and CCG hairpins formed by odd number triplets. Unpaired bases are colored. (**b**) CAG, CTG, and CGG hairpins formed by an even number of triplets. (**c**) Triple helix formed by GAA repeat tract. Watson–Crick pairings are shown by double lines, Hoogsteen pairings by single lines. (**d**) Tetraplex structure formed by CCG repeats. Guanosine quartets are shown in black. (Figure originally published by G.-F. Richard and reprinted with permission from the American Society for Microbiology [1])

a test tube [15, 16]. Subsequent studies showed that GAA/TTC repeats, involved in Friedreich's ataxia, were shown to form a triple helix, containing both Watson–Crick and Hoogsteen bonds (Fig. 2c) [17, 18], a specific structure common to all polypurine-polypyrimidine tracts, as demonstrated by Sergei Mirkin more than 30 years ago [19]. In addition, CGG as well as GCC triplet repeats are able to fold into DNA tetraplex (or G4, or quadruplex), similar to structures formed at the end of human telomeres [20, 21]. Formation of a CAG or CTG hairpin on one DNA strand leads to a slipped-stranded structure in which one or more mung bean nuclease-sensitive hairpin(s) are visible as bulges by electron microscopy [22]. More recently, atomic force microscopy showed that very long CAG trinucleotide repeats of various lengths (111–415 triplets) exhibited unusual structural features such as convolutions as well as single and multiple protrusions, suggesting that these structures were most probably multiple hairpins [23]. In all the above cases, the stability of the repeat-containing secondary structure increased with repeat length, making long trinucleotide repeats more prone to fold than shorter ones. Since the propensity to expansion was known to be tightly correlated to repeat size (the formerly called "Sherman paradox" [3]), soon emerged the idea that secondary structures could be triggering the expansion process [24].

3 Secondary DNA Structures and Mismatch Repair

The mismatch-repair system (hereafter abbreviated MMR), is conserved from bacteria to man [25] and is involved in detecting synthesis mistakes made by polymerases and signaling them to the repair machinery. In its absence, microsatellite instability exhibits several hundredfold to thousandfold increases in *Saccharomyces cerevisiae* [26–28] and *Schizosaccharomyces pombe* [29]. Two kinds of damage are recognized by the MMR: base substitution and insertions or deletions (indels). They are processed by two slightly different machineries. The MSH2-MSH6 heterodimeric complex (MutSα) recognizes single base mismatches and small indels of 1–2 nucleotides, whereas the MSH2-MSH3 heterodimer (MutSβ) recognizes larger indels. Bound MutS complexes subsequently recruit MutL complexes, the EXO1 exonuclease and the DNA synthesis machinery to repair the error (reviewed in [30]). When the first trinucleotide repeat disorders were discovered, mismatch repair became the first obvious candidate for a possible role in large repeat expansions. Soon, experimental assays were designed in yeast to detect large trinucleotide repeat length alterations. Very surprisingly, it was shown that short CAG or CTG repeat tracts (25 triplets) were not significantly more expanded or contracted in an *msh2* mutant as compared to wild type [31]. When slightly longer

CAG repeat tracts were assayed, a modest twofold increase in contractions was observed in an *msh2* strain, far from the thousandfold destabilization of microsatellites in the absence of MMR [32, 33]. It must be noted here that trinucleotide repeats, like all microsatellites, exhibit small length changes in MMR mutants, mainly +1 or −1 triplet [34], but larger expansions or contractions did not seem to be significantly more elevated in MMR-deficient backgrounds. However, when it comes to trinucleotide repeats, things are often more complicated than they seemed at first. In 1997, Christopher Pearson and Richard Sinden published a remarkable article in which they showed that purified MSH2 protein bound in vitro to CAG/CTG slipped-stranded structured DNA [35]. It was subsequently established that the MSH2-MSH3 complex bound CAG hairpins [36, 37], and that CAG and CTG repeats when more prone to contractions in transgenic mice deficient for the MSH2 protein [38, 39]. It was later demonstrated that the MSH2 ATPase activity was essential to generate repeat expansions, strongly suggesting that a functional MMR was indeed required to promote them [40]. Reinvestigation of CAG/CTG repeat tract dynamics in yeast showed that these sequences accumulated small incremental expansions over time, that were suppressed in an *msh3Δ* mutant background [41]. Finally, Msh2p was shown to be enriched in yeast cells at a CAG or CTG long repeat tract, in an *MSH3*-dependent manner [42]. All these data point to a role for the MutSβ complex in CAG/CTG repeat expansions. Similar results were observed for CGG/CCG repeats in a fragile X premutation mouse model [43] and for GGA/TTC repeats in a Friedreich's ataxia mouse model [44], but several questions remain open. Does MutSβ hairpin binding plays a stabilizing role, protecting them from degradation or repair by the cellular machinery? Is the MMR also involved in repeat expansion for other microsatellites? How do MutSβ-bound secondary structures interact with histones and with replication, recombination, and repair machineries? Is the expansion mechanism promoted by MutSβ iterative or saltatory? In other words, does it happen once or more than once in a short period of time? In any case, it seems that trinucleotide repeat-forming secondary structures activate the mismatch-repair machinery in such a way that it promotes their expansion, by a mechanism that still needs to be clarified.

4 Technical Issues to Be Considered When Trying to Amplify CAG/CTG Trinucleotide Repeats by PCR

A convenient way to analyze trinucleotide repeat length is by using two flanking primers to amplify the repeat tract by PCR. However, this approach might be laborious due to possible slippage of the newly synthesized strand over its template during the PCR reaction

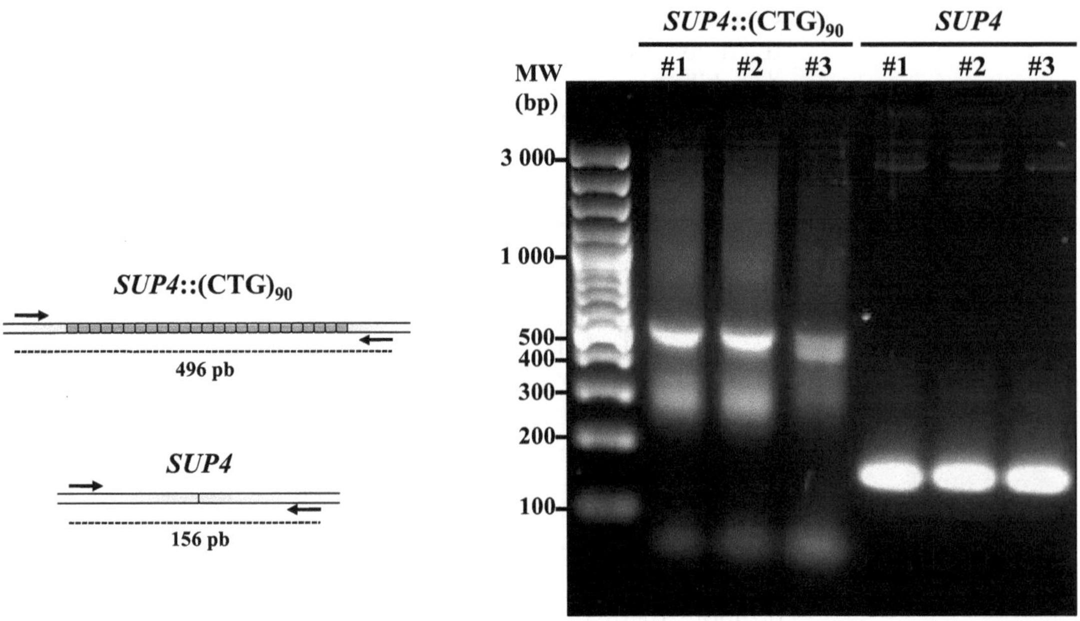

Fig. 3 PCR amplification of wild-type and CTG repeat-containing locus. The same genomic DNA was used as a template in triplicate PCR reactions (labeled 1, 2, and 3). A sharp unique band was obtained when the locus that does not contain a CTG repeat was amplified (*SUP4*). Nonreproducible bands and a smear were obtained when the CTG repeat-containing locus was amplified (*SUP4*::CTG_{90}). Similar results were obtained with other primer sets located close to the repeat tract

itself, leading to amplification products of aberrant apparent sizes. One such example is shown in (Fig. 3). A $(CTG)_{90}$ repeat was integrated into a yeast chromosome, at the *SUP4* locus, and amplified by PCR using primers located upstream and downstream, close to the repeat tract. The PCR reaction was run in triplicate using the same genomic DNA as a template. In the three reactions, shorter products around 300 bp were detected as a smear migrating below the expected size of 496 bp. In addition, in reaction #3 an additional band was visible below the main product, suggesting that slippage of a few repeat units occurred in one of the earliest PCR cycles (Fig. 3). This very frequent problem could be reduced by designing primers further away from the repeat tract, but in that case the total length of the final PCR product would become the limiting factor. With very large expansions, such as those observed in DM1, DM2, Friedreich's ataxia, or ALS, the repeat tract length itself may be too large to be amplified by PCR, independently of the position of flanking primers and one has to use alternative methods such as Southern blot [42] or exotic PCR reactions [45] to estimate tract length. An example of a Southern blot used to analyzed trinucleotide repeat length is shown in (Fig. 4).

Another caveat of PCR amplification of trinucleotide repeat tracts results from allele length heterogeneity in template genomic DNA. This is specially an issue if DNA was extracted from a tissue

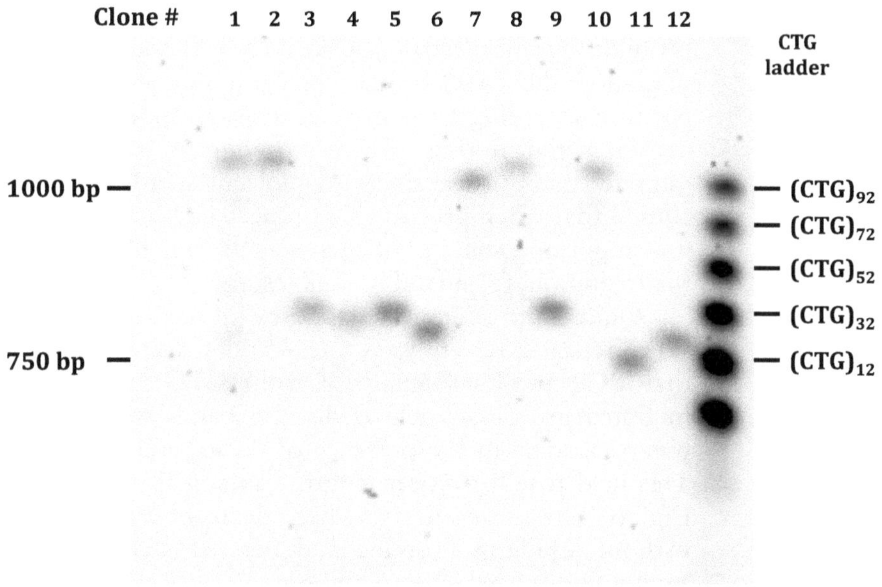

Fig. 4 Southern blot to determine CTG repeat tract length. DNA was prepared and the gel was run, transferred, and hybridized as previously described [42]. The repeat tract length of 12 independent yeast clones was analyzed (#1 to 12). To the right is a molecular weight ladder corresponding to the number of expected triplets. In this strain, the CTG repeat tract should normally be around 100 triplets. This is the case for clones #1, 2, 8, and 10, all other clones exhibiting contractions of variable lengths. Note that clone #1 shows a number of faint discrete bands of lower molecular weight, indicating repeat tract mosaicism

or a mix of tissues, and was not amplified clonally from a single cell (or a very small number of cells). In that case, one particular allele may be preferentially amplified, usually but not necessarily the shortest one, most often the most frequent allele in the population considered. This tends to underrepresent rare alleles present in the population and therefore gives a biased picture of trinucleotide repeat tract instability in the corresponding tissue or culture. To palliate this problem, small-pool PCR protocols were designed and optimized to amplify trinucleotide repeat tracts. In short, template DNA is diluted to a small number of genomes per reaction (typically ~5–10) and PCR is carried out on many individual reactions at the same time. This allows to determine more precisely the amount of trinucleotide repeat length variability within a DNA sample [46, 47].

5 Aberrant Trinucleotide Repeat Tract Mobility on Agarose Gels

In addition to artifacts due to PCR slippage, trinucleotide repeats may show abnormal mobility in agarose gels. This has been known for a long time, since more than 20 years ago it was shown that migration of an expanded CGG allele from a fragile X patient (>200 CGG triplets) in an agarose gel was aberrant when the gel and running buffer were supplemented with 5 μg/ml ethidium bromide during electrophoresis. When the gel was stained after migration the CGG-containing band migrated at the expected position according to its molecular weight. However, when staining occurred during gel electrophoresis, the expected band migrated as a diffuse smear of molecules [48]. The author concluded that when precise CGG repeat tract length determination was important, staining of agarose gels should be performed after the migration, for unambiguous results.

Quite surprisingly, the opposite observation was made with CTG repeats. Recently, Gomes-Pereira and Monckton showed that PCR products amplified from CTG-containing templates migrated in agarose gels as discrete bands when electrophoresis was performed in the presence of 0.2 μg/ml ethidium bromide. This held true for repeat lengths ranging from five to 200 CTG triplets. On the contrary, when electrophoresis was performed without ethidium bromide and the gel was stained afterward, smeary additional bands of higher molecular weights were detected above the expected repeat size [49]. Additional experiments supported the hypothesis that these smears corresponded to slipped-stranded molecules formed during sequential cycles of denaturation-polymerization performed during the PCR reaction. It was not completely clear, though, how the presence of ethidium bromide during electrophoresis completely suppressed the detection of such molecules. Nevertheless, the authors concluded that precise repeat tract length determination by electrophoresis in agarose gels of CTG trinucleotide repeats should always be performed in the presence of ethidium bromide, to avoid such artifacts.

GAA trinucleotide repeats form triple helices (Fig. 2c) and plasmids carrying such repeats were shown to exhibit aberrant mobility in agarose gels, a retarded band of high molecular weight being detected at different ethidium bromide concentrations [50]. At the present time, it is unclear whether other microsatellites expanded in human disorders also exhibit similar properties, but it should be kept in mind that precise size determination of trinucleotide repeat tract length by agarose gel electrophoresis should be considered with extreme care.

In conclusion, all studies on trinucleotide repeats had to face these technically challenging features: frequent repeat size changes, stable secondary structure formation, and aberrant mobility in agarose gels. Most of the analytical molecular methods developed to study trinucleotide repeats aimed at circumventing these obstacles. Several of them are extensively described in the present book and will hopefully be useful to researchers in the many areas of this fascinating field.

Acknowledgments

Work in my lab is generously supported by the Centre National de la Recherche Scientifique (CNRS) and by the Institut Pasteur.

References

1. Richard G-F, Kerrest A, Dujon B (2008) Comparative genomics and molecular dynamics of DNA repeats in eukaryotes. Microbiol Mol Biol Rev 72:686–727
2. Brook JD et al (1992) Molecular basis of myotonic dystrophy: expansion of a trinucleotide (CTG) repeat at the 3′ end of a transcript encoding a protein kinase family member. Cell 68:799–808
3. Fu Y-H et al (1991) Variation of the CGG repeat at the fragile X site results in genetic instability: resolution of the Sherman paradox. Cell 67:1047–1058
4. Fu YH et al (1992) An unstable triplet repeat in a gene related to myotonic muscular dystrophy. Science 255:1256–1258
5. McMurray CT (2010) Mechanisms of trinucleotide repeat instability during human development. Nat Rev Genet 11:786–799
6. Mirkin SM (2007) Expandable DNA repeats and human disease. Nature 447:932–940
7. Mosbach V, Poggi L, Richard G-F (2018) Trinucleotide repeat instability during double-strand break repair: from mechanisms to gene therapy. Curr Genet. https://doi.org/10.1007/s00294-018-0865-1
8. Pearson CE, Edamura KN, Cleary JD (2005) Repeat instability: mechanisms of dynamic mutations. Nat Rev Genet 6:729–742
9. Usdin K, House NC, Freudenreich CH (2015) Repeat instability during DNA repair: insights from model systems. Crit Rev Biochem Mol Biol. https://doi.org/10.3109/10409238.2014.999192
10. Gacy AM, Goellner G, Juranic N, Macura S, McMurray CT (1995) Trinucleotide repeats that expand in human disease form hairpin structures in vitro. Cell 81:533–540
11. Mitas M et al (1995) Hairpin properties of single-stranded DNA containing a GC-rich triplet repeat: (CTG)15. Nucleic Acids Res 23:1050–1059
12. Yu A, Mitas M (1995) The purine-rich trinucleotide repeat sequences d(CAG)15 and d(GAC)15 form hairpins. Nucleic Acids Res 23:4055–4057
13. Yu A et al (1995) The trinucleotide repeat sequence d(GTC)15 adopts a hairpin conformation. Nucleic Acids Res 23:2706–2714
14. Nadel Y, Weisman-Shomer P, Fry M (1995) The fragile X syndrome single strand d(CGG)n nucleotide repeats readily fold back to form unimolecular hairpin structures. J Biol Chem 48:28970–28977
15. Pinheiro P et al (2002) Structures of CUG repeats in RNA. J Biol Chem 277:35183–35190
16. Sobczak K, de Mezer M, Michlewski G, Krol J, Krzyzosiak WJ (2003) RNA structure of trinucleotide repeats associated with human neurological diseases. Nucleic Acids Res 31:5469–5482
17. Mariappan SV, Catasti P, Silks LA 3rd, Bradbury EM, Gupta G (1999) The high-resolution structure of the triplex formed by the GAA/TTC triplet repeat associated with Friedreich's ataxia. J Mol Biol 285:2035–2052
18. Suen IS et al (1999) Structural properties of Friedreich's ataxia d(GAA) repeats. Biochim Biophys Acta 1444:14–24
19. Mirkin SM et al (1987) DNA H form requires a homopurine-homopyrimidine mirror repeat. Nature 330:495–497
20. Fojtik P, Vorlickova M (2001) The fragile X chromosome (GCC) repeat folds into a DNA tetraplex at neutral pH. Nucleic Acids Res 29:4684–4690
21. Fry M, Loeb LA (1994) The fragile X syndrome d(CGG)n nucleotide repeats form a stable tetrahelical structure. Proc Natl Acad Sci U S A 91:4950–4954
22. Pearson CE et al (2002) Slipped-strand DNAs formed by long (CAG)*(CTG) repeats: slipped-out repeats and slip-out junctions. Nucleic Acids Res 30:4534–4547
23. Duzdevich D et al (2011) Unusual structures are present in DNA fragments containing super-long huntingtin CAG repeats. PLoS One 6:e17119
24. McMurray CT (1999) DNA secondary structure: a common and causative factor for expansion in human disease. Proc Natl Acad Sci U S A 96:1823–1825

25. Larrea AA, Lujan SA, Kunkel TA (2010) SnapShot: DNA mismatch repair. Cell 141:730 e1
26. Harfe BD, Jinks-Robertson S (2000) Sequence composition and context effects on the generation and repair of frameshift intermediates in mononucleotide runs in Saccharomyces cerevisiae. Genetics 156:571–578
27. Strand M, Prolla TA, Liskay RM, Petes TD (1993) Destabilization of tracts of simple repetitive DNA in yeast by mutations affecting DNA mismatch repair. Nature 365:274–276
28. Tran HT, Keen JD, Kricker M, Resnick MA, Gordenin DA (1997) Hypermutability of homonucleotide runs in mismatch repair and DNA polymerase proofreading yeast mutants. Mol Cell Biol 17:2859–2865
29. Mansour AA, Tornier C, Lehmann E, Darmon M, Fleck O (2001) Control of GT repeat stability in Schizosaccharomyces pombe by mismatch repair factors. Genetics 158:77–85
30. Jiricny J (2006) The multifaceted mismatch-repair system. Nat Rev Mol Cell Biol 7:335–346
31. Miret JJ, Pessoa-Brandão L, Lahue RS (1998) Orientation-dependent and sequence-specific expansions of CTG/CAG trinucleotide repeats in Saccharomyces cerevisiae. Proc Natl Acad Sci U S A 95:12438–12443
32. Miret JJ, Pessoa-Brandao L, Lahue RS (1997) Instability of CAG and CTG trinucleotide repeats in Saccharomyces cerevisiae. Mol Cell Biol 17:3382–3387
33. Richard G-F, Dujon B, Haber JE (1999) Double-strand break repair can lead to high frequencies of deletions within short CAG/CTG trinucleotide repeats. Mol Gen Genet 261:871–882
34. Schweitzer JK, Livingston DM (1997) Destabilization of CAG trinucleotide repeat tracts by mismatch repair mutations in yeast. Hum Mol Genet 6:349–355
35. Pearson CE, Ewel A, Acharya S, Fishel RA, Sinden RR (1997) Human MSH2 binds to trinucleotide repeat DNA structures associated with neurodegenerative diseases. Hum Mol Genet 6:1117–1123
36. Owen BA et al (2005) (CAG)(n)-hairpin DNA binds to Msh2-Msh3 and changes properties of mismatch recognition. Nat Struct Mol Biol 12:663–670
37. Tian L et al (2009) Mismatch recognition protein MutSbeta does not hijack (CAG)n hairpin repair in vitro. J Biol Chem 284:20452–20456
38. Manley K, Shirley TL, Flaherty L, Messer A (1999) Msh2 deficiency prevents in vivo somatic instability of the CAG repeat in Huntington disease transgenic mice. Nat Genet 23:471–473
39. Savouret C et al (2003) CTG repeat instability and size variation timing in DNA repair-deficient mice. EMBO J 22:2264–2273
40. Tome S et al (2009) MSH2 ATPase domain mutation affects CTG*CAG repeat instability in transgenic mice. PLoS Genet 5:e1000482
41. Williams GM, Surtees JA (2015) MSH3 promotes dynamic behavior of trinucleotide repeat tracts in vivo. Genetics 200:737–754
42. Viterbo D, Michoud G, Mosbach V, Dujon B, Richard G-F (2016) Replication stalling and heteroduplex formation within CAG/CTG trinucleotide repeats by mismatch repair. DNA Repair 42:94–106
43. Lokanga RA, Zhao XN, Usdin K (2014) The mismatch repair protein MSH2 is rate limiting for repeat expansion in a fragile X premutation mouse model. Hum Mutat 35:129–136
44. Ezzatizadeh V et al (2012) The mismatch repair system protects against intergenerational GAA repeat instability in a Friedreich ataxia mouse model. Neurobiol Dis 46:165–171
45. Dandelot E, Gourdon G (2018) The flash-small-pool PCR: how to transform blotting and numerous hybridization steps into a simple denatured PCR. BioTechniques 64:262–265
46. Gomes-Pereira M, Bidichandani SI, Monckton DG (2004) Analysis of unstable triplet repeats using small-pool polymerase chain reaction. In: Kohwi Y (ed) Trinucleotide repeat protocols. Humana Press, New York, pp 61–76. https://doi.org/10.1385/1-59259-804-8:061
47. Tome S, Nicole A, Gomes-Pereira M, Gourdon G (2014) Non-radioactive detection of trinucleotide repeat size variability. PLoS Curr 6. PLOS Currents Muscular Dystrophy https://doi.org/10.1371/currents.md.ad50113b899fa1352ce70c087eead706
48. Cummins JH (1997) The unique alteration of electrophoretic mobility of fragile-X-expanded fragments in the presence of ethidium bromide. Tech Tips Online 2:84–86
49. Gomes-Pereira M, Monckton DG (2017) Ethidium bromide modifies the agarose electrophoretic mobility of CAG·CTG alternative DNA structures generated by PCR. Front Cell Neurosci 11:153
50. Sakamoto N et al (1999) Sticky DNA: self-association properties of long GAA.TTC repeats in R.R.Y triplex structures from Friedreich's ataxia. Mol Cell 3:465–475

Chapter 2

Fast Assays to Detect Interruptions in CTG.CAG Repeat Expansions

Stéphanie Tomé and Geneviève Gourdon

Abstract

Different interrupted repeat expansions have been found in several trinucleotide repeat (TNR) diseases such as fragile X syndrome (FXS), spinocerebellar ataxias (SCAs), and myotonic dystrophies (DMs). Their origins and roles remain poorly understood, especially in myotonic dystrophy type 1 (DM1). We present here the triplet repeat primed polymerase chain reaction (TP-PCR) and restriction enzyme-digested PCR to detect and identify interrupted triplet repeat alleles in DM1. TP-PCR consists of a PCR amplification using a fluoresceinated (FAM) primer flanking the repeat region and a primer pair in CTG.CAG repeats. A detailed analysis of interrupted triplet repeat tracts is essential to fully understand the role of interruptions in the pathogenesis and molecular mechanisms observed in TNR diseases.

Key words Trinucleotide repeats, Interrupted repeat expansions, Myotonic dystrophy type 1, Polymerase chain reaction, Triplet repeat prime PCR (TP-PCR), Restriction enzyme-digested PCR

1 Introduction

Among repeated DNA sequences described in the human genome, pure expanded trinucleotide repeats have been associated to several neurological and neuromuscular disorders such as FXS and DM1 [1]. Triplet repeat expansions are genetically highly unstable in both the germ line and soma with an instability biased toward expansions. In the FXS locus, interrupted CGG repeat alleles were first described in the 1990s [2]. Many alleles (<200 repeats) usually contain 1 to 3 AGG interruptions interspersed between repeats every 9–10 CGG repeats at the 5′ end of the repeat. The presence of AGG interruptions reduces repeat instability in FXS patients. In the FXS locus, the number and location of AGG interruptions are constant between individuals compared to those described in DM1 patients [2–5]. Various types of interruptions in the CTG repeat expansions are found in around 3–8% of the DM1 population depending of the ethnic group [6, 7]. The number, type, and

Guy-Franck Richard (ed.), *Trinucleotide Repeats: Methods and Protocols*, Methods in Molecular Biology, vol. 2056, https://doi.org/10.1007/978-1-4939-9784-8_2, © Springer Science+Business Media, LLC, part of Springer Nature 2020

location of interruptions within the CTG repeat expansions are highly variable between individuals but also among patients in the same DM1 family. CCG, GGC, and CTC interruptions have been reported at the 3′ and/or 5′ end of the CTG repeat expansion in DM1 [7–14]. More recently, a single CAG interruption at the 5′ end of CTG repeat expansion has been described in an unusual DM1 family suggesting that other types of interruptions may occur in DM1 families [7]. All these interruptions are essential modifiers of triplet repeat instability and clinical features in DM1. The origin and role of these different interruptions observed in the DM locus remain poorly understood. Thus, the ability to detect and identify the interruptions located in TNR sequence is important to improve our knowledge of DM1 pathogenesis and instability. The molecular genetic testing of the DM locus is commonly carried out by conventional PCR amplification (typically using 15 ng DNA) of the CTG.CAG repeats or by Southern blot analysis (typically 10 μg DNA) to estimate the size of normal and expanded alleles. However, these two approaches do not detect the presence or absence of interruptions in the CTG.CAG repeat tracts and result in data loss. First, Warner et al. described the TP-PCR assay to replace Southern blotting as a new test that detect CTG expanded allele in 1 day instead of a week, resulting in reduced costs of the experiment [15]. The improvement of this method allows to detect interruptions and to identify them. We report here a combination of TP-PCR assays and restriction enzyme-digested PCR to reveal the presence of interrupted triplet repeat DM allele by reducing the time of experiment as well as the cost of testing in research and diagnostic laboratories.

2 Materials

2.1 Reagents

1. 1 M Tris–HCl, pH 8.5.
2. 0.5 M EDTA, pH 8.
3. 5 M NaCl.
4. 20% SDS solution.
5. Lysis buffer: 100 mM Tris–HCl pH 8.5, 5 mM EDTA pH 8, 0.2% SDS, 200 mM NaCl.
6. Proteinase K solution (20 mg/mL).
7. Phenol–chloroform–isoamyl alcohol.
8. Chloroform (stabilized with ethyl alcohol).
9. 100% ethanol.
10. Qubit dsDNA high-sensitivity kit.
11. Qubit dsDNA broad-range kit.
12. Mineral oil.

13. Deionized H_2O.
14. Taq DNA polymerase.
15. Oligonucleotide Primers (Table 1).
16. 1× polymerase chain reaction buffer (ThermoFisher scientific, Ref: SM0005) (*see* **Note 1**).
17. TBE 10× solution.
18. Ultrapure agarose.
19. 25 mM ethidium bromide stock solution.
20. Generuler 1 kb DNA ladder (or another similar DNA ladder).
21. DNA-loading dye (Orange G and 60% glycerol).
22. Formamide.
23. GeneScan 600 LIZ dye size standard v2.0 (or similar).
24. SsiI (AciI) restriction enzyme.
25. AluI restriction enzyme.
26. NucleoSpin Gel and PCR cleanup columns (Macherey-Nagel) or similar purification columns from another provider.

2.2 Equipment

1. 20 μL, 200 μL, and 1 mL Filter pipetman tips.
2. 1.5 mL screw-top Eppendorf tubes.
3. Qubit 3 fluorometer (ThermoFisher scientific).
4. Qubit assay tubes (ThermoFisher scientific, Ref: Q32856).
5. PCR tubes.
6. Thermal cycler.
7. Agarose gel electrophoresis trays, tanks, and power packs.
8. Ultraviolet (UV) transilluminator.
9. 3500 XL analyzer (ThermoFisher scientific, Ref: 4406016).
10. GeneMapper Software (ThermoFisher scientific).

3 Methods

3.1 DNA Extraction and Quantification

Genomic DNAs are extracted from cells and tissues according to standard DNA extraction protocols. Good quality genomic DNAs are obtained by standard phenol–chloroform extraction and ethanol precipitation techniques (*see* **Note 2**).

1. Lyse cells or tissues with 500 μL of lysis buffer (100 mM Tris–HCl pH 8.5, 5 mM EDTA pH 8, 0.2% SDS, and 200 mM NaCl).

Table 1
Primers used to assess TP-PCR and CTG repeat amplification [7, 10, 15–17]

Name	Primers	References
Forward TP-PCR		
DM-C-FAM	5′-A AC GGG GCT CG A AGG GTC CTT-3′	Tomé et al. [7]
P4CAG	5′-TAC GCA TCC CAG TTT GAG ACG CAG CAG CAG CAG CAG CA-3′	Warner et al. [15]
P3R	5′-TAC GCA TCC CAG TTT GAG ACG-3′	Warner et al. [15]
Reverse TP-PCR		
Somy4R-FAM	5′-CGG GTT TGG CAA AAG CAA ATT TCC CGA-3′	Musova et al. [10]
P4CTG	5′-TAC GCA TCC CAG TTT GAG ACG TGC TGC TGC TGC TGC T-3′	Warner et al. [15]
P3R	5′-TAC GCA TCC CAG TTT GAG ACG-3′	Warner et al. [15]
Forward specific TP-PCR		
DM-C-FAM	5′-A AC GGG GCT CG A AGG GTC CTT-3′	Tomé et al. [7]
ST-P4-5′CAG(CTG)i; (ST-P4-5′)	5′-TAC GCA TCC CAG TTT GAG ACG CAG CAG CAG CAG CAG **CTG**-3′	Tomé et al. [7]
ST-P4-5′CAG(CCG)i; (ST-P4–5′)	5′-TAC GCA TCC CAG TTT GAG ACG CAG CAG **CGG** CAG CAG C-3′	Tomé et al. [7]
P3R	5′-TAC GCA TCC CAG TTT GAG ACG-3′	Warner et al. [15]
Reverse specific TP-PCR		
Somy4R-FAM	5′-CGG GTT TGG CAA AAG CAA ATT TCC CGA-3′	Musova et al. [10]
ST-P4-3′CTG(CCG)i; (ST-P4-3′)	5′-TAC GCA TCC CAG TTT GAG ACG CTG CTG **CCG** CTG CTG C-3′	Unpublished
P3R	5′-TAC GCA TCC CAG TTT GAG ACG-3′	Warner et al. [15]
CTG repeat amplification		
101	5′- CTT CCC AGG CCT GCA GTT TGC CCA TC-3′	Seznec et al. [17]
102	5′- GAA CGG GGC TCG AAG GGT CCT TGT AGC-3′	Seznec et al. [17]
CTG repeat amplification		
DM-C	5′-AAC GGG GCT CGA AGG GTC CT-3′	Monckton et al. [16]
DM-BR	5′-CGT GGA GGA TGG AAC ACG GAC-3′	Monckton et al. [16]

2. Add 200 μg/mL of Proteinase K.
3. Incubate at 55 °C overnight.
4. Centrifuge for 10 min at 12,700 rpm in a microcentrifuge (*see* **Note 3**).
5. Take out 400 μL of supernatant and put it in the new tube of 1.5 mL.
6. Add 400 μL phenol–chloroform.
7. Shake the tube.
8. Centrifuge for 3 min at 12,700 rpm.
9. Take 400 μL of the upper phase and put it in a new tube of 1.5 mL.
10. Add 400 μL of chloroform and shake the tube.
11. Centrifuge for 3 min at 12,700 rpm.
12. Take 300–400 μL of the upper phase and put it in a new tube of 1.5 mL.
13. Add 2 volumes of 100% cold ethanol and gently shake tube.
14. Centrifuge for 15 min at 12,700 rpm to obtain one pellet.
15. Remove the supernatant.
16. Add 400 μL of 70% cold ethanol.
17. Remove the supernatant and dry the pellet (*see* **Note 4**).
18. Resuspend the pellet in 50–200 μL of water (*see* **Note 5**).

3.2 dsDNA Quantification (See Note 6)

The concentration of DNA in solution is estimated using the Qubit fluorometer. This assay is fast and uses selective dyes for dsDNA. Quantification is more sensitive and gives a more accurate value than spectrophotometer quantification, which determines the concentration of all nucleic acids and nucleotides. If no Qubit is available, alternative quantification methods may be used.

1. Prepare sufficient Qubit working solution to analyze the two standards provided by the suppliers and all samples.
2. Dilute the Qubit dsDNA reagent 1:200 in Qubit dsDNA buffer (= Qubit working solution).
3. Add 10 μL of each standard in 190 μL of Qubit working solution and add 1 μL of each sample in 199 μL Qubit working solution.
4. Mix tubes by vortexing 2 s. Avoid bubbles.
5. Incubate for 2 min at room temperature in the dark.
6. Read standards and samples using the program dsDNA quantification with the Qubit fluorometer.

3.3 Triplet Repeat Prime PCR (TP-PCR) and Fragment Size Analysis (See Note 7)

TP-PCR is usually performed on both strands of the CTG repeat using one fluorescent labelled oligonucleotide flanking the CTG. CAG repeat region (P1-FAM) and two other P4 and P3 oligonucleotides (Fig. 1a). Primer P4 is complementary to the five pure CTG.CAG repeats and contains a 5′ random sequence recognized by primer P3. The P3 primer and the high concentration of P3 and P1-FAM compare to a low concentration of repeat unit specific P4 (10:1 molar ratio) prevent progressive shortening of the amplified products during the PCR. TP-PCR generates a mixture of PCR fragments that are analyzed by capillary electrophoresis using Applied Biosystems model 3500XL genetic analyzer (Short or long fragment analysis program). The data is analyzed using GeneMapper software. Each amplicon of increasing length and diminishing yield is displayed as typical traces (Fig. 2). Each peak differs in the size of one triplet repeat. The pattern of trace enables to determine an expanded CTG repeat allele that cannot be obtained by conventional PCR and to detect the presence of interruptions at the 5′ (TP-PCR using P1-FAM forward primer) or 3′ (TP-PCR using P1-FAM reverse primer) end of the repeat region (*see* **Notes 8** and **9**). TP-PCR using the P1-FAM forward primer generates a first amplicon containing 5 CTG repeats with a size of 69 bp. In parallel, TP-PCR using the P1-FAM reverse primer generates a first amplicon containing 5 CTG repeats with a size of 271 bp. Based on the same principle of the TP-PCR described by Warner et al. [15], we performed PCR assay using specific primers that bind to CCG or CAG repeat interruptions (Fig. 1b). Forward TP-PCR is performed using DM-C-FAM, P3 primers and a specific interrupted ST-P4-5′ oligonucleotide to detect nonconsecutive interruptions at the 5′ end of the CTG repeat. In contrast, reverse TP-PCR is performed using Somy4R-FAM, P3 primers, and a specific interrupted ST-P4-3′ oligonucleotide to detect nonconsecutive interruptions at the 3′ end of the CTG repeat. Specific interrupted ST-P4 primers are complementary to the five-six interrupted CTG repeats located at the 5′ or 3′ end of the CTG repeat. The size of the amplicons will depend on the location of the interruptions (*see* **Note 10**). This method enables to quickly identify CCG interruptions and CAG repeat interruptions without sequencing a difficult triplet repeat region.

1. Determine dsDNA concentration by Qubit fluorometer (*see* Subheading 3.2).
2. Dilute DNA to obtain a concentration range around 20–100 ng/μL.
3. Amplify 20–100 ng of DNA in a final volume of 25 μL with 0.06 U of Taq polymerase, 1 μM of P1-FAM and P3R primers, and 0.1 μM of P4 or ST-P4 primer (Table 1), in 1× PCR buffer. Each final reaction can be covered with one drop of mineral oil to avoid evaporation. The PCR amplification con-

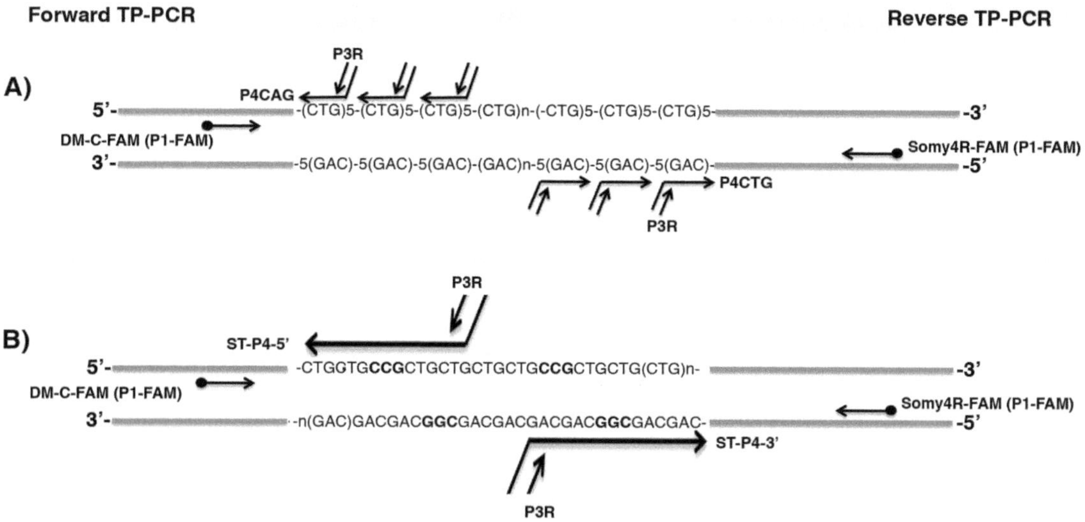

Fig. 1 Schematic diagram depicting the location of repeat-primed PCR primers used to amplify either the 5′ end of the CTG repeat expansion (Forward TP-PCR) or the 3′ end of the CTG repeat expansion (Reverse TP-PCR). (**a**) TP-PCR with P4 primers binding five-six pure CTG repeats. (**b**) TP-PCR with ST-P4 primers binding five interrupted CTG repeats. Interruptions are represented in bold

ditions comprised an initial denaturation step at 94 °C for 5 min, then 30 cycles of denaturation at 94 °C for 1 min, annealing at 68 °C for 90 s, and extension at 72 °C for 2 min followed by a final extension at 72 °C for 10 min (*see* **Notes 11–13**).

4. For fragment size analysis, add 0.3 μL of GeneScan 600 LIZ dye size standard v2.0 to 1–3 μL of each PCR product.
5. Complete with 99.5% formamide to obtain a final volume of 20 μL.
6. Install the PCR tubes without cap in 3500 Genetic Analyzer and run the fragment analysis program (From 30 to 60 min).
7. Analyze the results using GeneMapper Software 5 from ThermoFisher scientific.

3.4 Restriction Enzyme-Digested PCR

We describe an alternative assay that takes advantage of the fact that CCG and CAG interruptions in the CTG-repeat tract generate cleavage sites for the restriction enzyme AciI (CCGC site) and AluI (AGCT site). The CTG repeat region obtained by PCR is digested with these enzymes and the digested and undigested products are loaded on agarose gel.

1. Amplify 5–20 ng of DNA in a final volume of 25 μL with 0.04 U of Taq polymerase, 0.4 μM of 101 and 102 primers, in 1× PCR buffer. Each final reaction is covered with one drop of mineral oil to avoid evaporation. The PCR amplification conditions comprised an initial denaturation of 96 °C for 5 min,

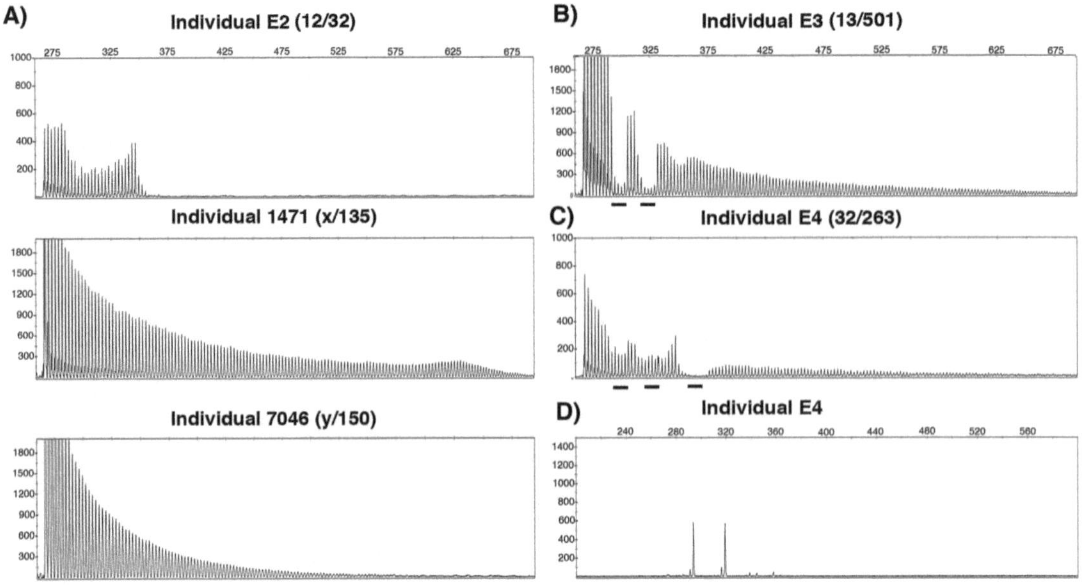

Fig. 2 Traces obtained after Reverse TP-PCR and fragment analysis. The *y*-axis represents the intensity of fluorescence (arbitrary unit), whereas the *x*-axis represents the size in bp of each PCR product. Each fragment obtained by TP-PCR is represented by one peak. The interruptions are represented by a line in the electropherograms **b** and **c** (the number of interruptions can not be determined by TP-PCR). The first peak represents an amplicon with 5 CTG repeats (electropherograms from **a** to **c**). The sizes of CTG repeat in normal and expanded alleles are represented in brackets when the size is known. The size of normal allele was determined by direct sequencing for individuals E2, E3, and E4. The size of expanded allele was determined by PCR for all individuals. The size of normal alleles is unknown for individuals 1471 and 7046. (**a**) Traces from non DM1 individual (Individual E2) and DM1 patients carrying pure CTG repeat expansions. (**b**) Trace from DM1 patient carrying interrupted CTG repeat expansion. Interruptions are usually represented by a clear gap in the electropherogram. (**c**) Trace from DM1 patient carrying interrupted CTG repeat expansion and a normal allele with 32 CTG repeats. The TP-PCR traces from expanded and normal allele overlap. If the interruptions are located in the first thirty CTG repeats, the interruptions will be represented by a decrease of the yield of amplicon generated from this region as observed in the electropherogram **c** from individual E4. No gap in the TP-PCR traces will be observed in this case. (**d**) Traces obtained after reverse specific TP-PCR using ST-P4-3′ primer that recognizes CCG interruptions. Each peak represents at least one interruption (***see*** **Note 10**)

then 30 cycles of denaturation at 96 °C for 45 s, annealing at 68 °C for 30 s, and extension at 72 °C for 3 min followed by a chase of annealing temperature of 1 min and a final extension at 72 °C for 10 min (*see* **Notes 14–16**).

2. Load PCR products on a 2% agarose gel stained with ethidium bromide and 1 kb ladder (*see* **Note 17**).
3. Separate very well both PCR products (from normal and expanded alleles).
4. Excise the DNA fragment corresponding to the expanded allele with a clean scalpel.
5. Weight the gel slice and transfer it in a tube of 1.5 mL.

6. Add 200 μL of buffer NTI for each 100 mg of agarose gel.
7. Incubate sample for 10 min at 50 °C (*see* **Note 18**).
8. Load up 600 μL of sample (NT1 plus dissolved gel) in a NucleoSpin PCR cleanup column into a collection tube.
9. Centrifuge for 30 s at 10,000 rpm and discard flow-through.
10. Place the column back in collection tube.
11. Repeat **steps 6–8** if necessary.
12. Add 700 μL of Buffer N3 to NucleoSpin PCR cleanup column.
13. Centrifuge for 30 s at 10,000 rpm and discard flow-through.
14. Place the column back in collection tube.
15. Repeat **steps 10–12**.
16. Centrifuge for 1 min at 10,000 rpm.
17. Place the NucleoSpin PCR cleanup column in a new tube of 1.5 mL.
18. Add 20–50 μL of water in the middle of NucleoSpin PCR cleanup column without touching the bottom of the column.
19. Incubate for 10 min at room temperature.
20. Centrifuge for 5 min at 8000 rpm.
21. Quantify dsDNA purified PCR product by Qubit fluorometer using standard methods.
22. 40–200 ng of purified PCR product is digested with 20 U of AluI or AciI *and* 1× buffer in a volume of 20 μL (complete the volume with sterilized water).
23. Incubate sample at 37 °C for 3–16 h.
24. Run 40–200 ng undigested PCR product and digested PCR product on a 2.5% agarose gel (*see* **Note 19**).

3.5 Alternative PCR Cleanup (*See* Note 20)

1. When the PCR (**step 1** above) is complete, mix PCR products with 2 V of buffer NT1 to obtain sample N1.
2. Load up 600 μL of N1 in a NucleoSpin PCR cleanup column into a collection tube.
3. Centrifuge for 30 s at 10,000 rpm and discard flow-through.
4. Place the column back in collection tube.
5. Repeat **steps 2–4** if necessary.
6. Add 700 μL Buffer N3 to NucleoSpin PCR cleanup column.
7. Centrifuge for 30 s at 10,000 rpm and discard flow-through.
8. Place the column back in collection tube.
9. Repeat **steps 6–8**.
10. Centrifuge for 1 min at 10,000 rpm.

11. Place the NucleoSpin PCR cleanup column in a tube of 1.5 mL.
12. Add 20–50 μL of water in the middle of NucleoSpin PCR cleanup column without touching the bottom of the column.
13. Incubate for 10 min at room temperature.
14. Centrifuge for 5 min at 8000 rpm.
15. Quantify dsDNA purified PCR product by Qubit fluorometer using standard methods.
16. 40–200 ng of purified PCR product is digested with 20 U of AluI or AciI *and* 1× buffer in a volume of 20 μL (complete the volume with sterilized water).
17. Incubate sample at 37 °C for 3–16 h.
18. Run 40–200 ng undigested PCR product and digested PCR product on a 2.5% agarose gel (*see* **Note 19**).

4 Notes

1. SM0005 buffer is sold by ThermoFisher Scientific and produced in Vilnius, Lithuania. This buffer is essential to amplify the expanded allele. Each tube contains a 10× working concentration (45 mM Tris–HCl (pH 8.8), 11 mM $(NH_4)_2SO_4$, 4.5 mM $MgCl_2$, 0.113 mg/mL BSA, 4.4 μM and 1 mM of each dNTP). Add 69 μM of β-mercaptoethanol in 10× buffer before use.
2. Triplet Prime PCR and Restriction enzyme-digested PCR are performed from genomic DNA extracted from cells, tissues, or blood. It is necessary to work with good-quality DNA which is generally obtained by phenol–chloroform assay as described herein. These two assays work well from genomic DNA extracted with Genomic DNA purification kits from different suppliers. However, the optimal yield and quality of DNA is generally observed with the phenol–chloroform method.
3. All centrifugation steps are performed in the 5427R microcentrifuge from Eppendorf (Rotor FA-45-48-11), but alternative microcentrifuges may be used. 12,700, 10,000 and 8000 rpm correspond to 18,210, 11,290 and 7230 × *g*, respectively.
4. Avoid traces of ethanol that could disrupt the next stage of the experiments.
5. The quality of the genomic DNA is assessed by resolving about 200 ng of DNA on a 0.8% agarose gel stained with ethidium bromide and Lamdba DNA/HindIII marker. Degraded DNA looks like a smear of smaller fragments.
6. The benchtop Qubit Fluorometer accurately measure dsDNA using Qubit dsDNA high-sensitivity (HS) and broad-range

(BR) assays are highly selective for dsDNA. Both assays can be used. HS Qubit DNA assay measures initial concentration from 10 pg/μL to 100 ng/μL, whereas BR Qubit DNA assay measures initial concentration from 100 pg/μL to 1000 ng/μL. The procedure is identical between both assays. If necessary, the Qubit 3.0 user manual from ThermoFisher scientific can provide more details on instructions and protocols.

7. TP-PCR is a fast method to identify the presence of an expanded allele in DM1 patients. However, the size of the CTG expansions cannot be determined by this method. A classical PCR or Southern blot should be performed.
8. The signal of the amplicons decreases with their size (Fig. 2). It is blindly difficult to see the interruptions within the repeated region at the end of the traces. To avoid misinterpretation of the TP-PCR traces, it is essential to assess forward and reverse TP-PCR.
9. Repeated sequences are difficult to amplify by PCR. It is difficult to amplify more than 200 CTG repeats by forward and reverse TP-PCR. Interruptions are difficult to observe in the middle of CTG.CAG repeats larger than 300 CTG repeats by TP-PCR. Single molecule, real time sequencing developed by PacBio can be used to sequence large CTG repeat from genomic DNA extracted from blood of DM1 patient [14]. However, this innovative technology remains very expensive and does not allow a wide utilization.
10. CCG and CAG interruptions within CTG repeated sequences are identified by TP-PCR using specific ST-P4 primers. This strategy has been validated in blood from several DM1 patients [7]. Here, the ST-P4-primers were designed to identity non-consecutive CCG and CAG interruptions by a fast method. This strategy can be extended to other motifs by designing new primers that will bind other types of interruptions. This strategy remains fast and low cost compared to the single-cell sequencing cited in **Note 9**.
11. The PCR amplification conditions change when reverse specific TP-PCR is performed (Table 1). The annealing temperature is 70 °C.
12. Troubleshooting: low yield after the fragment analysis. The amplicon mixture obtained by TP-PCR is low. Check the efficiency of TP-PCR by loading 10 μL of PCR products on a 1.5% agarose gel stained with ethidium bromide and 1 kb ladder. The PCR looks like a smear of larger amplicons [13]. Adjust the quantity of PCR product added on formamide and GeneScan 600 LIZ dye Size standard v2.0 to obtain a usable TP-PCR trace.

13. Troubleshooting: no signal. Make sure that each step of the TP-PCR and fragment analysis was correctly performed. Repeat reaction set up. It is suggested to add controls for each TP-PCR experiment.
14. PCR will be performed to amplify CTG repeat and will generate two amplicons containing normal CTG repeat or expanded CTG repeat with a size of 112 bp + (xCTG).
15. Another PCR, compatible with the restriction enzyme digestion, can be performed to amplify CTG repeat. Amplify 5–20 ng of DNA in a final volume of 25 μL with 0.04 U of Taq polymerase, 0.4 μM of DM-C and DM-BR primers, in 1× PCR buffer. Each final reaction is covered with one drop of mineral oil to avoid evaporation. The PCR amplification conditions comprised an initial denaturation of 96 °C for 5 min, then 28 cycles of denaturation at 96 °C for 45 s, annealing at 68 °C for 30 s, and extension at 70 °C for 3 min followed by a chase of annealing temperature of 1 min and a final extension at 70 °C for 10 min [16, 18]. PCR will generate two amplicons containing normal CTG repeat or expanded CTG repeat with a size of 147 bp + (xCTG).
16. In order to optimize the quantity of purified PCR product to assess digestion in the good condition, multiple replicate reactions are performed.
17. If the size of the CTG repeat is less than 500 CTG, gel extraction is assessed using NucleoSpin Gel according to the manufacturer's recommendation from Macherey-Nagel.
18. Agarose gel has to be completely dissolved after incubation. If necessary, increase the incubation time to achieve this.
19. The digestion can be incomplete and result from somatic instability observed in DM1 patient.
20. If the size of the CTG repeat is more than 500 CTG, gel extraction is assessed using PCR cleanup according to the manufacturer's recommendation from Macherey-Nagel.

Acknowledgments

The authors would like to thank Anchel González Barriga for helpful discussion and comments. This work was supported by Institut National de la Santé et de la recherche Médicale (INSERM), Université Paris Descartes, and AFM-Téléthon (project number 16331 and 19757). This program received a state subsidy managed by the National Research Agency under the "Investments for the Future" program bearing the reference ANR-10-IAHU-01.

References

1. Paulson H (2018) Repeat expansion diseases. Handb Clin Neurol 147:105–123
2. Eichler EE, Holden JJ, Popovich BW, Reiss AL, Snow K et al (1994) Length of uninterrupted CGG repeats determines instability in the FMR1 gene. Nat Genet 8:88–94
3. Nolin SL, Sah S, Glicksman A, Sherman SL, Allen E et al (2013) Fragile X AGG analysis provides new risk predictions for 45-69 repeat alleles. Am J Med Genet A 161A:771–778
4. Yrigollen CM, Martorell L, Durbin-Johnson B, Naudo M, Genoves J et al (2014) AGG interruptions and maternal age affect FMR1 CGG repeat allele stability during transmission. J Neurodev Disord 6:24
5. Domniz N, Ries-Levavi L, Cohen Y, Marom-Haham L, Berkenstadt M et al (2018) Absence of AGG interruptions is a risk factor for full mutation expansion among Israeli FMR1 premutation carriers. Front Genet 9:606
6. Santoro M, Masciullo M, Silvestri G, Novelli G, Botta A (2016) Myotonic dystrophy type 1: role of CCG, CTC and CGG interruptions within DMPK alleles in the pathogenesis and molecular diagnosis. Clin Genet 92(4):355–364
7. Tome S, Dandelot E, Dogan C, Bertrand A, Genevieve D et al (2018) Unusual association of a unique CAG interruption in 5′ of DM1 CTG repeats with intergenerational contractions and low somatic mosaicism. Hum Mutat 39(7):970–982
8. Botta A, Rossi G, Marcaurelio M, Fontana L, D'Apice MR et al (2017) Identification and characterization of 5′ CCG interruptions in complex DMPK expanded alleles. Eur J Hum Genet 25:257–261
9. Braida C, Stefanatos RK, Adam B, Mahajan N, Smeets HJ et al (2010) Variant CCG and GGC repeats within the CTG expansion dramatically modify mutational dynamics and likely contribute toward unusual symptoms in some myotonic dystrophy type 1 patients. Hum Mol Genet 19:1399–1412
10. Musova Z, Mazanec R, Krepelova A, Ehler E, Vales J et al (2009) Highly unstable sequence interruptions of the CTG repeat in the myotonic dystrophy gene. Am J Med Genet A 149A:1365–1374
11. Pesovic J, Peric S, Brkusanin M, Brajuskovic G, Rakocevic-Stojanovic V et al (2017) Molecular genetic and clinical characterization of myotonic dystrophy type 1 patients carrying variant repeats within DMPK expansions. Neurogenetics 18(4):207–218
12. Santoro M, Masciullo M, Pietrobono R, Conte G, Modoni A et al (2013) Molecular, clinical, and muscle studies in myotonic dystrophy type 1 (DM1) associated with novel variant CCG expansions. J Neurol 260:1245–1257
13. Dryland PA, Doherty E, Love JM, Love DR (2013) Simple repeat-primed PCR analysis of the myotonic dystrophy type 1 gene in a clinical diagnostics environment. J Neurodegener Dis 2013:857564
14. Cumming SA, Hamilton MJ, Robb Y, Gregory H, McWilliam C et al (2018) De novo repeat interruptions are associated with reduced somatic instability and mild or absent clinical features in myotonic dystrophy type 1. Eur J Hum Genet 26:1635–1647
15. Warner JP, Barron LH, Goudie D, Kelly K, Dow D et al (1996) A general method for the detection of large CAG repeat expansions by fluorescent PCR. J Med Genet 33:1022–1026
16. Monckton DG, Wong LJ, Ashizawa T, Caskey CT (1995) Somatic mosaicism, germline expansions, germline reversions and intergenerational reductions in myotonic dystrophy males: small pool PCR analyses. Hum Mol Genet 4:1–8
17. Seznec H, Lia-Baldini AS, Duros C, Fouquet C, Lacroix C et al (2000) Transgenic mice carrying large human genomic sequences with expanded CTG repeat mimic closely the DM CTG repeat intergenerational and somatic instability. Hum Mol Genet 9:1185–1194
18. Gomes-Pereira M, Bidichandani SI, Monckton DG (2004) Analysis of unstable triplet repeats using small-pool polymerase chain reaction. Methods Mol Biol 277:61–76

Chapter 3

Tracking Expansions of Stable and Threshold Length Trinucleotide Repeat Tracts In Vivo and In Vitro Using *Saccharomyces cerevisiae*

Gregory M. Williams, Athena K. Petrides, Lata Balakrishnan, and Jennifer A. Surtees

Abstract

Trinucleotide repeat (TNR) tracts are inherently unstable during DNA replication, leading to repeat expansions and/or contractions. Expanded tracts are the cause of over 40 neurodegenerative and neuromuscular diseases. In this chapter, we focus on the $(CAG)_n$ and $(CTG)_n$ repeat sequences that, when expanded, lead to Huntington's disease (HD) and myotonic dystrophy type 1 (DM1), respectively, as well as a number of other neurodegenerative diseases. TNR tracts in most individuals are relatively small and stable in terms of length. However, TNR tracts become increasingly prone to expansion as tract length increases, eventually leading to very long tracts that disrupt coding (e.g. HD) or noncoding (e.g., DM1) regions of the genome. It is important to understand the early stages in TNR expansions, that is, the transition from small, stable lengths to susceptible threshold lengths. We describe PCR-based in vivo assays, using the model system *Saccharomyces cerevisiae*, to determine and characterize the dynamic behavior of TNR tracts in the stable and threshold ranges. We also describe a simple in vitro system to assess tract dynamics during 5′ single-stranded DNA (ssDNA) flap processing and to assess the role of different DNA metabolism proteins in these dynamics. These assays can ultimately be used to determine factors that influence the early stages of TNR tract expansion.

Key words Trinucleotide repeat, Expansion, Contraction, Polymerase chain reaction, *Saccharomyces cerevisiae*, DNA replication, Repeat tract dynamics, Microsatellite instability

1 Introduction

Trinucleotide repeat (TNR) sequences lead to many neurodegenerative diseases once they expand beyond a threshold length. A major mechanism by which these tracts are thought to expand is through DNA replication, particularly during Okazaki fragment processing [1–3], which involves 5′ ssDNA flap cleavage by Rad27 (FEN1 in humans), creating nick at the base of the flap that is sealed by ligation by Cdc9 (Lig1 in humans) [4]. Rad27 and Cdc9 also play an important role in long patch base excision repair

Guy-Franck Richard (ed.), *Trinucleotide Repeats: Methods and Protocols*, Methods in Molecular Biology, vol. 2056, https://doi.org/10.1007/978-1-4939-9784-8_3, © Springer Science+Business Media, LLC, part of Springer Nature 2020

(LP-BER), which is another mechanism by which TNR tracts are thought to expand [5, 6]. In *Saccharomyces cerevisiae*, loss of Rad27 (*rad27Δ*) leads to an increase in dinucleotide and trinucleotide repeat expansions [7–11].

Repetitive sequences (i.e., mono-, di-, tri-, tetra-, etc.), or microsatellites, are inherently difficult to replicate accurately and are consequently hotspots for genetic mutation due to the increased frequency of replicative polymerase slippage events that can occur during synthesis of these regions [12–15]. This leads to microsatellite instability and an elevated rate of change in the number of repeats. If left unrepaired, these slippage events are mutagenic and can be detrimental to the cell. $(CNG)_n$ TNR sequences present an additional hurdle to accurate DNA replication because of their propensity to form secondary structure (due to C-G base pairing) when the DNA is single-stranded, as can happen during replication, particularly during lagging strand synthesis [3, 16]. While the mismatch repair (MMR) system, particularly Msh2-Msh3, typically directs repair of these slippage events, particularly in repetitive DNA sequences [17–19], these TNR structures are refractory to MMR [20]. In fact, Msh2 and Msh3 have been shown to promote TNR expansions in a variety of systems [16, 21–28].

TNR tract expansions can occur in small or large increments and it appears to depend on the initial size of the tract [29, 30]. Shorter stable and threshold length tracts expand incrementally [16, 27, 30] and are predicted to occur during replication through replication slippage events or altered flap ligation during lagging strand synthesis [3, 16, 30–33]. These smaller expansions may also occur via misalignment of repeats during homologous recombination and double-strand DNA break repair [32] or during repair of oxidation damage of CNG repeats through base excision repair [5, 32, 34]. Notably, Msh2-Msh3 has been implicated in each of these mechanisms. Transcription-coupled repair has also been implicated in incremental expansions [32]. Larger scale expansions of TNR tracts appear to occur via homologous recombination, template switching, and break-induced replication [30, 32]. Overall, expansions can occur within a coding region or a noncoding region of DNA, with noncoding regions tending to accumulate larger expansions [30].

Expansions of TNR sequences are associated with several hereditary neurological diseases, including Huntington's disease (HD), myotonic dystrophy (DM1), and Friedrich's ataxia (FRDA) [28, 30, 32, 33, 35, 36]. As the tract size increases, the expression and/or function of a protein is increasingly compromised, eventually leading to disease (Fig. 1). The transition from a stable repeat tract to an expanded, pathogenic tract is a critical step in the development of TNR-mediated disease. However, small changes in tract size can mean the difference between stability and instability. Furthermore, tract length has been strongly correlated with

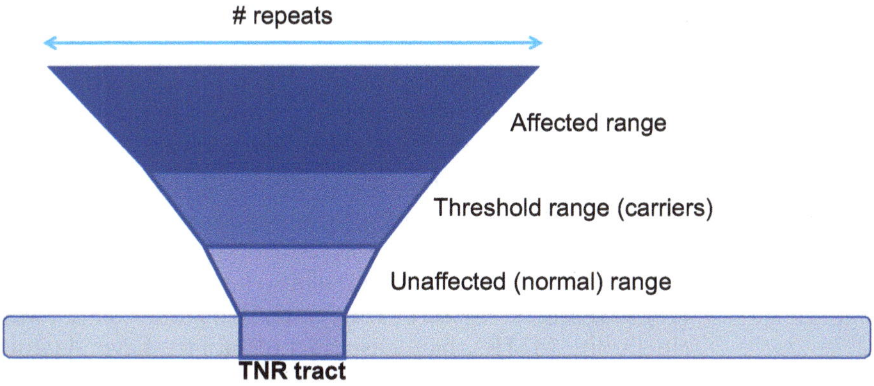

Fig. 1 TNR tracts within the normal range (which is tract-dependent) are stably maintained. Through a variety of mechanisms in DNA metabolism, a TNR tract can expand, bringing the tract into a "threshold-length" range, in which these somewhat longer tracts are not pathogenic, but are increasingly susceptible to expansion; these individuals are carriers for disease. Further tract expansion crosses the disease-specific threshold; tracts above this threshold are pathogenic and cause disease. As the TNR tract length increases, the tract is increasingly unstable and prone to changes in length, particularly expansions

heritability of TNR expansion diseases, age of onset of disease, penetrance of disease, and severity of disease [37–46]. Variant repeats and repeat interruptions reduce the propensity to expand and result in milder phenotypes [45, 47]. Therefore, even small reductions in tract length, or in the probability of expansion, have significant implications for the prevention and treatment of human disease.

Small expansions within a stable TNR bring the tract into a "threshold-range" in which the tracts are not pathogenic but are increasingly prone to expansions [25, 27, 37, 48] (Fig. 1). Such intermediate alleles for HD (~27–35 CAG repeats) have recently been reported in ~6% of the general population [40], suggesting that these individuals are potential HD carriers. As a result, it is of interest to understand the dynamic behavior of TNR tracts within the threshold or intermediate range as well as the mechanisms driving these changes in tract length. Historically, end-point experiments, including single sperm typing [49–53] have been used to assess changes in tract length, although induced pluripotent cells derived from patients have been used to assess tract-length changes over time [54]. The single sperm typing studies facilitated important modeling experiments that predicted that threshold-length TNR tracts will preferentially increase in increments smaller than the repeats themselves [55–57]. Using the dynamic in vivo system described in this chapter, we demonstrated that threshold length tracts are highly dynamic, they increase (or decrease) in increments as small as a single repeat unit and the changes in tract length are biased toward expansion in vivo [27]. These observations were consistent with our in vitro observations [16], which allowed us to assess the mechanistic contribution of potential modifiers of tract length such as Msh2-Msh3.

Here we describe a set of in vivo in *S. cerevisiae* and in vitro assays using *S. cerevisiae* purified proteins, designed to assess repeat tract length with one repeat resolution under different conditions and in the presence of different protein factors. In this protocol, we focus specifically on $(CAG)_n$ and $(CTG)_n$ repeat tracts within the stable and threshold ranges, that is, those poised to expand—or contract. Using these approaches, we can detect dynamic tract length changes and start to understand the underlying mechanism(s) (including MMR) that cause tract instability. Several genetic modifiers of TNR expansions disease have been identified in human populations [33, 44, 58–60]. These assays can be used to determine the effect of these modifiers as well as therapeutic drugs on repeat tract dynamics.

2 Materials

Make up all buffers with deionized water (dIH_2O). Store at room temperature unless otherwise noted.

2.1 General Reagents for In Vivo Assays

1. 10× TBE: For 1 L: 108.0 g Tris base, 55.0 g boric acid, 7.44 g Ethylenediaminetetraacetic acid (EDTA). The 0.5× TBE solution is 45 mM Tris-borate, 1 mM EDTA.
   (a) Add each of the measured components into a beaker containing a stir bar and 500 mL of deionized water and place beaker onto a stir plate.
   (b) Allow components to dissolve in solution (~1 h). Heat can be used to assist components into solution (not to exceed 60 °C).
   (c) Bring dissolved solution up to a final volume of 1 L with dIH_2O. Store at room temperature.
   (d) To make polyacrylamide gel running buffer, dilute the 10× TBE buffer down to 0.5× TBE (950 mL dIH_2O + 50 mL 10× TBE).
2. Solutions for Lithium acetate transformations.
   (a) 1 M Lithium acetate (LiAc), pH 7.5 (adjusted with a few drops of diluted acetic acid). Autoclave.
   (b) 10× TE (100 mM Tris–HCl pH 7.5, 10 mM EDTA, pH 7.5). Autoclave.
   (c) 50% PEG (50% w/v). Filter-sterilize.
   (d) LiAC/TE Mix: 1 mL of 1 M LiAc, 1 mL of 10× TE, 8 mL of sterile dIH_2O. Make fresh.

(e) 40% PEG Mix: 1 mL of LiAc, 1 mL 1× TE, 8 mL of 50% PEG. Make fresh.

3. Chromosome Preparation Buffer.
   (a) 8.68 mL of H_2O/Triton X solution: 8.48 mL of H_2O + 200 μL Triton X-100.
   (b) 1 mL of 10% SDS.
   (c) 200 μL of 5 M NaCl.
   (d) 100 μL of 1 M Tris–HCl, pH 8.0.
   (e) 20 μL of 0.5 M EDTA, pH 8.0.
4. 1× Amino acid drop-out mix (powder)—for this protocol we use mixes lacking histidine OR histidine and uracil: 800 mg adenine, 800 mg uracil, 800 mg tryptophan, 800 mg histidine, 800 mg arginine, 800 mg methionine, 1.2 g tyrosine, 1.2 g lysine, 2.4 g leucine, 2.0 g phenylalanine, 8.0 g threonine.

2.2 Polymerase Chain Reaction (PCR)

PCR Reaction Mixture: 2 mM $MgCl_2$, 10 × Taq Buffer (200 mM Tris–HCl pH 8.8, 100 mM $(NH_4)_2SO_4$, 100 mM KCl, 1% Triton X-100), dNTP mix (2.5 mM each), *Taq* Polymerase (*see* **Note 1**), Primers SO295 and SO296 (Table 1).

2.3 Expansion Assays and Time Courses

1. Synthetic Complete (SC) plates (1 L): 7.0 g Yeast Nitrogen Base without amino acids (+ammonium sulfate), 0.87 g amino acid drop-out mix (−histidine OR −histidine and −uracil), 20.0 g agar, 950 mL sterile dIH_2O.
   (a) Add stir bar and all measured contents into a 2 L flask, capping the top with aluminum foil.
   (b) Autoclave at 121 °C for 40 min.
   (c) Remove from autoclave and add 50.0 mL of sterile 40% glucose to flask.
   (d) Allow flask to cool before pouring into plates. Store at room temperature or at 4 °C.
2. Liquid Synthetic Complete medium (1 L): 7.0 g Yeast Nitrogen Base without amino acids (+ammonium sulfate), 0.87 g of −histidine amino acid drop-out mix, 950 mL sterile dIH_2O.
   (a) Add all contents into a 1 L screw-cap bottle.
   (b) Autoclave at 121 °C for 40 min.
   (c) Remove from autoclave, add 50.0 mL of sterile 40% glucose to bottle and allow media to cool to room temperature before use.
   (d) Liquid media can be stored for long periods of time without addition of 40% glucose.
3. Synthetic Complete (SC) plates containing 5-FOA (1 L).

Table 1
List of oligonucleotide sequences. *All oligonucleotides are in the 5'–3' orientation*

In vivo TNR expansion assay	
SO295	AAACTCGGTTTGACGCCTCCCATG
SO296	AGCAACAGGACTAGGATGAGTAGC
A: Flap substrates (in vitro)	
T1	GCC CAG TCA CGT CGT TGT AAA ACG GGT CGT GAC TGG GAA AAC CCT GGC G
U1	CGC CAG GGT TTT CCC AGT CAC GAC CA
D5	GCC GCT GTT TTA CAA CGA CGT GAC TGG G
D10	CAC TGG CCG TCG TTT TAC AAC GAC GTG ACT GGG
D20	TTA GTT AAT TCA CTG GCC GTC GTT TTA CAA CGA CGT GAC TGG G
D30	TTC ACG CCT GTT AGT TAA TTC ACT GGC CGT CGT TTT ACA ACG ACG TGA CTG GG
B: Bubble substrates (in vitro)	
T2	GCC CAG TCA CGT CGT TGT AAA ACG GGT CGT GAC TGG GAA AAC CCT GGC
U2	CAC GCT ACC GAA TTC TGA
D4	CTT GAA GAT CTG GTA ATG CCC ACG TTG ACC CCA GTC
D6	CTT GCT TAG GGG CGC CAA CCC ACG TTG ACC CCA GTC

C: Polymerase substrate (in vitro)	
T3	CCC ACC TAA CTT TAA ATC CGA CCG TGC CAG CCG TGA CCG GCA GCA TAG GCC TTA AGC AGA ACC AAC ATC CTA GGG TCG TGT AAC TTC CGT CCT CCA CCG CAG CCC ACC TG
U3	GTCCACCCGACGCCACCTCCTGCCTTCAATGTGCTGGGATCCTA
D3	AGACGAATTCCGGATACGACGGCCAGTGCCGACCGTGCCAGCCTAAATTTCAATCCACCC
D: Equilibrating flap substrates (in vitro)	
T4	GCC CAG TCA CGT CGT TGT AAA ACG GGT CGT GAC TGG GAA AAC CCT GGC
UR4	CGA CCG TGC CAG CCT AAA TTT CAA TTT CTA CTT CCA ATT GAT ACG CGC TAT AAC C
UE4	TTC CCA GTC ACG ACC CTT AGC TGC TGC TGC TGC TGC TGC TGC TGC TGC TG
DR4	/p/TTC TAC TTC CAA TTG ATA CGC GCT ATA ACC CCG TCC ACC CGA CGC CAC CTC CTG C
DE4	/p/CTG CTG CTG CTG CTG CTG CTG CTG CTG CTG CAC GAG GTA AAA CGA CGG CCA GTG

(a) In a 2 L flask, add a stir bar, 700 mL of deionized water, 20.0 g of agar, and 20.0 g of glucose. Autoclave at 121 °C for 40 min.

(b) In a separate beaker containing a stir bar and 200 mL of deionized water, add 7.0 g Yeast Nitrogen Base without amino acids (+ammonium sulfate), 0.87 g of –histidine –uracil amino acid drop-out mix, 50 mg of uracil, 1.0 g 5-FOA (0.1%).

(c) Stir contents of beaker on a stir plate until dissolved (~1–2 h). Bring the total volume up to 300 mL using dIH_2O.

(d) Filter-sterilize the 5-FOA solution using a 0.2 μm filter.

(e) Once the flask of agar and glucose cools to approximately 80 °C, add the 5-FOA solution to the flask, allowing it to completely mix on the stir plate. Immediately pour into plates.

(f) Allow the plates to cool, then store at 4 °C in the dark (*see* **Note 2**).

4. 12% Polyacrylamide, 0.5× TBE Gels.

(a) Acrylamide–bisacrylamide solution (29:1).

(b) 10× TBE.

(c) 10% ammonium persulfate (APS).

(d) TEMED.

(e) Horizontal gel apparatus, 16 cm × 14 cm glass plates, 0.75 mm spacers and a 20 well comb.

(f) 10× polyacrylamide loading dye (0.25% bromophenol blue, 0.25% xylene cyanol, 30% glycerol).

(g) Low-molecular weight DNA marker.

(h) Plastic staining tray.

(i) Ethidium bromide.

2.4 Southern Blotting

1. Denaturation buffer: 0.5 N NaOH, 1.5 M NaCl.
2. Neutralization buffer: 0.5 M Tris–HCl pH 7.0, 3.0 M NaCl. Start with ~700 mL dIH_2O, bring Tris and NaCl into solution. Adjust pH to 7.0 with concentrated HCl and then bring final volume (1 L) with dIH_2O.
3. 10× SSC: dissolve 87.7 g of NaCl and 44.1 g of sodium citrate in ~800 mL dIH_2O. Adjust pH to 7.0 with a few drops of 10 N NaOH and adjust to 1 L dIH_2O. This concentrated stock of NaOH is required to quickly adjust the pH.
4. 1.85 MBq (50 μCi) [α-^{32}P] dCTP (~111TBq/mmol, 370 MQq/mL).

5. Random Priming DNA labeling kit.
6. Stratalinker or equivalent UV cross-linker.
7. Hybridization buffer: 0.5 M phosphate, 7% SDS, 1 mM EDTA pH 8.0, 10 mg/mL BSA.
8. Wash buffer: 40 mM phosphate, 5% SDS, 1 mM EDTA pH 8.0.
9. HYBAID hybridization oven, or similar.
10. Hybridization bottles.
11. STORM PhosphorImager, or equivalent phosphor imaging technology.
12. Storage phosphor screen.

2.5 Reagents for In Vitro Oligonucleotide Labeling

1. Oligonucleotides (Table 1).
2. Labeling Reaction Buffer: 1 M Tris–HCl (pH 8.0), 1 M $MgCl_2$, 1 M NaCl.
3. dIH_2O.
4. α-^{32}P dCTP (6000 Ci/mmol).
5. DNA Polymerase I, large *Klenow* fragment (2 U/μL).
6. 10× TBE (Stock Buffer): 1 M Tris–borate, 0.02 M EDTA, dissolved in 1 L of dIH_2O.
7. 1× TBE (Electrophoresis buffer): Dilute 100 mL of 10× TBE in 900 mL of dIH_2O.
8. 10% ammonium persulfate (APS).
9. Tetramethylethylenediamine (TEMED).
10. 12% Polyacrylamide sequencing gel: 45 mL acrylamide–bisacrylamide (40% w/v), 63 g urea, 15 mL 10× TBE, 300 μL 10% APS, 30 μL TEMED and 37.5 mL dIH_2O. Sequencing gel is made using 0.8 mm thick spacers and a 26-well comb.
11. Ethanol: 95% and 70%.
12. Duplex Annealing buffer: 100 mM potassium acetate, 30 mM HEPES pH 7.5.
13. Micro Bio-Spin P-30 column.
14. Whatman filter paper.
15. Scintillation vials.
16. Scintillation fluid.
17. Spin-X filter column 0.22 μm.
18. Autoradiography markers.
19. Glycogen.

2.6 Enzyme Assays

1. 1× TBE (Electrophoresis buffer): 0.1 M Tris–borate, 0.002 M EDTA, dissolved in 1 L of dIH_2O.

2. Nuclease reaction buffer: 50 mM Tris–HCl (pH 8.0), 2 mM DTT, 0.25 mg/mL bovine serum albumin (BSA), 30 mM NaCl, 4 mM $MgCl_2$, 2 mM ATP and 5% glycerol.
3. Ligation reaction buffer: 30 mM Tris–HCl (pH 7.6), 2 mM DTT, 0.25 mg/mL bovine serum albumin (BSA), 40 mM NaCl, 8 mM $MgCl_2$, 1 mM ATP and 5% glycerol.
4. Polymerase reaction buffer: 50 mM Tris–HCl (pH 7.5), 2 mM DTT, 0.25 mg/mL bovine serum albumin (BSA), 75 mM NaCl, 4 mM $MgCl_2$, 1 mM ATP, 50 μM dNTPs, and 5% glycerol.
5. Electromobility gel shift assay (EMSA) reaction buffer: 50 mM Tris–HCl (pH 8.0), 2 mM DTT, 0.25 mg/mL BSA, 30 mM NaCl, 20 μM EDTA, and 5% glycerol.
6. Termination dye: 90% formamide (v/v), 10 mM EDTA, 0.1% xylene cyanol, and 0.1% bromophenol blue.
7. 6% polyacrylamide native gel: 15 mL acrylamide–bisacrylamide (40% w/v), 10 mL 10× TBE, 550 μL 10% APS, 55 μL TEMED, and 74.5 mL dIH_2O. 24-well combs and 1.55 mm thick spacers are used to make native gel.
8. 15% polyacrylamide sequencing gel: 22.5 mL acrylamide–bisacrylamide (40% w/v), 33.8 g urea, 8 mL 10× TBE, 300 μL 10% APS, 30 μL TEMED, and 29.2 mL dIH_2O. 26-well combs and 0.35 mm thick spacers are used to make denaturing gel.

2.7 Recombinant Proteins

1. Msh2-Msh3 (*see* **Note 3**).
2. $Rad27^{FEN1}$ (*see* **Note 4**).
3. $Cdc9^{Lig1}$ (*see* **Note 5**).
4. DNA Polymerase Delta Pol δ (*see* **Note 6**).

2.8 Equipment

1. OPTIMAX™ X-ray processor.
2. Scintillation counter.
3. Sequencing S2 gel electrophoresis apparatus for 30 cm × 40 cm vertical glass plates.
4. Polyacrylamide gel electrophoresis apparatus for 17 cm × 15 cm vertical glass plates.
5. 30 cm × 40 cm (W × L) vertical glass plates, 0.35 mm spacers and 26-well comb for polyacrylamide gel electrophoresis (PAGE) gels.
6. 17 cm × 15 cm (W × L) vertical glass plates, 1.55 mm spacers, and 24-well comb for native electrophoresis gels.
7. Power supply.
8. Typhoon™ FLA 9500 phosphorimager or similar phosphor imaging technology.

3 Methods

3.1 Construction of Strains Containing TNR Tracts

1. Use a *URA3* reporter system construct to select for expansion events in vivo [61–64]. TNR substrates are integrated into each strain of interest, using plasmids that contain the reporter construct, repeat tract sequences, and sequences to integrate the system at the *LYS2* locus [16, 27, 63]. Plasmids encoding $(CAG)_{25}$, $(CTG)_{25}$, scrambled $(C,A,G)_{25}$ or $(C,T,G)_{25}$ are used [62, 63]. Each repeat tract is cloned into the regulatory region controlling expression of the *URA3* reporter gene. When the distance between the TATA box and the initiator ATG for the *URA3* gene is increased beyond 29 repeats, *URA3* is no longer expressed, making the cells resistant to 5-FOA (*see* **Note 7**) (Fig. 2).
2. Linearize each plasmid by digestion with *Bsu*36I and then transform the appropriate yeast strain using the lithium acetate method [65], to allow integration at the *LYS2* locus by homologous recombination.
3. For each transformation, set up a 5 mL culture in liquid medium from a single colony. Incubate overnight in a 30 °C shaker.

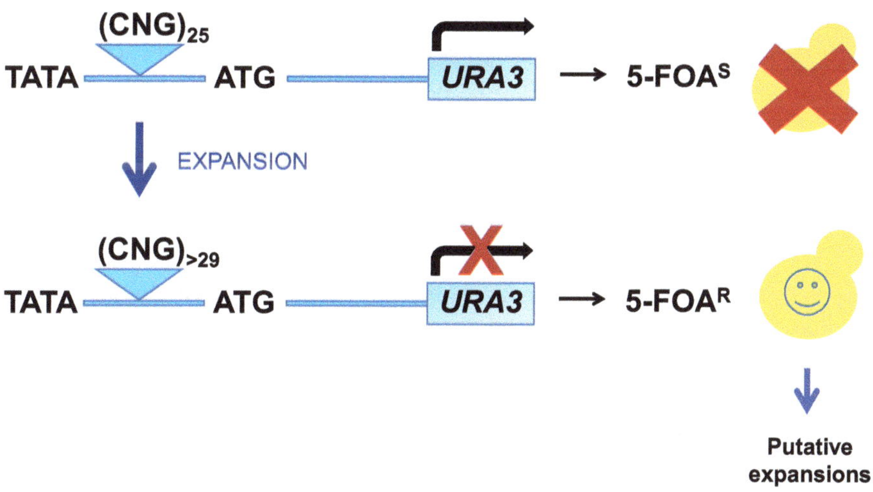

Fig. 2 TNR reporter system used to select expansions. This construct is integrated on the lagging strand at the chromosomal *LYS2* locus by homologous recombination with *HIS3* as a selectable marker. Single integration is confirmed by Southern blotting. The *URA3* gene is used as a reporter gene to select for expansions [62]. The *Schizosaccharomyces pombe adh1* promoter is used to drive *URA3* expression. This promoter is sensitive to the distance between TATA and ATG; 55–125 bp is optimal for function. Insertion of a trinucleotide repeat $(CNG)_{25}$ between TATA and ATG allows *URA3* expression and results in sensitivity to the drug 5-FOA, which is toxic to the cell in the presence of the Ura3 gene product. Expansion of the TNR tract beyond 29 repeats alters the transcriptional start site, inactivating *URA3* expression and leading to 5-FOA resistance. These events are selected on plates containing 5-FOA

4. From the saturated culture, dilute 1:30 to start a new 20–30 mL liquid culture in a 125 mL sterile flask. Incubate in a 30 °C shaker until the culture reaches mid-logarithmic growth (OD_{600} ~0.5–0.8).
5. Collect the cells by centrifugation (3000 × *g*). Wash the pellet in 1 mL sterile dIH_2O. Transfer to a microcentrifuge tube.
6. Collect the cells by centrifugation (16,000 × *g*) and discard the supernatant. Wash the cells with 1 mL LiAc/TE mix. Collect the by centrifugation again and resuspend the pellet in 250 μL LiAc/TE mix.
7. For each transformation, mix 50 μL of the yeast suspension, ~150 ng digested plasmid and 10 μL sonicated salmon sperm DNA (10 mg/mL). Always do a negative control with no plasmid DNA added.
8. After mixing, add 600 μL 40% PEG mix.
9. Incubate reactions in a 30 °C shaker for at least 30 min.
10. Incubate the reactions in a 42 °C water bath for 15 min to heat shock.
11. Briefly centrifuge the reaction (30 s), discarding the supernatant. Resuspend the cells in 200 mL 1× TE, pH 7.5. Select for integrants by plating on SC –histidine. Incubate in 30 °C incubator for ~3 days.
12. Individual transformants are struck out to single colonies on SC histidine plates. A single colony from each candidate is frozen down for storage in 20% glycerol until ready to test for single integration of the reporter construct.
13. Perform Southern blotting (*see* below) to ensure that a *single* copy of the reporter construct has been integrated at the correct chromosomal locus [63].

3.2 TNR Expansion Assay: Selecting for Expansions

1. From a frozen glycerol (20%) stock of the strain that is to be tested, streak cells out to single colonies on a SC-histidine. Place plate into the 30 °C incubator for 3–4 days allowing the single cells to grow into ~2 mm colonies (Fig. 3a).
2. Select and mark three individual colonies to test for unexpanded tracts, labeling them 1, 2, and 3.
3. Perform colony PCR on these colonies to confirm that the repeat tract size is 25 repeats (75 bp). Perform PCR as follows:
   (a) For each reaction, combine 12.3 μL sterile dIH_2O, 1.6 μL 25 mM $MgCl_2$, 2 μL 10× Taq Buffer, 2 μL dNTP mix (2.5 mM each), 0.8 μL of 5 pmol/μL SO295, 0.8 μL of 5 pmol/μL SO296, 0.5 μL *Taq* Polymerase (*see* **Note 1**).

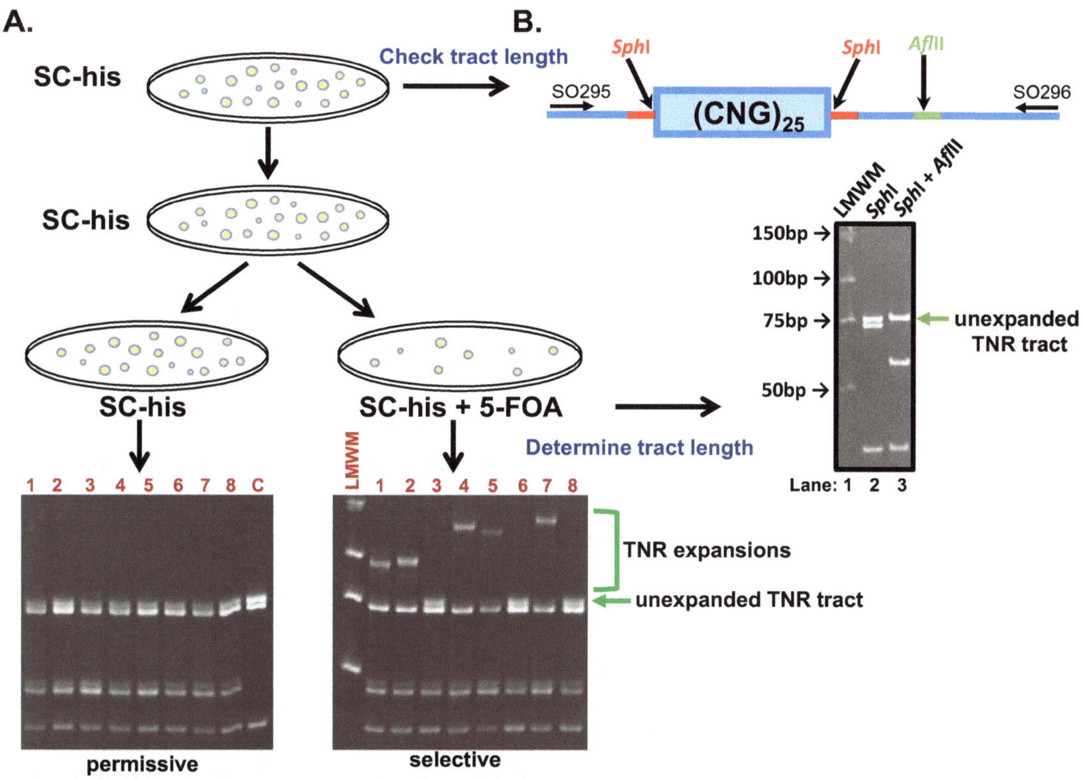

Fig. 3 Selection for TNR expansion events. (**a**) Cells with an integrated reporter construct are diluted and plated on SC-his (to maintain the construct) to form single colonies. The TNR tract size of individual colonies is assessed (*see* **b**). Colonies with unexpanded tracts are selected for the expansion assay. The colonies are resuspended, diluted and plated on permissive plates (SC-his) to allow expansions to occur during the growth of the colony. Ten colonies are selected, resuspended, diluted and plated on permissive (SC-his) and selective (SC-his+5-FOA) plates. Colony counts on permissive and selective plates are used to calculate mutation rates, or apparent TNR expansion rates. The TNR tract size of a subset of colonies is assessed to determine a false positive rate and to assess the range in expansion sizes observed in different genetic backgrounds and with different TNR tract sequences. These gels show amplified tracts digested with *Sph*I, which results in the doublet observed in permissive plate lanes when the tract is unexpanded. The majority of colonies grown on selective plates exhibit TNR tract expansions. (**b**) The TNR tract length can be determined by PCR, using primers upstream and downstream of the repeat sequence (S0295 and S0296), resulting in a PCR fragment of 188 bp. The amplified regions of DNA immediately upstream and downstream of the repeat tract can be digested with *Sph*I, freeing the TNR tract. Lane 2 shows that *Sph*I digestion results in three distinct bands, with a doublet at 79 bp (the 25 repeat TNR tract) and 73 bp and a 41 bp fragment. To eliminate the doublet for easier assessment of the TNR tract size, the 73 bp fragment is further digested with *Afl*II, resulting in a 59 bp fragment, as seen in Lane 3. A 14 bp fragment is not visible on this gel. Lane 1 shows a portion of the low molecular weight marker (LMWM, NEBiolabs)

(b) Using a sterile 200 μL pipette tip, take a very small sample of the colony by barely touching the tip to the colony to obtain a small number of cells on the tip. Resuspend the cells in 20 μL of your PCR mix, making sure to put the tip directly into the PCR mix and twirl. Make sure all liquid that makes its way into the pipette tip through capillary action is cleared back into the PCR tube, by pushing down on the top of the tip with your finger.

(c) 5 min. Incubation at 95 °C; 35 cycles of 2 min. at 95 °C; 1 min. at 53 °C, 1 min. at 72 °C. End with a 10 min incubation at 72 °C.

4. Digest the PCR reactions using *Sph*I and *Afl*II. Make a master digestion mix to be added directly to the 20 μL PCR reaction, as follows. The 10 μL mix to be added to 1 PCR reaction is: 0.2 μL *Sph*I (NEB), 0.2 μL *Afl*II (NEB), 3.0 μL NEB Buffer 2.1, and 6.4 μL sterile dIH_2O.

   (a) Add 10 μL of digestion mix to each 20 μL PCR reaction.

   (b) Incubate digestion reaction for 1 h and 30 min in a 37 °C water bath.

   (c) Store digested reactions at −20 °C, if necessary.

5. Run the digested reaction on a 12% polyacrylamide, 0.5× TBE gel to confirm the tract size (Fig. 3b):

   (a) Add 3 μL of 10× polyacrylamide loading dye (0.25% bromophenol blue, 0.25% xylene cyanol, 30% glycerol) to each sample. Mix well.

   (b) Load 10 μL of your digested sample into each well. You should have ~20 μL remaining, which can be stored at −20 °C.

   (c) Make sure to load a plasmid control (last lane) as well as the Low Molecular Weight Marker (10 μL of loading dye, 1–2 μL of marker).

   (d) Run gels for 2 h at 250 v.

   (e) Stain the gel for 10 min in 250 mL of deionized water containing 0.5 μg/μL ethidium bromide.

6. Remove a colony with an unexpanded tract from the plate using a sterile flat-ended toothpick and resuspend it in 100 μL of sterile dIH_2O in a microcentrifuge tube. Vortex the tube to resuspend the colony, and serial dilute the resuspension to 10^{-4} (10 μL of undiluted resuspension into 990 μL of sterile deionized water, vortex, 10 μL of 10^{-2} dilution into 990 μL of sterile deionized water to get 1 mL of 10^{-4} dilution), vortexing between dilutions.

7. Plate 20 μL of the 10^{-4} dilution onto a SC −histidine plate and incubate at 30 °C for 3–4 days, allowing the colonies to grow to ~2 mm in diameter.

8. Select ten colonies that are ~2 mm in diameter to test in the TNR expansion assay. It is important to make sure all of your selected colonies are approximately the same size; colonies of

similar size will have undergone roughly the same number of cell divisions.

9. Remove each colony from the plate using a sterile flat-ended toothpick and resuspend in 100 μL of sterile deionized water, twirling the toothpick in the water to get as many cells as possible. Label the tube and vortex to further resuspend the colony. Dilute the resuspension to 10^{-4} (*see* **step 3**). Each resuspended colony will be plated on both selective and permissive plates to determine expansion rates.
10. Plate 20 μL of the 10^{-4} dilution onto SC –histidine and spread using sterile glass beads, making sure that the resuspension is evenly spread on each plate (*see* **Note 8**). These are the permissive plates; all cells will grow. These plates reflect the total number of cells tested.
11. Plate 75 μL of the undiluted resuspension onto SC –histidine plates containing 5-FOA. These are the selective plates, only allowing growth of cells that lack *URA3* expression, presumably due to TNR tract expansion (*see* **Note 9**). Spread the resuspension on the plate using sterile glass beads.
12. Place selective and permissive plates into a 30 °C incubator and allow them to grow for 3–4 days until the majority of colonies on the plates reach a diameter of ~1–2 mm so that they are easy to count. It may be necessary to allow the selective plates to grow a day longer to allow for sufficient growth in the presence of 5-FOA.
13. Remove plates from the incubator and count the number of colonies on all plates. With colony counts from selective and permissive plates, apparent expansion (or mutation) rates are calculated (*see* below).

3.3 Fluctuation Analysis Calculations

1. To calculate apparent expansion rates in the TNR expansion assay, colonies on selective and permissive plates are counted. Expansion rates are calculated by iterative formulas [66]. The 95% confidence intervals are determined from tables of confidence intervals for the median [67, 68].
2. To calculate the mutation rates for the time course experiments (*see* Subheadings 3.5–3.7), the probability of a change in tract size was treated as a binomial distribution with p = the proportion of tracts with a change in length and q = the proportion of tracts with no length change.
3. The rate of tract change was defined as the number of changes observed/the number of cells examined per generation. It is therefore important to determine the doubling time (or generation time) of each strain prior to calculating mutation rates. Growth curve experiments in both liquid medium and on plates are used to determine the number of generations for

these calculations (*see* Subheading 3.9). To calculate 95% confidence intervals (95% C.I.) on the mutation rates, the F statistic are used [69, 70].

3.4 Assessing Tract Length

1. Determining TNR tract size following the expansion assay allows the assessment of spontaneous repeat lengths and the impact of genetic background or growth conditions on the size of these changes (Figs. 3 and 4).
2. After running digested PCR reaction on a 12% polyacrylamide gel, stain and image gel (*see* Subheading 3.2). The digested TNR sequences should be clearly visible. Image the gel as straight as possible, making sure to have a level bottom edge.
3. From a predetermined point on the gel (i.e. the bottom of each well), measure the distance, in millimeters (mm), between the bands of known size in the low molecular weight marker used on the gel. These measurements (*Y*-axis) are plotted versus the known size of each band (*X*-axis) to generate a standard curve from which tract lengths can be interpolated.
4. Using the same starting point of reference that was used in **step 2**, measure the known TNR tract band in each lane of the gel. Use the standard curve graph to determine the tract length in base pairs of each fragment. Divide this number by three to report the number of repeats within the tract.
5. These measurements can be done with a ruler or with imaging software, as illustrated in Fig. 4.

3.5 Time Courses

1. Time courses are performed from different starting material, depending on the goal of the study. The first step in each type is to select expansion events and determine expansion sizes, as described in Subheading 3.2.
2. Time courses can be performed in large *liquid* cultures, in different types of media to measure the effect of carbon source and to measure expansions in actively replicating versus stationary phase cells. This allows the examination of a broad population of cells and the number of generation times can be modulated. For liquid time courses:
   (a) Resuspend confirmed expanded colonies in 106 mL of liquid SC- histidine (*see* **Note 10**) and grow the culture to saturation in a 30 °C shaker for 3 days (72 h) (Fig. 5).
   (b) From this saturated culture, remove 5 mL to isolate genomic DNA (*see* Subheading 3.6) that will be used as a template for PCR to determine the average tract size in the culture. This is the Day 0 time point. At the same time, take 10 μL of the culture to dilute to 10^{-4} and plate 100 μL on SC-histidine plates to generate individual colonies from the starting population. Incubate the plates at 30 °C for

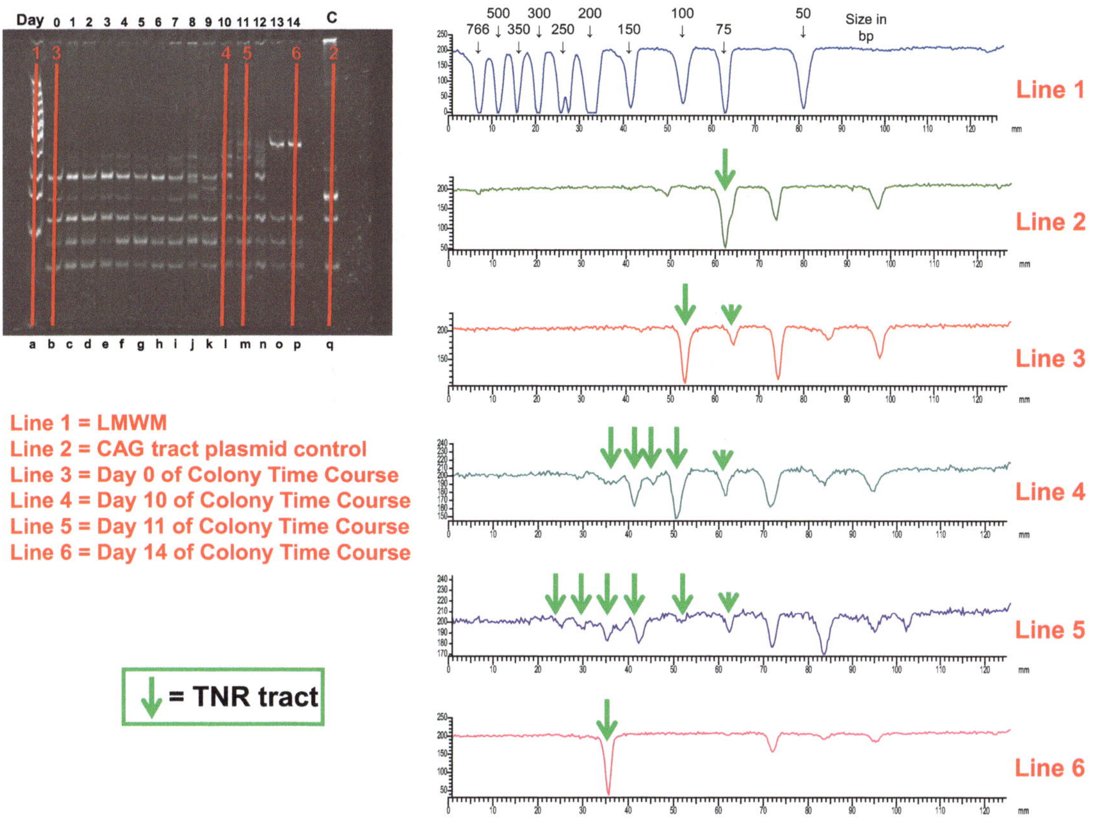

Fig. 4 Assessing tract length changes. The distance a DNA fragment migrates through the gel is used to assess the size of the fragment. Gels are all stained after electrophoresis so that ethidium bromide will not affect DNA migration. The migration through the gel can be measured by hand or using software, such as ImageQuant, as illustrated here. It is critical that the measurements start at the same point on the gel for each lane. The software generates a series of peaks along each line that correspond to bands of DNA. Left side: a colony time course experiment with an expanded tract at Day 0 (lane b). Vertical lines (red) are drawn through the middle of several lanes, including one containing a molecular weight marker, to assess fragment sizes. A standard curve is generated from the low molecular weight marker (LMWM, lane a). Tract sizes are determined by interpolating from the standard curve. In this time course, multiple expansion events are observed, as indicated by the vertical green arrows. The plasmid control defines the unexpanded tract and is marked C on the gel panel (lane q). A time course starting from a single colony is shown here

3 days. Colony PCR can be performed to determine the starting tract sizes within the population.

(c) Use 200 μL of the saturated culture to inoculate a fresh flask containing 10 mL of liquid SC- histidine (1:50 dilution) to propagate the next time point. Place this flask in the 30 °C shaker for 24 h. This is your logarithmic phase, or replicative culture. The cells will grow and divide in this culture (Fig. 5 left).

(d) To start a stationary phase culture, collect the remainder of the cells in the saturated culture by centrifugation at

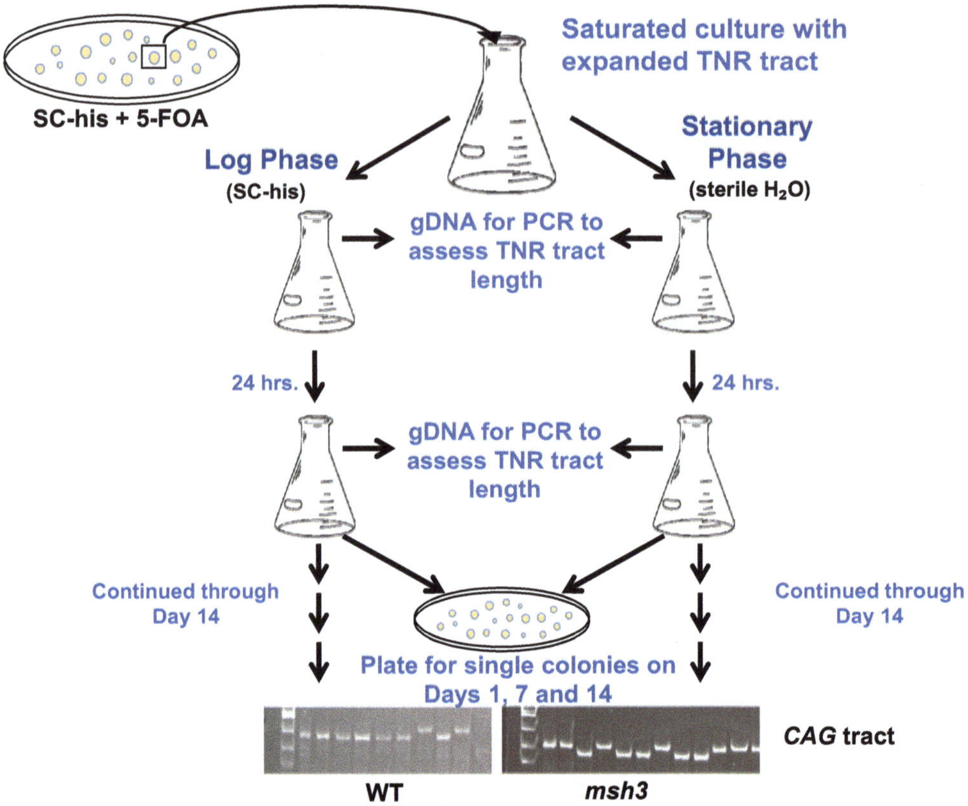

Fig. 5 Schematic of the liquid time course experiment protocol. A colony with a confirmed expanded tract is used to inoculate a liquid culture in SC–his, which is grown to saturation in a 30 °C shaker. The saturated culture is used to inoculate two fresh cultures, one that is maintained in logarithmic (log) phase, that is, actively replicating, in SC–his (left side) and one that is maintained in stationary phase, that is, senescent or non-replicating, in water (right side). For the log phase culture, every 24 h, a sample was taken to prepare genomic DNA for downstream analysis and a fresh culture (in SC–his) was inoculated. For the stationary phase culture, the cells were maintained in sterile water. Every 48 h the cells were washed and resuspended in fresh water. Every 24 h a sample was taken to prepare genomic DNA. For both cultures, cells were diluted and plated to generate single colonies. The tract length of these colonies was determined to assess the range of tract size changes within the population and how it might depend on genetic background. Tract lengths are determined by PCR amplification of the tract followed by digestion with *SphI* or *SphI/AflII*. The digested DNA is separated by gel electrophoresis on 12% native acrylamide gels and then stained with ethidium bromide. In this panel, the PCR products were digested with *SphI/AflII*. We note more contractions than expansions in the *msh3Δ* background (bottom gels)

3000 × *g* for 5 min. Remove the supernatant, making sure to keep the pellet formed at the bottom of the tube. Add 10 mL of sterile dIH$_2$O to the tube, pipetting the pellet back into solution. Collect the resuspended cells by centrifugation (3000 × *g*, 5 min) and remove the supernatant. Repeat this wash step with 10 mL of sterile dIH$_2$O. Resuspend the pellet in 10 mL of sterile dIH$_2$O and add to 90 mL of sterile dIH$_2$O in a 500 mL sterile flask. This will serve as your stationary phase culture. The cells will survive but will exhibit very little growth or division without nutrients. Incubate this stationary phase culture at 30 °C for 24 h (Fig. 5 right).

(e) Every 24 h, remove both logarithmic phase and stationary phase cultures from the 30 °C shaker. Remove 5 mL from each culture to extract genomic DNA, which will be used as template for PCR to determine TNR tract size. If desired, remove 10 μL to dilute and plate as described above. Incubate plates at 30 °C for 3 days. To determine the range of expansions within the population, as opposed to the average, colony PCR can be performed on colonies to determine tract sizes from individual colonies from the liquid culture. We typically plate cells on days 1, 7 and 14 to monitor the health of the culture as well as tract size (Fig. 5).

(f) Take 200 μL of your newly saturated logarithmic phase cultures and add them to a flask containing 10 mL of fresh SC-histidine and incubate in a 30 °C shaker for 24 h.

(g) The cells in the stationary phase cultures should be washed and resuspended in fresh sterile dIH_2O as described above every 48 h to reduce cell death. Resuspend each pellet in fresh sterile dIH_2O, making sure to keep the total volume accurate: (100 mL)–(days × 5 mL) = current volume.

(h) Repeat **steps 7–9** throughout the entirety of the time course.

(i) Throughout the time course, use the isolated genomic DNA (gDNA) as a template for PCR to determine the average tract size in the culture (Fig. 5).

3. Time courses can also be performed starting with *individual colonies* that are allowed to continue to grow over time. Colonies are moved to non-selective plates for the time course, to allow expansion and contraction events to happen in an unbiased way. For colony time courses:

(a) After confirming the size of the initial TNR tract expansion, select colonies for the time course experiment. Different sized expansions can be selected to test, that is, threshold length tracts or affected range tracts. Mark these colonies on the back of the plate.

(b) Using a sterile flat end toothpick, swipe the entire colony off from selective plate containing 5-FOA and deposit it onto a new SC–histidine plate and label the colony appropriately. It is important to remove confirmed colonies from the selective plate to allow for dynamic expansion *and* contraction events.

(c) Perform colony PCR on each of the colonies to obtain the "time point zero" for the time course experiment (*see* Subheading 3.2). Place the plates back into the 30 °C incubator for 24 h.

(d) After 24 h, remove the plates and perform colony PCR on each individual colony (*see* Subheading 3.2). When taking a small amount of the colony with a sterile tip for colony PCR, you may sample from either the same portion of the colony (i.e., 12 o'clock), or different portions of the colony (i.e., 3, 6, and 9 o'clock) at different time points. Because the cells are always sampled from the perimeter of the colony, the cells from the colony continue to grow and fill in the sampled space. The growth rate on solid media can be determined (*see* Subheading 3.12) to find the generation time of each strain on these plates (*see* **Note 11**).

(e) Return plates to the 30 °C incubator for 24 h.

(f) Repeat **steps 6** and **7** for 14 days. If necessary, transfer colonies to new plates by swiping the entire colony off of the old plate and depositing it onto a fresh synthetic medium plate lacking histidine.

(g) Colony PCR reactions for each time point should be digested with *Sph*I and *Afl*II to assess tract length over time (Figs. 4 and 6).

(h) Time courses can also be started from single cells that are allowed to go through a few cell divisions prior to propagating a new microcolony to continue the time course.

4. Time courses can also be started from *single cells* that are allowed to go through a few cell divisions prior to propagating a new microcolony to continue the time course.

   (a) After confirming the size of the initial TNR tract expansion, select a 2 mm colony from the selective plate and resuspend it in 200 μL of sterile dIH_2O.

   (b) Plate 50 μL of this resuspension onto the top left side of a fresh SC-histidine. Tilt the plate so that the resuspension drips down towards the bottom of the plate in a straight line. Tilt the plate back and forth so that the cells are evenly distributed along the streak. Allow this streak to dry for approximately 5–7 min (Fig. 7).

   (c) Using a tetrad dissection microscope, i.e. a microscope with a micromanipulator (*see* **Note 12**), focus on individual cells under 30× magnification. Switch to 150× magnification and identify single cells within the streak of cells. Choose unbudded cells so that you are starting with a homogeneous/single tract.

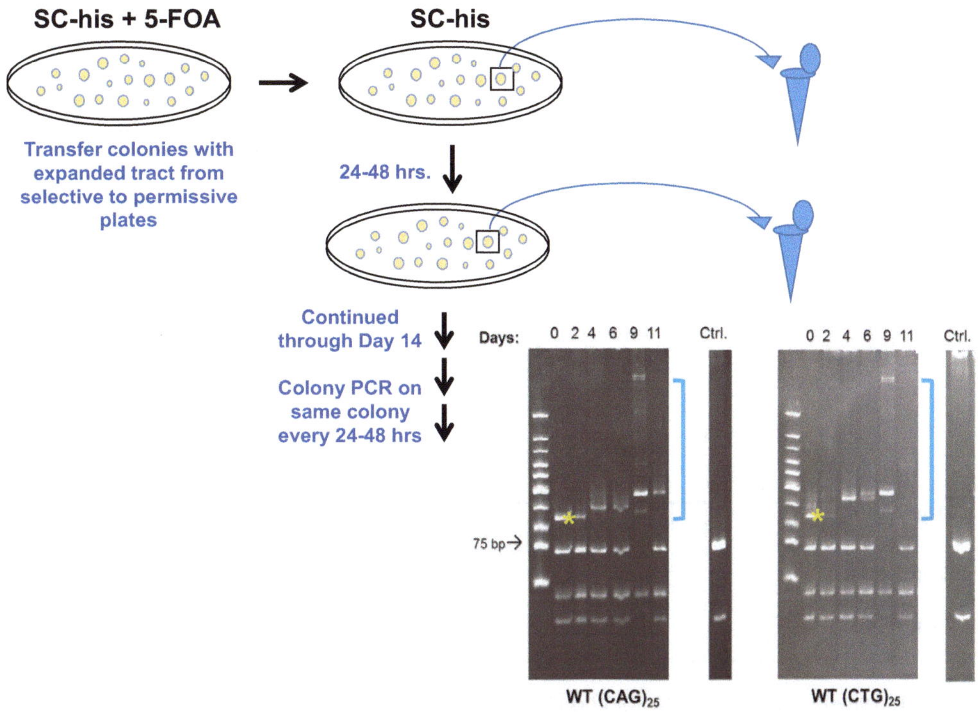

Fig. 6 Schematic of the colony time course experiment protocol. A colony with a confirmed expanded tract is transferred to a nonselective plate (SC−his) to allow both expansions and contractions to occur as the colony continues to grow. Colony PCR is performed with individual colonies. The TNR tract of each colony is amplified and digested with *SphI* or *SphI/AflII*. The digested DNA is separated by gel electrophoresis on 12% native acrylamide gels and then stained with ethidium bromide. The plate is replaced in the 30 °C incubator and is resampled every 24 to 48 h. At each time point the colony is subjected to colony PCR and restriction digestion to assess tract length. The gel panels illustrate tract length changes over time with both *CAG* and *CTG* tracts in the wild-type background. These PCR products were digested with *SphI*. The control lanes are amplified and digested plasmid DNA containing the unexpanded TNR tract

(d) Carefully swipe the single cell off the plate with the micromanipulator and place it at a defined location on the plate. Repeat with two additional cells from the same colony. Do not puncture the plate with the cell and glass rod; this will deposit the cell into the agar where it will not grow (Fig. 7). Use a fresh plate for each colony from which you are taking single cells.

(e) Incubate plates at 30 °C, allowing cells to undergo 8–10 rounds of replication, resulting in a microcolony of approximately 250–1000 cells. Determination of the generation time for each strain (*see* below) will reveal how long the cells should be incubated. Typically 15–20 h are required for 8–10 generations in our strain background, on synthetic media [27].

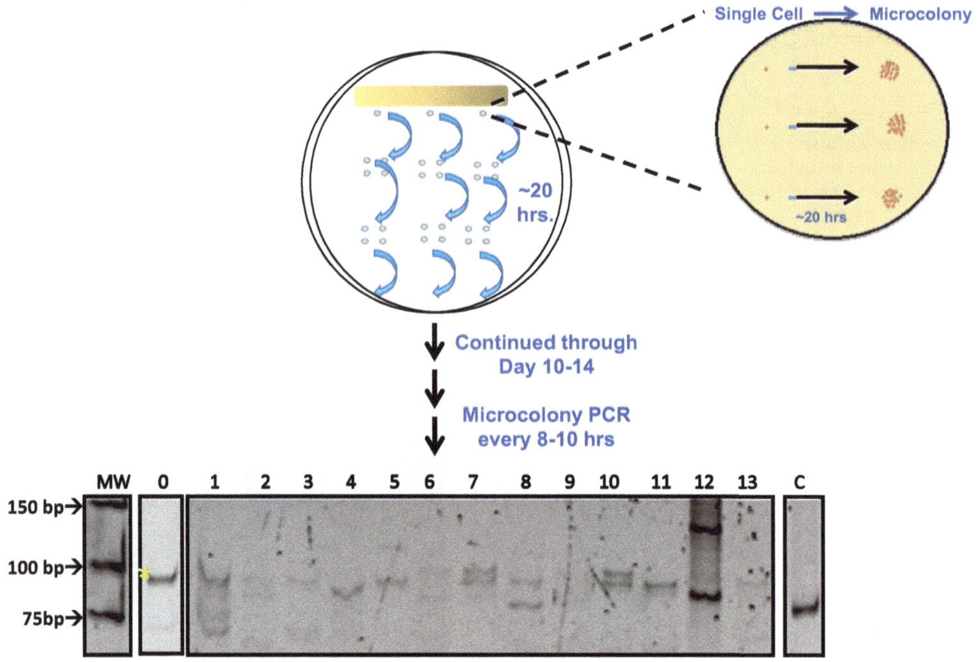

Fig. 7 Dynamic changes in TNR tracts starting from a single cell. A colony with a confirmed expanded tract is resuspended, applied to a permissive (SC−his) plate and individual cells are spread by tilting the plate back and forth to separate the cell suspension. Using a microscope with a micromanipulator, individual cells from each colony are isolated and allowed to undergo 8–10 rounds of replication, to generate a microcolony that contains approximately 250–1000 cells. A single cell from the microcolony is taken to propagate another microcolony for the time course. In fact, this is repeated three more times for each microcolony to ensure that at least one of the four cells generates a microcolony. The remainder of the microcolony is used in a PCR reaction to determine tract length. This process is repeated every ~20 h throughout the time course. PCR reactions are digested with *SphI*/*AflI* and resolved on a 12% polyacrylamide gel and stained with ethidium bromide. The lanes marked C in each panel indicate the 75-base-pair tract amplified from the TNR plasmid control. The numbers across the top of the gels indicate the time point. In this microcolony time course, the initial expansion is shown at time point zero and is marked with a yellow asterisk. Dynamic changes in the length of the TNR tract are observed as a function of time. Multiple bands are observed at some time points, likely due to cellular heterogeneity. The gel image is inverted to ease observation of faint DNA bands

(f) After 8–10 generations, select four individual cells for your next time point from each microcolony. You may have to disrupt the microcolony, spreading it a little, to capture individual cells. Transfer the four cells to a new, defined location on the plate, for example the four corners of a square. Four cells are necessary to ensure you have at least one microcolony that grows for your next time point (Fig. 7).

(g) Return to the original microcolony and puncture the agar around the smeared microcolony to mark the location of the microcolony on the plate; this should be visible without the microscope. This will be useful removing the microcolony from the plate for PCR (Fig. 7).

(h) Repeat **steps 9–11** for the rest of your time courses, making sure to mark each microcolony that will be swiped off the plate and used for template in PCR.

(i) Use a sterile 200 μL pipette tip to harvest each microcolony and resuspend it in 20 μL of the colony PCR mix (*see* Subheading 3.2).

(j) Using the microscope, check that each microcolony was harvested. There will be a small number of cells that did not make it onto the tip; this is ok. If there appears to be a substantial number of cells still present on the plate, mark the area surrounding the microcolony again and re-swipe the plate using a sterile 200 μL pipette tip (*see* **Note 13**).

(k) Place plates back into the 30 °C incubator for another 8–10 generations.

(l) After incubation, examine the propagated microcolonies and observe their size. Out of the four microcolonies that you have grown, chose the single microcolony that fits the criteria the best (250–1000 cells in size, *see* **Note 14**).

(m) Repeat **steps 10–15** for each microcolony for the duration of the time course (Fig. 7).

(n) Microcolony PCR reactions for each time point should be digested with *Sph*I and *Afl*II (*see* Subheading 3.2) to assess dynamic tract behavior (Fig. 7).

3.6 Genomic DNA Preparation

1. Collect cells by centrifugation a 3000 × *g* and discard supernatant. You should have a pellet at the bottom of the tube.
2. Add 500 μL of sterile dIH_2O to each tube and vortex to resuspend the pellet. Transfer resuspension to a microcentrifuge tube.
3. Centrifuge for 30 s at 16,000 × *g*.
4. Remove tubes from microfuge and pour out the supernatant. Vortex the pellet in the residual liquid to resuspend.
5. Add 200 μL Chromosome Preparation Buffer.
6. Add 200 μL of well-mixed phenol–chloroform (1 part phenol and 1 part chloroform), vortex to mix, and spin down at 16,000 × *g* for 5 min. (Store phenol-chloroform at 4 °C and cover tube with aluminum foil, it is light sensitive).
7. Add 0.3 g of acid-washed glass beads (*see* **Note 15**).
8. Vortex tubes at 2000 rpm (6.71 × *g*) in a multivortex (Eppendorf Mixmate for example) in cold room for 3 min.
9. Add 200 μL of 1× TE, pH 8.0 to each vortexed tube.
10. Centrifuge for 5 min at 16,000 × *g*.

11. While waiting for your samples, set up clean microcentrifuge tubes and add 10 μL of 4 M ammonium acetate to each tube.
12. After centrifugation, transfer the supernatant into ammonium acetate-containing tubes. Add 1 mL of 95% ethanol to each tube and invert twice. Your reactions are stable at this point.
13. Spin down your samples for 2 min in a microfuge at 16,000 × *g*.
14. Pour out ethanol, making sure not to pour out the pellet at the bottom of the tube. Add 1 mL of 70% ethanol to wash each pellet. Gently invert your tubes a few times.
15. Briefly centrifuge your samples for 30 s at 16,000 × *g*. Remove residual ethanol with your micropipette.
16. Dry DNA pellets for 15–30 min at room temperature or use a vacuum apparatus. Ensure that all ethanol is evaporated from your samples, since its presence can affect downstream applications.
17. Resuspend dried pellets in 50 μL of 1× TE (pH 8.0) with 50 μg/mL RNAse A. Never vortex your gDNA. This gDNA can be used as a template for PCR, using 1 μL of genomic DNA sample, instead of a colony, in each 20 μL PCR reaction (*see* Subheading 3.2).

3.7 Probe Labeling for Southern Blotting

Southern blotting is used to confirm single integration of the TNR reporter construct at the correct chromosomal location. It is also used to confirm that the PCR products obtained following PCR in each of the different time course experiments actually contain a TNR tract.

Two different probes are used.

1. For a probe to determine proper integration of the reporter construct, a plasmid preparation of pBL94 [16, 63] is used. The plasmid is digested with *Bam*HI to release a 1.2 kb fragment that contains *lys2* [63]. Gel purify the 1.2 kb fragment after electrophoresis through a 1% agarose gel.
2. For a tract specific probe to confirm the presence of the TNR tract following PCR of time course samples, a plasmid preparation of pBL169 [27, 62] is used. PCR amplify the TNR tract in 2 or more 50 μL PCR reactions using primers SO295 and SO296 (*see* Table 1). Digest each of the PCR reactions with the restriction enzyme *Sph*I to isolate the repeat tract. Gel purify the 75 bp PCR product after electrophoresis through a 12% polyacrylamide, 0.5 × TBE gel, and staining with ethidium bromide (*see* Subheading 3.2). Collect the DNA from multiple bands on a single column to increase the concentration of your final extracted DNA fragment.
3. For both probes, elute with a small volume of sterile dIH_20 (30 μL) to increase the overall DNA content of the extraction.

Sterile dIH_2O is used instead of the provided elution buffer to assure proper labeling using a random primer DNA labeling kit.

4. Radiolabel the purified probes with the Random Primer DNA Labeling kit, following the protocol provided in the kit. Once radiolabeled, the probes can be stored in a designated radioactivity approved freezer at −20 °C until it is ready to be used.

3.8 Southern Blotting: Gel Transfer

1. (a) For confirmation of integration, isolate gDNA and digest with *Bam*HI. Run through a 0.8%, 0.5× TBE agarose gel.
   (b) For time course tract confirmation, digest PCR reactions with *Sph*I and *Afl*II and run the products through a 12% polyacrylamide, 0.5× TBE gel and stain the gel with ethidium bromide (*see* Subheading 3.2). Take a picture of the gel to orient you later.
2. In a clean Pyrex dish, denature the gel at room temperature for 60 min in 500 mL of denaturation buffer. Completely immerse the gel in buffer to ensure the entire gel is at high pH to uniformly denature the DNA.
3. Neutralize the gel in 500 mL of neutralization buffer at room temperature for 30 min. Remove the buffer and repeat the neutralization step. After two washes, the gel pH should be 8 or less. This can be tested by touching a pH strip to the side of the gel.
4. Place a raised, weighted platform in the middle of a clean Pyrex dish. Fill reservoir with 1× SSC to ½ in. deep, to below the surface of the platform.
5. Cut two sheets of Whatman 3 MM paper the width of the gel and drape them over the platform with the ends hanging into the 1× SSC-filled reservoir. Wet the entire wick with 1× SSC and remove any trapped air bubble by rolling a Pasteur pipette across the surface.
6. Cut a piece of neutral Nytran membrane to fit the size of the gel and label the back of the membrane that is not in contact with the gel. Wet the membrane briefly in deionized water and then soak it in 1× SSC for 5 min.
7. Notch one corner of the gel and of the neutral Nytran membrane to determine the orientation following transfer. The notches should be aligned for transfer. Carefully invert and lay gel on top of the wick. Remove any air bubbles between gel and the wick (*see* **Note 16**).
8. Place plastic wrap on all four sides of the gel to prevent lateral diffusion of your DNA.

9. Flood the gel surface with 1× SSC and carefully lay the neutral Nytran membrane on top of the gel, aligning the gel notch with the membrane notch, removing any air bubble.
10. Cut four pieces of Whatman paper to the exact size of the gel. Soak these pieces for 5 min in 1× SSC, before laying them on top of the gel. Once again, make sure that all bubbles are removed by rolling a Pasteur pipette over top of the transfer set up.
11. Place a stack of paper towels (4″ tall) cut slightly larger than the gel to cover the gel transfer area. Place a weight on top of the paper towels. Wrap the entire reservoir and transfer setup with plastic wrap to help prevent evaporation of the 1× SSC buffer. Allow the transfer to proceed overnight (~15–20 h) [63].
12. After overnight transfer, unwrap the reservoir and remove the gel. Image the gel to make sure that all of the DNA has transferred from the gel to the Nytran membrane.
13. Dry the membrane between to pieces of filter paper under the fume hood.
14. Wrap the membrane in plastic wrap.
15. Crosslink the wrapped blot at 1600 μJ, using a Stratalinker or equivalent UV crosslinker. The DNA should be stably maintained on the neutral Nytran membrane and can be stored at 4 °C until ready to hybridize with a tract specific probe.

3.9 Southern Blotting: Hybridization Protocol Using α^{32}P-dCTP Labeled Tract-Specific Probe

1. Following the transfer, remove the radiolabeled probe from the radioactive materials freezer and let it thaw on ice behind a plexiglass shield.
2. Heat the thawed probe to 95 °C for 5 min and then place on ice for 5 min.
3. Add 5 μL of radiolabeled probe [≈0.008 mCi] to 10 mL of hybridization buffer in a 250 mL screw-cap bottle that contains the neutral Nytran membrane blot that is to be probed.
4. Screw the bottle cap on tight and wrap the top several times with Parafilm to prevent any leaking.
5. Add the sealed Southern blotting tube into a rotating hybridization oven at 65 °C and allow it to incubate overnight (~15–20 h).
6. Remove the screw-cap bottle form the oven and discard the hybridization buffer and unbound radiolabeled probe into an appropriate radioactive liquid waste container, making sure the blot itself stays within the screw-cap bottle.
7. Add 250 mL of wash buffer to the bottle. Screw the cap on tight and once again wrap the top of the bottle several times

with Parafilm to prevent leaking. Put the sealed tube back into the oven at room temperature for 20 min.

8. Remove the bottle from the oven and discard the wash buffer into an approved radioactive liquid waste container.
9. Repeat **steps 6–8** for a second wash. Survey the oven with the Geiger counter to assure there is no radioactivity present in or around the oven.
10. Remove the washed blot from the screw-cap bottle and air dry on a piece of Whatman paper on the radioactivity bench behind plexiglass.
11. Wrap the blot with plastic wrap and expose it to a phosphor imaging screen. Note the orientation of the blot on the screen so it can be correctly interpreted later. Radioactive label that has undergone less than one half-life can be exposed for 4–8 h and will show clear resolution when imaged using a PhosphorImager (Fig. 8). After the blot is imaged and the results obtained, the blot should be disposed in an approved dry radioactive waste container.

3.10 Generation Time in Liquid Culture

To calculate rates of change and to normalize and compare individual time courses, it is necessary to determine the number of generations a culture or colony has undergone during a particular time period. Generation times, or doubling times, can be determined in liquid media or upon growth on agar plates.

1. Streak out the TNR-containing strain of interest on SC-histidine plates to generate single colonies. SC-histidine ensures that the colonies maintain the TNR reporter system. Place plates in the 30 °C incubator and allow them to grow for ~3 days, until colonies are ~2 mm in diameter.
2. Select ~2 mm colony using a sterile wooden stick and resuspend the colony in 10 mL of liquid SC–histidine in a 125 mL sterile flask. Place the flask in a 30 °C shaker overnight to allow saturation of the culture.
3. After ~16 h, remove the flask from the shaker and measure the density of the culture. Dilute the saturated culture 1:10 (100 μL of culture + 900 μL of media) in SC-histidine in a microcentrifuge tube (*see* **Note 17**). Using a spectrophotometer, measure and record the optical density at 600 nm (OD_{600}) of the dilution. Multiply this number by 10 (to account for the dilution) to determine the OD_{600} of the saturated culture.
4. Dilute the saturated culture to an OD_{600} of 0.1 with liquid SC-histidine in fresh 250 mL flask. The final culture volume should be 50 mL.
5. Remove 1 mL from the newly diluted culture and measure the OD_{600}. This is the zero time point.

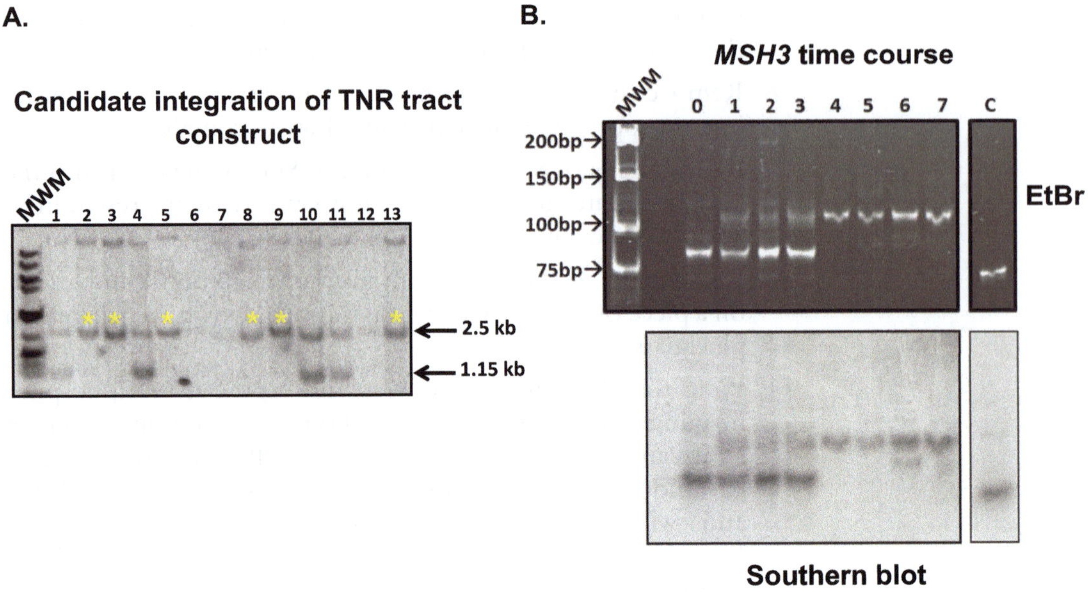

Fig. 8 Southern blotting to assess construct integration and tract identity. (**a**) Following transformation with the reporter construct, candidate integrants were assessed by Southern blot, to confirm integration and to select single reporter construct integrants. Genomic DNA was digested with *Bam*HI, electrophoresed, denatured and transferred to neutral Nytran membrane. Using the reporter specific probe, single integration events result in a single band at 2.5 kb (indicated by the yellow asterisks on the gel). No integration (or integration elsewhere in the chromosome) results in a 1.15 kb band. Double integrants result in a band at both 2.5 and 1.15 kb (lanes 1, 4, 10, 11). (**b**) Using a tract specific probe to confirm TNR identity. A wild-type $(CTG)_{25}$ colony PCR time courses is performed as described above. Digested PCR samples were resolved on a 12% polyacrylamide gel, stained with ethidium bromide and imaged (*top panel*). DNA from the gel was then transferred to a neutral Nytran membrane, cross-linked, and subjected to Southern blot using a tract-specific TNR probe (*bottom panel*). Wild-type Southern blot confirms progressive expansion of the TNR tract over time. Numbers across the top indicate days of the time course. The lanes marked C indicate the 75-base-pair tract amplified from the TNR plasmid control

6. Place the diluted culture in the 30 °C shaker. Measure the optical density of the culture (OD_{600}) every 45 min for 10 h.
7. At the end of the 10 h period, allow cultures to saturate overnight in the 30 °C shaker.
8. The next morning, **steps 1–10** can be repeated for a second set of time points. At the end of the 2 day period, optical density measurements can be plotted on a graph as a function of time to extrapolate a generation (or doubling) time.

3.11 Generation Time on Solid Media

1. Streak out the strain of interest to single colonies on SC-histidine plates and allow the colonies to grow to ~2 mm in a 30 °C incubator. Select a 2 mm colony from the plate using a sterile flat end toothpick and resuspend it in 200 μL of sterile deionized water.

2. Plate 50 μL of this resuspension onto the top left side of a fresh synthetic medium plate lacking histidine. Tilt the plate so that the resuspension drips down towards the bottom of the plate in a straight line. Tilt the plate back and forth so that the cells are evenly distributed along the streak. Allow this streak to dry for approximately 5–7 min.
3. Using a microscope equipped with a micromanipulator, select individual cells as described above (Subheading 3.7), placing cells in defined locations so they can be monitored over time.
4. Incubate each plate at 30 °C.
5. Monitor the individual cells closely to observe budding of daughter cells. When division is complete, the daughter cell is easily removed from the mother cell with the needle.
6. As soon as possible, remove the daughter cell and place it just below the mother cell on the plate. The single cells selected for the growth curve experiment are unlikely to be at precisely the same stage of the cell cycle. The time required to complete the first cell division should not be included in the growth curve because the cells initially selected may not be a precisely the same stage of the cell cycle. Once the first daughter cell is separated from the mother, start the growth curve (*see* **Note 13**).
7. Every 30 min, for 10 h, remove the plates from the incubator to monitor daughter cell budding and cell division. Note the amount of time it took for the daughter cell to completely separate from the mother and restart the timer. In order to record doubling times accurately, it is best to follow fewer cells at a time, and repeat the experiment several times with different starting colonies.
8. At the end of the 10 h period, median and mean doubling times can be calculated.

3.12 Preparing DNA Substrates for In Vitro Biochemical Enzyme Assays

1. Labelling of oligonucleotides.
   (a) Pre-Anneal Step: Anneal 2 μL of 10 μM primer to be labeled to 5 μL of 10 μM complementary primer in the presence of 10 μL of dIH_2O and 3 μL of 10× labeling reaction buffer.
   (b) Incubate reaction at 95 °C for 5 min and transfer to 70 °C heat block. Turn off heat block to slowly cool down the reaction to room temperature for a minimum of 1.5 h (*see* **Note 18**).
   (c) To the pre-annealed reaction, add 4 μL of α-^{32}P dCTP, 1 μL of Klenow fragment and 5 μL of dIH_2O to make a final volume of 30 μL. Incubate reaction for ~ 1.5 h at 37 °C (*see* **Notes 19** and **20**).

(d) Add 10 μL of dIH_2O to incubated samples to bring the final volume up to 40 μL.

(e) Pipette the radiolabeled oligonucleotide (total 40 μL volume) into the spin column and centrifuge for 5 min at 1,000 × *g* to remove the unincorporated radiolabel. Save the eluate (radiolabeled oligonucleotide) and discard the spin column (*see* **Note 21**).

(f) In triplicates, spot 0.5 μL of radiolabeled oligonucleotide on a piece of Whatman filter paper and place in the scintillation vials filled with 4 mL of scintillation fluid. Measure the amount of radionucleotide incorporated using the scintillation counter. Readings should be saved as "*after counts*".

(g) To the remaining radiolabeled oligonucleotide sample, add 20 μL of 2× termination dye and heat at 95 °C for 5 min.

(h) Load the samples on the pre-run sequencing gel and electrophorese for 1 h 45 min at 80 W (*see* **Note 22**).

(i) Subsequent to completion of electrophoresis, one plate of the sequencing gel needs to be removed and the gel on the other plate needs to be covered with saran wrap. Use autorad markers to ensure proper orientation of radiolabeled oligonucleotides for gel extraction in later steps.

(j) In a dark room, expose the gel to an autoradiography film for about a minute and develop in the X-ray processor.

(k) Position the developed film on the gel and cut out the bands containing the radiolabeled oligonucleotide. Put the gel piece in 500 μL of TE and allow for end-over-end rotation overnight.

(l) Transfer the gel pieces and DNA in TE to a Spin-X filter column and centrifuge for 2 min at 1,000 × *g* to separate the gel pieces from the DNA. Discard the column, but retain the flow through.

(m) To the tube containing the flow through, add 1500 μL 90% Ethanol, 1 μL of glycogen. Incubate for at least 1 h in −80 °C.

(n) Centrifuge at 15,000 × *g* for 20 min. Discard supernatant and ensure pellet is not disturbed in the process.

(o) Add 500 μL of 70% ethanol and centrifuge at 15,000 × *g* for 10 min to wash the pellet. Discard supernatant.

(p) Allow the pellet to dry in the 37 °C heat block for 10 min (*see* **Note 23**).

(q) Resuspend pellet in 30 μL of TE.

(r) In triplicates, spot 0.5 µL of sample on precut filter paper and place in scintillation vials (similar to **step 6**). Reading should be saved as "*recovery counts*".

(s) Calculate the volume of labelled primer that accounts for 1 µM or 1 pmol/µL (*see* **Note 24**).

2. Annealing radiolabeled substrates.

In order to generate an enzyme substrate that mimics an intermediate found during DNA transactions, the downstream radiolabeled oligonucleotide is annealed to a complementary template. An upstream primer is also annealed to the same template. Annealing is done in a 1:2:4 ratio of radiolabeled oligonucleotide, template, and upstream primer. The reaction is carried out in 100 µL of duplex annealing buffer. Annealing is initiated by heating the microcentrifuge tube containing the reaction mixture at 95 °C for 5 min and then subsequently switching off the heat block to gradually lower the temperature to allow for maximal annealing overnight (*see* **Notes 25** and **26**). Since the radiolabeled primer stock concentration is 1 µM or 1 pmol/µL, the concentration of the desired annealed substrate will be 10 nM or 10 fmol/µL. An example of an annealing reaction with a final volume of 100 µL and concentration of 10 nM:

Labelled primer = 3.6 µL (calculated volume required for 1 µM).

Template (1 µM) = 2 µL.

Upstream (1 µM) = 4 µL.

Duplex buffer = 90.4 µL.

Total = 100 µL of 10 nM annealed substrate.

3. Assaying substrate annealing efficiency.

(a) Prepare 6% native gel and allow to polymerize. Once polymerized, set up native gel on the electrophoresis apparatus and pre-run gel in 1× TBE buffer.

(b) Add 1 nM of labeled primer or annealed substrate to 15 µL of reaction buffer.

(c) Load 15 µL of sample to the native gel and run for 1 h at 180 V.

(d) Transfer gel to Whatman filter paper and cover with plastic wrap.

(e) Using vacuum, dry gel in the gel dryer for ~1 h.

(f) Expose dried gel to the phosphor screen overnight (*see* **Note 27**).

(g) Scan and image results using Typhoon™ FLA 9500 laser scanner.

(h) Evaluate annealing efficiency by assessing the shift in the annealed substrate compared to labeled primer (*see* **Note 28**).

4. Detecting Msh2-Msh3 substrate interaction using electromobility gel shift assay (EMSA).
   (a) Prepare 6% native gel and allow to polymerize. Once polymerized, set up native gel on the electrophoresis apparatus and pre-run gel in 1× TBE buffer.
   (b) Initial binding reactions should test optimum substrate–protein binding concentrations. Binding reactions should be set up on ice.
   (c) Add 0.5 μL of annealed substrate (10 nM) to 9.5 μL of 1× EMSA buffer (*substrate mix*).
   (d) Increasing concentrations of recombinant Msh2-Msh3 should be added to 1× EMSA buffer to make a final volume of 10 μL (*enzyme mix*).
   (e) To initiate the reaction, add 10 μL of *substrate mix* and 10 μL of *enzyme mix* and allow to incubate at 30 °C for 10 min.
   (f) Set up one reaction in the absence of *enzyme mix*. This will serve as the "*substrate only*" control.
   (g) After incubation, directly load 18 μL of the reaction onto the pre-run gel and electrophorese for 1 h at 180 V (*see* **Note 29**).
   (h) Follow **steps 4–7** from Subheading 3.12.
   (i) Use ImageQuant software to quantitate the substrate and protein-bound substrate bands.
   (j) Binding efficiency is calculated by the following: % Bound product = $\{(b)/(b + a)\} \times 100$, where "*b*" is the protein-bound substrate and "*a*" is the remaining unbound substrate.
   (k) On determination of optimum protein concentration that shows ~40–50% Msh2-Msh3 binding to substrate, repeat **steps 3–10** by titrating in a smaller range of protein concentration.
   (l) Similarly, a time-course experiment can be performed wherein a fixed concentration of Msh2-Msh3 (at a concentration which shows ~40–50% binding to substrate) is incubated with the substrate for 0, 1, 2.5, 5, 10, 15, 20 and 30 min, following the same steps as outlined above (**steps e–j**). This experiment will inform us about the kinetics of Msh2-Msh3 binding to a cognate substrate.
   (m) A binding competition assay can also be performed by adding in a fixed amount of a particular enzyme and then titrating in Msh2-Msh3. This experiment will show if Msh2-Msh3 can outcompete another protein from the substrate and will provide information about binding

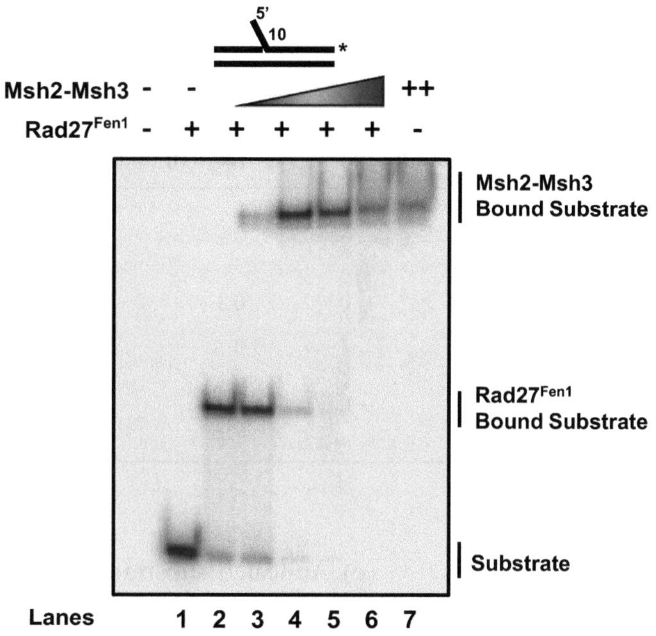

Fig. 9 Msh2-Msh3 binding efficiency in the presence of $Rad27^{Fen1}$. Substrate binding efficiency was assessed using EMSA. A10 nt flap substrate was preincubated with 2.5 nM $Rad27^{Fen1}$ for 10 min before adding increasing concentrations of Msh2-Msh3 (0, 2.5, 12.5, 25, and 37.5 nM) and further incubating for 10 min. Lane 3 represents Msh2-Msh3 and FEN1 at equal molar concentrations (2.5 nM). The labeled substrate is illustrated above with the asterisk indicating the site of the ^{32}P label. The complexes formed are indicated beside the gel, which correspond to the particular band shift. (*Reproduced with permission from* [16])

affinities of one protein over the other. An example of Msh2-Msh3 outcompeting $Rad27^{Fen1}$ is shown in Fig. 9. Annealed substrate used for the reactions is a 10 nt flap. This substrate was made by annealing the D10: T1: U1 (Table 1a).

3.13 Assessing the Influence of Msh2-Msh3 on the Enzymatic Activities of DNA Replication Proteins

1. Rad27Fen1 cleavage in the presence of Msh2-Msh3.
   (a) Prepare 15% PAGE gel and allow to polymerize. Once polymerized, set up PAGE gel on the S2 sequencing apparatus and pre-run the gel for ~20 min at 80 W in 1× TBE buffer (*see* **Notes 30** and **31**).
   (b) Setup reaction by adding 0.5 μL of annealed substrate (10 nM) to 9.5 μL of 1× nuclease buffer (*substrate mix*).
   (c) Add increasing concentrations of Msh2-Msh3 and a fixed concentration of $Rad27^{Fen1}$ to 1× nuclease buffer and bring up the total to 10 μL (*enzyme mix*).
   (d) An example of reaction setup is outlined in Table 2.

Table 2
Nuclease assay reaction setup

Reaction #	$Rad27^{FEN1}$ (2.5 nM) (in μL)	Msh2-Msh3 (25 nM) (in μL)	1× Buffer (in μL)	Substrate mix (in μL)
1	–	–	10	10
2	1.0	–	9	10
3	1.0	0.1	8.9	10
4	1.0	0.5	8.5	10
5	1.0	1.0	8.0	10
6	1.0	1.5	8.5	10

(e) Annealed substrates used for the reactions are 5, 10, 20 and 30 nt flaps. These substrates are made by annealing the D5 (or D10, D20, D30): T1: U1 (Table 1a).

(f) After incubating the reactions for 10 min at 30 °C, add 20 μL of termination dye and incubate for 5 min at 95 °C. Directly load 20 μL of the reaction onto the pre-run gel and electrophorese for 1 h and 30 min at 80 W (*see* **Note 32**).

(g) Follow **steps d–g** from section "Assaying substrate annealing efficiency".

(h) Compare the amount of nuclease activity by quantifying the intensity of each band produced (*see* **Note 33**) (Fig. 10).

2. Cdc9LigI ligation in the Presence of Msh2-Msh3.

(a) Follow **steps a–e** from Subheading 3.13, **step 1**.

(b) Setup reactions similar to the example outlined in Table 2. Use $Cdc9^{Lig1}$(12.5 nM) instead of $Rad27^{Fen1}$in 1× ligation buffer.

(c) Annealed substrates used for the reactions are bubble substrates containing either a 4 nt or 6 nt gap between the upstream and downstream primers. The 4 nt gap bubble substrate is made by annealing D4:T2:U2 and the 6 nt gap bubble substrate is made by annealing D6:T2:U2 (Table 1b).

(d) Compare the amount of ligated product by quantifying the intensity of each band produced (*see* **Note 34**) (Fig. 11).

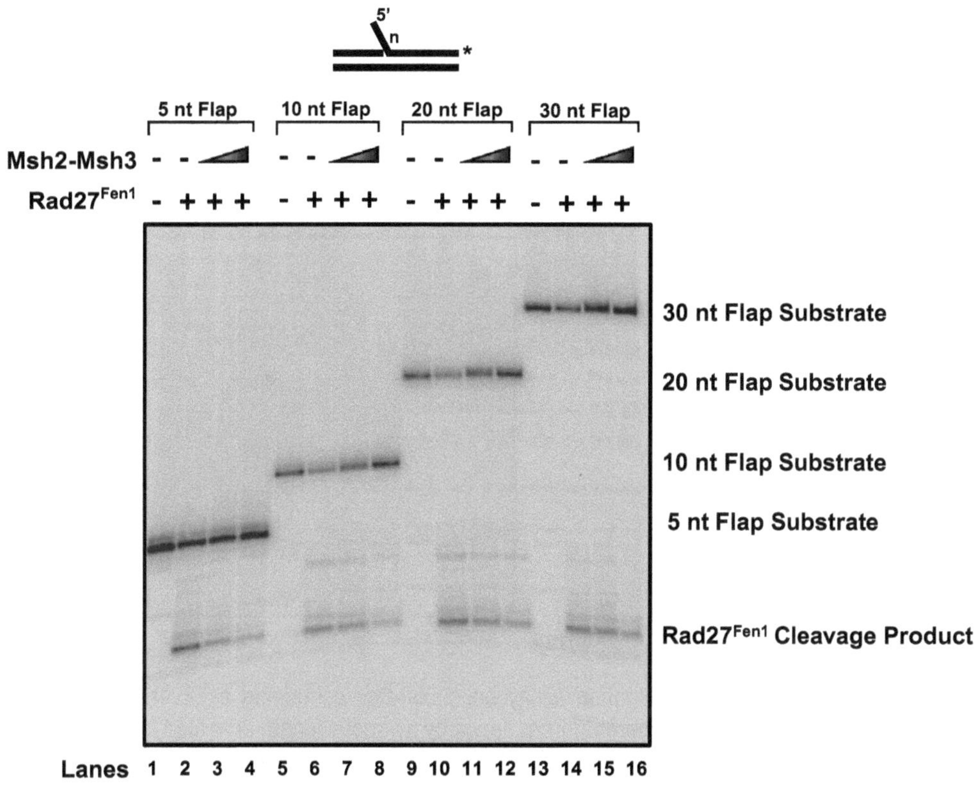

Fig. 10 Nuclease Assay: Rad27^{Fen1} cleavage assay on substrates with 5′ flaps of various lengths (5, 10, 20, and 30 nt). Substrates were incubated with Rad27^{Fen1} (2.5 nM) and increasing concentrations of Msh2-Msh3 (0, 12.5, and 25 nM). The labeled substrate is illustrated above with the asterisk indicating the site of the ^{32}P label. Nuclease products are indicated beside the gel. (*Reproduced with permission from* [16])

3. DNA Polymerase delta (Pol δ) synthesis in the presence of Msh2-Msh3.
   (a) Follow **steps a–e** from Subheading 3.13, **step 1**.
   (b) Setup reactions similar to that outlined in Table 2. Use Pol δ (25 nM) instead of Rad27^{Fen1} in 1× polymerase buffer.
   (c) Compare the amount of fully synthesized product by quantifying the intensity of each band produced (*see* **Note 35**) (Fig. 12).
   (d) Annealed substrates used for the reactions are bubble substrates containing either a 4 nt or 6 nt gap between the upstream and downstream primers. The 4 nt gap bubble substrate is made by annealing D4:T2:U2 and the 6 nt gap bubble substrate is made by annealing D6:T2:U2 (Table 1c).
4. Assaying the role of Msh2-Msh3 in contributing to TNR expansions.
   (a) Follow **steps a–e** from Subheading 3.13, **step 1**.

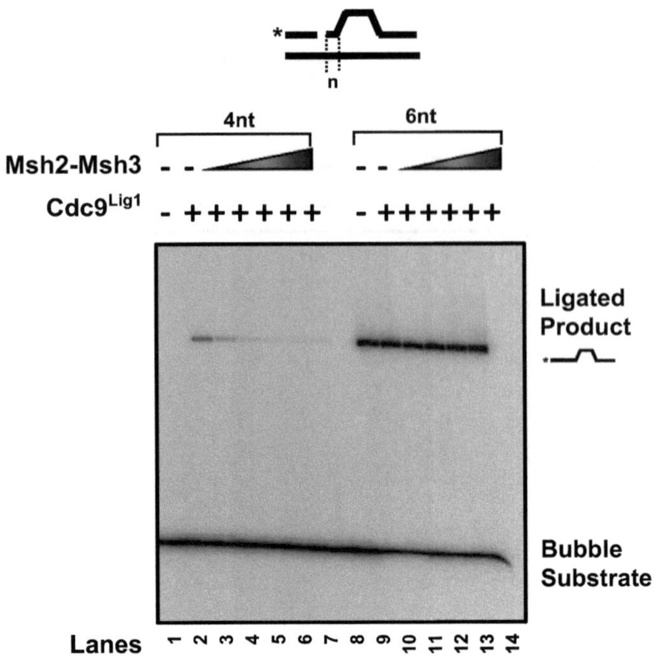

Fig. 11 Ligation assay on substrates containing a 12 nt unannealed bubble region separated from a nick by a various length annealed DNA regions (4, 6 nt). Substrates were incubated with Cdc9^{Ligl} (12.5 nM) and increasing concentrations of Msh2-Msh3 (0, 2.5, 5, 12.5, 25, and 37.5 nM). The labeled substrate is illustrated above with the asterisk indicating the site of the ^{32}P label. Ligation products are indicated beside the gel. (*Reproduced with permission from* [16])

(b) In **step c** from Subheading 3.13, **step 1**, to make the enzyme mix add all three enzymes, Msh2-Msh3 (increasing concentrations), Rad27^{Fen1} and Cdc9^{Lig1}.

(c) TNR expansions are measured on a random equilibrating flap substrate (DR4:T4:U4) and on a TNR repeat (CTG_{10}) equilibrating flap substrate (DE4:T4:UE4) (Table 1d).

(d) If no expansions are introduced, one will observe a single ligated product, however if repeats are generated, one will observe multiple ligated products (Fig. 13).

4 Notes

1. We use lab-purified *Thermus aquaticus* (*Taq*) polymerase. Briefly, *Taq* is overexpressed in *Escherichia coli* (BL21), harvested by centrifugation and the pellet is frozen in liquid nitrogen. The pellet is thawed and resuspended in Buffer A (50 mM HEPES pH 8.0, 50 mM glucose, 1 mM EDTA) containing lysozyme (4 mg/mL) and then incubated at room temperature for at least 15 min, until the cells are lysed and

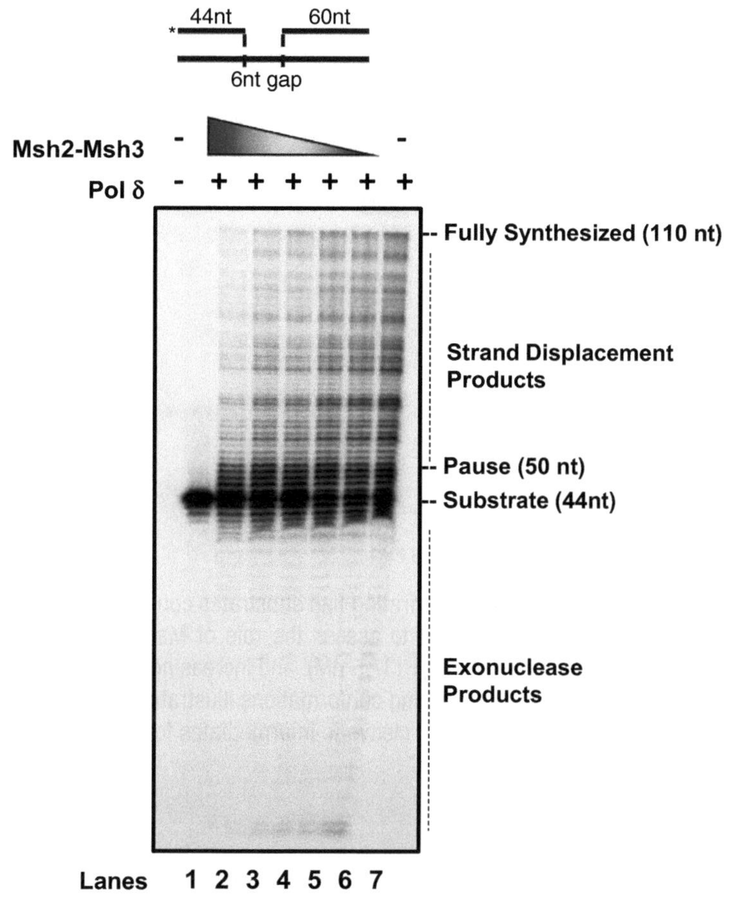

Fig. 12 Strand displacement synthesis assay: The effect of Msh2-Msh3 binding on the strand displacement synthesis of Pol δ was tested using a substrate mimicking a lagging strand intermediate. Substrates were incubated with Pol δ (25 nM) and differing concentrations of Msh2-Msh3 (37.5, 25, 12.5, 5, 2.5, and 0 nM). The labeled substrate is illustrated above with the asterisk indicating the site of the ^{32}P label. Strand displacement, exonuclease and fully synthesized products are indicated beside the gel

appear gooey. Buffer B (10 mM HEPES pH 8.0, 50 mM KCl, 1 mM EDTA, 0.5% Tween 20, 0.5% NP-40) was added and the lysate incubated in a 75 °C water bath for 45 min, with periodic inversion. The lysate was centrifuged at 20,000 × *g* and the supernatant transferred to a new tube. The supernatant was treated with DNaseI, in the presence of $MgCl_2$ and $MnCl_2$, at 75 °C for 45 min, centrifuged and the supernatant kept. The supernatant was dialyzed again three changes of dialysis buffer (20 mM Tris pH 7.5, 200 mM KCl, 1 mM EDTA), then diluted 2× with storage buffer (50 mM Tris pH 7.5, 50 mM KCl, 1 mM DTT, 0.5% Tween 20, 0.5% NP-40) containing 50% glycerol and then 2× again with stor-

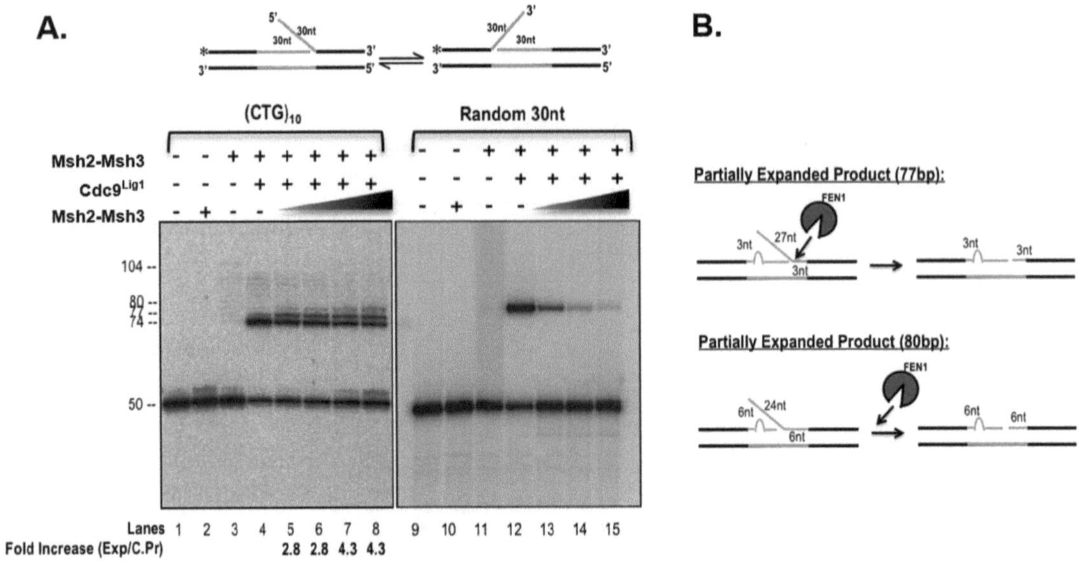

Fig. 13 (**a**) Expansion Assay: Equilibrating flap substrates containing either a ten CTG repeat of thirty randomly generated nucleotides were used to assess the role of Msh2-Msh3 in repeat expansion. Substrates were incubated with FEN1 (2.5 nM), Lig1 (37.5 nM), and increasing concentrations of Msh2-Msh3 (0, 12.5, 25, and 37.5 nM). Top: substrate equilibrating conformations illustration with asterisk indicating site of ^{32}P label, TNRs in gray. (**b**) Illustration of Rad27^{Fen1} cleavage intermediates for equilibrating flap substrates. (*Reproduced with permission from* [16].)

age buffer containing 75% glycerol. The final protein was aliquoted and stored at −80 °C.

2. 5-FOA is light-sensitive.
3. Msh2-Msh3 was overexpressed as a complex in a protease-deficient strain of *S. cerevisiae* (EAY33) and purified as previously described [71] and modified [72].
4. Rad27^{FEN1} was overexpressed in *E. coli* strain BL21 (DE3) codon plus and purified as previously described [73].
5. Cdc9^{Lig1} was overexpressed in a protease-deficient strain of *S. cerevisiae* (BJ2168) and purified as previously described [74].
6. DNA Pol delta (Pol δ) was overexpressed as a complex in *E. coli* strain BL21 (DE3) codon plus and purified as previously described [75].
7. This elegant system was developed, verified and characterized by the Lahue lab [61, 62, 76] and is comprehensively described in previous *Methods in Molecular Biology* publications [63, 64].
8. Pour 8–10 spreading glass beads on each plate. Shake/rotate the plate, keeping it on the benchtop surface to move the beads around to cover the plate. It may be helpful to add 50 μL

of sterile dIH_2O to each plate before adding the glass beads. A stack of ~5 plates can be plated at the same time.

9. Mutations in the *URA3* locus will also result in resistance to 5-FOA [63]. It is therefore necessary to check for false positives by performing colony PCR, digesting the DNA and electrophoresing the DNA to image the gel, as described above.
10. Synthetic media lacking histidine is used throughout all the time courses to ensure that the TNR reporter construct is maintained. [63].
11. It is advisable to perform a few colony PCR reactions per colony per time point in case one or more colony PCR reactions are not successful for technical reasons.
12. A 25 μm or 50 μm glass needle is attached to the dissection arm using putty. This is what will be used to move cells around on the plate.
13. Removing marked microcolonies from plates with pipette tips is easiest and most efficient when the pipette tip is held and swiped across the plate at a low angle, i.e. close to parallel to the plate.
14. Although tedious, it is best to only have 4 and 5 single cells per plate. Observing too many cells on a single plate, each with potentially different starting times, may result in the plate being out of the incubator for too long. Ideally, the plate should be incubating at 30 °C for 30 min at a time.
15. For acid-washed beads, we purchase unwashed Sigma 425–600 micron beads (G9268) and acid-wash in the laboratory. Pour the beads into a 1 L beaker containing 5 M nitric acid in the fume hood. Stir occasionally for 1–2 days. Wash with ~5 volumes of dIH_2O and then with 5 volumes of 18 Ω dIH_2O. Remove as much liquid as possible and bake at 450 °F for ~2 h. Store the beads in a – 20 °C freezer.
16. It is helpful to continuously wet the gel with 1× SSC. Invert the gel because the DNA is often more concentrated near the bottom.
17. A 1:10 dilution is necessary to get an accurate reading of your saturated culture.
18. This step can also be done overnight to improve annealing efficiency.
19. Proper protective equipment (laboratory coats and gloves) should be worn at all times while handling radioactive material. Reactions should be set up behind plexiglass shields. All pipette tips and microcentrifuge tubes that have come in contact with radioactive material should be carefully discarded in a radioactive waste container.

20. During the incubation period, prepare sequencing gel and allow for polymerization. Prepare Bio-Spin columns according to manufacturer's protocol.
21. Set up the sequencing gel in 1× TBE buffer for "prerun" at 80 W.
22. Sequencing gels should be electrophoresed behind plexiglass shield in an area designated for radioactive work.
23. Keep lid of microcentrifuge tube open to allow for evaporation. However, the tube should be kept under a plexiglass cover for protection.
24. Specific Activity = [{Average After Count × 3) × (40 μL {volume onto spin column})/(20 {pmol of starting material})]. Recovery = (average recovery counts × 3)/specific activity.
25. Always keep the radiolabeled primer in limiting quantity compared to the unlabeled primers being added to make the substrate.
26. Annealing can also be done in a step gradient PCR block to control the various temperatures.
27. Freshly labeled substrates need to be exposed to the phosphor screen for approximately only 2 h prior to imaging.
28. Substrates should be annealed with 100% efficiency, that is, in the annealed substrate lane you should not observe any unannealed labeled primer. If you observe unannealed primer, you can increase the ratio of annealing to 1:4:8 of radiolabeled olig onucleotide:template:upstream primer.
29. Reactions can be loaded onto the gel with the power on. This allows the substrate bound protein complex to enter the gel matrix easily and will prevent retention in the wells.
30. When making a sequencing or denaturing gel, add distilled water, TBE and urea to a container with a stir bar. Microwave for 20 s to aid in dissolving urea. Place container on the stir plate and add the other components until all the urea is completely dissolved and the solution is clear.
31. Use a syringe to wash off the wells before pre-running the gel. This step should be repeated after pre-run and before loading the reactions.
32. Save the remainder of the reaction at −20 °C to rerun the reactions in case, the gel rips during transfer to the Whatman paper or during the drying process.
33. Nuclease activity calculation: $\{(b)/(b + a)\} \times 100$. For % cleavage, b is the cleaved product and a is the uncleaved substrate remaining.

34. Ligase activity calculation: $\{(b)/(b + a)\} \times 100$. For % ligation, *b* is the ligated product and *a* is the unligated substrate remaining.
35. Synthesis activity calculation: $\{(b)/(b + c + a)\} \times 100$. For % fully synthesized product, *b* is the fully synthesized product, *c* are the intermediate products and *a* is the remaining unsynthesized substrate.

Acknowledgments

We are particularly grateful for the generosity of Dr. Robert Lahue in providing reagents and for many useful discussions and comments in developing this protocol. We are also grateful for discussions with Dr. Catherine Freudenreich, Dr. Robert Bambara, and Dr. Eric Alani. Work in the Balakrishnan laboratory is supported by the National Institutes of Health (GM0938328 to L.B.) Work in the Surtees laboratory is supported by the National Institutes of Health (GM087459 to J.A.S.) and the American Cancer Society (RSG-14-235-01 to J.A.S.). J.A.S. is an ACS Research Scholar.

References

1. Ireland MJ, Reinke SS, Livingston DM (2000) The impact of lagging strand replication mutations on the stability of CAG repeat tracts in yeast. Genetics 155(4):1657–1665
2. Schweitzer JK, Livingston DM (1997) Destabilization of CAG trinucleotide repeat tracts by mismatch repair mutations in yeast. Hum Mol Genet 6(3):349–355
3. Gordenin DA, Kunkel TA, Resnick MA (1997) Repeat expansion [mdash] all in flap? Nat Genet 16(2):116–118
4. Balakrishnan L, Bambara RA (2013) Flap endonuclease 1. Annu Rev Biochem 82(1): 119–138
5. Kovtun IV et al (2007) OGG1 initiates age-dependent CAG trinucleotide expansion in somatic cells. Nature 447:447
6. Zhao X-N, Usdin K (2015) The repeat expansion diseases: the dark side of DNA repair. DNA Repair 32:96–105
7. Tishkoff DX et al (1997) A novel mutation avoidance mechanism dependent on *S. cerevisiae* RAD27 is distinct from DNA mismatch repair. Cell 88:253–263
8. Yang J, Freudenreich CH (2007) Haploinsufficiency of yeast FEN1 causes instability of expanded CAG/CTG tracts in a length-dependent manner. Gene 393(1): 110–115
9. Liu Y et al (2004) *Saccharomyces cerevisiae* flap endonuclease 1 uses flap equilibration to maintain triplet repeat stability. Mol Cell Biol 24(9):4049–4064
10. Callahan JL et al (2003) Mutations in yeast replication proteins that increase CAG/CTG expansions also increase repeat fragility. Mol Cell Biol 23(21):7849–7860
11. Daee DL, Mertz T, Lahue RS (2007) Postreplication repair inhibits CAG {middle dot} CTG repeat expansions in *Saccharomyces cerevisiae*. Mol Cell Biol 27(1):102–110. https://doi.org/10.1128/MCB.01167-06
12. Arana ME, Kunkel TA (2010) Mutator phenotypes due to DNA replication infidelity. Semin Cancer Biol 20(5):304–311
13. Ellegren H (2004) Microsatellites: simple sequences with complex evolution. Nat Rev Genet 5(6):435–445
14. Umar A, Kunkel TA (1996) DNA-replication fidelity, mismatch repair and genome instability in cancer cells. Eur J Biochem 238(2): 297–307
15. Strand M et al (1993) Destabilization of tracts of simple repetitive DNA in yeast by mutations

affecting DNA mismatch repair. Nature 365(6443):274–276
16. Kantartzis A et al (2012) Msh2-Msh3 interferes with Okazaki fragment processing to promote trinucleotide repeat expansions. Cell Rep 2(2):216–222
17. Sia E et al (1997) Microsatellite instability in yeast: dependence on repeat unit size and DNA mismatch repair genes. Mol Cell Biol 17(5):2851–2858
18. Romanova NV, Crouse GF (2013) Different roles of eukaryotic MutS and MutL complexes in repair of small insertion and deletion loops in yeast. PLoS Genet 9(10):e1003920
19. Kunkel TA, Erie DA (2015) Eukaryotic mismatch repair in relation to DNA replication. Annu Rev Genet 49(1):291–313
20. Crouse GF (2016) Non-canonical actions of mismatch repair. DNA Repair 38:102–109
21. Owen BAL et al (2005) $(CAG)_n$-hairpin DNA binds to Msh2-Msh3 and changes properties of mismatch recognition. Nat Struct Mol Biol 12(8):663–670
22. Manley K, Pugh J, Messer A (1999) Instability of the CAG repeat in immortalized fibroblast cell cultures from Huntington's disease transgenic mice. Brain Res 835(1):74–79
23. van den Broek WJAA et al (2002) Somatic expansion behaviour of the (CTG)n repeat in myotonic dystrophy knock-in mice is differentially affected by Msh3 and Msh6 mismatch–repair proteins. Hum Mol Genet 11(2): 191–198
24. Foiry L et al (2006) Msh3 is a limiting factor in the formation of intergenerational CTG expansions in DM1 transgenic mice. Hum Genetics 119(5):520–526
25. Gannon A-MM et al (2012) MutSβ and histone deacetylase complexes promote expansions of trinucleotide repeats in human cells. Nucleic Acids Res 40(20):10324–10333
26. Halabi A et al (2012) DNA mismatch repair complex MutSβ promotes GAA·TTC repeat expansion in human cells. J Biol Chem 287(35):29958–29967
27. Williams GM, Surtees JA (2015) MSH3 promotes dynamic behavior of Trinucleotide repeat tracts in vivo. Genetics 200(3):737–754
28. Schmidt MHM, Pearson CE (2016) Disease-associated repeat instability and mismatch repair. DNA Repair 38:117–126
29. Kim JC, Mirkin SM (2013) The balancing act of DNA repeat expansions. Curr Opin Genet Dev 23(3):280–288
30. Neil AJ, Kim JC, Mirkin SM (2017) Precarious maintenance of simple DNA repeats in eukaryotes. BioEssays 39(9):1700077
31. Kang S et al (1995) Pausing of DNA synthesis in vitro at specific loci in CTG and CGG triplet repeats from human hereditary disease genes. J Biol Chem 270(45):27014–27021
32. Usdin K, House NCM, Freudenreich CH (2015) Repeat instability during DNA repair: insights from model systems. Crit Rev Biochem Mol Biol:1–26
33. McGinty RJ, Mirkin SM (2018) Cis- and trans-modifiers of repeat expansions: blending model systems with human genetics. Trends Genet 34(6):448–465
34. Polyzos AA, McMurray CT (2017) Close encounters: moving along bumps, breaks, and bubbles on expanded trinucleotide tracts. DNA Repair 56:144–155
35. Mirkin SM (2007) Expandable DNA repeats and human disease. Nature 447(7147): 932–940
36. Kovtun IV, McMurray CT (2008) Features of trinucleotide repeat instability in vivo. Cell Res 18(1):198–213
37. Paulson HL, Fischbeck KH (1996) Trinucleotide repeats in neurogenetic disorders. Annu Rev Neurosci 19(1):79–107
38. Veitch NJ et al (2007) Inherited CAG·CTG allele length is a major modifier of somatic mutation length variability in Huntington disease. DNA Repair 6(6):789–796
39. Groh WJ et al (2011) Survival and CTG repeat expansion in adults with myotonic dystrophy type 1. Muscle Nerve 43(5):648–651
40. Kay C et al (2016) Huntington disease reduced penetrance alleles occur at high frequency in the general population. Neurology 87(3): 282–288
41. Langbehn DR, Hayden MR, Paulsen JS (2010) CAG-repeat length and the age of onset in Huntington disease (HD): a review and validation study of statistical approaches. Am J Med Genet B Neuropsychiatr Genet 153B(2):397–408
42. Keum JW et al (2016) The HTT CAG-expansion mutation determines age at death but not disease duration in Huntington disease. Am J Hum Genet 98(2):287–298
43. Chao T-K, Hu J, Pringsheim T (2017) Risk factors for the onset and progression of Huntington disease. Neurotoxicology 61:79–99
44. Long JD et al (2018) Genetic modification of Huntington disease acts early in the prediagnosis phase. Am J Hum Genet 103(3):349–357
45. Cumming SA et al (2018) De novo repeat interruptions are associated with reduced somatic instability and mild or absent clinical features in myotonic dystrophy type 1. Eur J Hum Genet 26(11):1635–1647

46. Zhao X-N, Usdin K (2018) Timing of expansion of fragile X premutation alleles during intergenerational transmission in a mouse model of the fragile X-related disorders. Front Genet 9:314
47. Braida C et al (2010) Variant CCG and GGC repeats within the CTG expansion dramatically modify mutational dynamics and likely contribute toward unusual symptoms in some myotonic dystrophy type 1 patients. Hum Mol Genet 19(8):1399–1412
48. Concannon C, Lahue RS (2014) Nucleotide excision repair and the 26S proteasome function together to promote trinucleotide repeat expansions. DNA Repair 13(0):42–49
49. Zhang L et al (1994) Studying human mutations by sperm typing: instability of CAG trinucleotide repeats in the human androgen receptor gene. Nat Genet 7(4):531–535
50. Leeflang EP et al (1995) Single sperm analysis of the trinucleotide repeats in the Huntington's disease gene: quantification of the mutation frequency spectrum. Hum Mol Genet 4(9):1519–1526
51. Leeflang EP et al (1999) Analysis of Germline mutation spectra at the Huntington's disease locus supports a mitotic mutation mechanism. Hum Mol Genet 8(2):173–183
52. Martorell L et al (2004) Germline mutational dynamics in myotonic dystrophy type 1 males: allele length and age effects. Neurology 62(2):269–274
53. Castel AL, Cleary JD, Pearson CE (2010) Repeat instability as the basis for human diseases and as a potential target for therapy. Nat Rev Mol Cell Biol 11(3):165–170
54. Du J et al (2013) Length-dependent CTG·CAG triplet-repeat expansion in myotonic dystrophy patient-derived induced pluripotent stem cells. Hum Mol Genet 22(25):5276–5287
55. Higham CF et al (2012) High levels of somatic DNA diversity at the myotonic dystrophy type 1 locus are driven by ultra-frequent expansion and contraction mutations. Hum Mol Genet 21(11):2450–2463
56. Morales F et al (2012) Somatic instability of the expanded CTG triplet repeat in myotonic dystrophy type 1 is a heritable quantitative trait and modifier of disease severity. Hum Mol Genet 21(16):3558–3567
57. Higham CF, Monckton DG (2013) Modelling and inference reveal nonlinear length-dependent suppression of somatic instability for small disease associated alleles in myotonic dystrophy type 1 and Huntington disease. J R Soc Interface 10(88)
58. Lee J-M et al (2015) Identification of genetic factors that modify clinical onset of Huntington's disease. Cell 162(3):516–526
59. Moss DJH et al (2017) Identification of genetic variants associated with Huntington's disease progression: a genome-wide association study. Lancet Neurol 16(9):701–711
60. Morales F et al (2016) A polymorphism in the MSH3 mismatch repair gene is associated with the levels of somatic instability of the expanded CTG repeat in the blood DNA of myotonic dystrophy type 1 patients. DNA Repair 40:57–66
61. Miret JJ, Pessoa-Brandão L, Lahue RS (1997) Instability of CAG and CTG trinucleotide repeats in *Saccharomyces cerevisiae*. Mol Cell Biol 17(6):3382–3387
62. Miret JJ, Pessoa-Brandão L, Lahue RS (1998) Orientation-dependent and sequence-specific expansions of CTG/CAG trinucleotide repeats in *Saccharomyces cerevisiae*. Proc Natl Acad Sci 95(21):12438–12443
63. Dixon M, Bhattacharyya S, Lahue R (2004) Genetic assays for triplet repeat instability in yeast. In: Kohwi Y (ed) Trinucleotide repeat protocols. Humana Press, pp 29–45
64. Williams GM, Surtees JA (2018) Measuring dynamic behavior of Trinucleotide repeat tracts in vivo in *Saccharomyces cerevisiae*. In: Muzi-Falconi M, Brown GW (eds) Genome instability: methods and protocols. Springer, New York, NY, pp 439–470
65. Gietz D et al (1992) Improved method for high efficiency transformation of intact yeast cells. Nucleic Acids Res 20(6):1425
66. Drake JW (1991) A constant rate of spontaneous mutation in DNA-based microbes. Proc Natl Acad Sci U S A 88(16):7160–7164
67. Dixon W, Massey F (1969) Introduction to statistical analysis. McGraw Hill, New York
68. Nair KR (1940) Table of confidence interval for the median in samples from any continuous population. SankhyÄ: The Indian Journal of Statistics (1933–1960) 4(4):551–558
69. Foster PL, Judith LC, Paul M (2006) Methods for determining spontaneous mutation rates. In: Methods in enzymology. Academic Press, pp 195–213
70. Zar JH (1999) Biostatistical analysis, fourth edition. Prentice Hall, Upper Saddle River, NJ
71. Surtees JA, Alani E (2006) Mismatch repair factor MSH2-MSH3 binds and alters the conformation of branched DNA structures predicted to form during genetic recombination. J Mol Biol 360(3):523–536

72. Kumar C et al (2014) ATP binding and hydrolysis by *Saccharomyces cerevisiae* Msh2–Msh3 are differentially modulated by mismatch and double-strand break repair DNA substrates. DNA Repair 18(0):18–30
73. Xie Y et al (2001) Identification of rad27 mutations that confer differential defects in mutation avoidance, repeat tract instability, and flap cleavage. Mol Cell Biol 21(15):4889–4899
74. Ayyagari R et al (2003) Okazaki fragment maturation in yeast. I. Distribution of functions between FEN1 AND DNA2. J Biol Chem 278(3):1618–1625
75. Langston LD, O'Donnell M (2008) DNA polymerase delta is highly processive with proliferating cell nuclear antigen and undergoes collision release upon completing DNA. J Biol Chem 283(43):29522–29531
76. Rolfsmeier ML et al (2001) Cis-elements governing Trinucleotide repeat instability in *Saccharomyces cerevisiae.* Genetics 157(4): 1569–1579

Chapter 4

Quantifying Replication Fork Progression at CTG Repeats by 2D Gel Electrophoresis

David Viterbo and Guy-Franck Richard

Abstract

Physical separation of branched DNA from linear molecules is based on the difference of mobility of linear versus branched DNA during two-dimensional agarose gel electrophoresis. Structured DNA migrates as slower species when compared to linear DNA of similar molecular weight. Metabolic processes such as S phase replication or double strand-break repair may generate branched DNA molecules. Trinucleotide repeats are naturally prone to form secondary structures that can modify their migration through an agarose gel matrix. These structures may also interfere in vivo with replication, by slowing down replication-fork progression, transiently stalling forks, possibly leading to secondary structure such as Holliday junctions or hemicatenanes. Alternatively, reversed replication forks may occur following fork stalling, disrupting replication dynamics and modifying DNA migration on agarose gel. So although two-dimensional agarose gel electrophoresis theoretically allows to resolve a mixture of structured DNA molecules and quantify them by radioactive hybridization, its practical application to trinucleotide repeats faces some serious technical challenges.

Key words Trinucleotide repeats, 2D gel, Replication fork, Reversed fork, Recombination, Phosphor screen technology

1 Introduction

Physical separation of branched DNA from linear molecules was developed by Bell and Byers in 1982 [1]. This method was based on the difference of mobility of linear versus branched DNA during two-dimensional agarose gel electrophoresis, in the presence of ethidium bromide. It was shown that structured DNA molecules migrate as slower species when compared to linear DNA of similar molecular weight. Since metabolic processes such as S phase replication or double strand-break repair may generate branched DNA molecules, this method was extensively used to study replication fork progression [2, 3] as well as meiotic recombination intermediates [4, 5]. In order to run a 2D gel, total genomic DNA must be extracted from replicating cells and digested with a restriction enzyme, to generate large DNA fragments, usually more than

Guy-Franck Richard (ed.), *Trinucleotide Repeats: Methods and Protocols*, Methods in Molecular Biology, vol. 2056,
https://doi.org/10.1007/978-1-4939-9784-8_4,

3–4 kb in size, since replication intermediates may be hard to visualize with smaller fragments. Digested DNA is then migrated in the first dimension at low voltage, in the absence of ethidium bromide, so that molecules are separated according to their size. In the second dimension, voltage is increased and ethidium bromide is added in order to rigidify molecules which are then separated according both to their size and to their structure. After the second dimension, the gel is transferred to a nylon membrane and hybridized with a radioactive ^{32}P-labeled probe, whose signal is subsequently quantified using phosphor screen technology (Fig. 1).

Trinucleotide repeat expansions are involved in many neurological pathologies like Huntington disease, myotonic dystrophy type 1 (Steinert disease), fragile-X syndrome, Friedreich's ataxia, or multiple spinocerebellar ataxias. These trinucleotide repeats are located in coding or noncoding sequences, depending on the disease [6–11]. CAG/CTG repeats form imperfect hairpins in vitro (*see* Chapter 1) and these secondary structures may interfere with DNA synthesis during replication, repair or recombination. Therefore, it was early postulated that such repeats may stall replication forks in vivo [12] and subsequently demonstrated by 2D gel

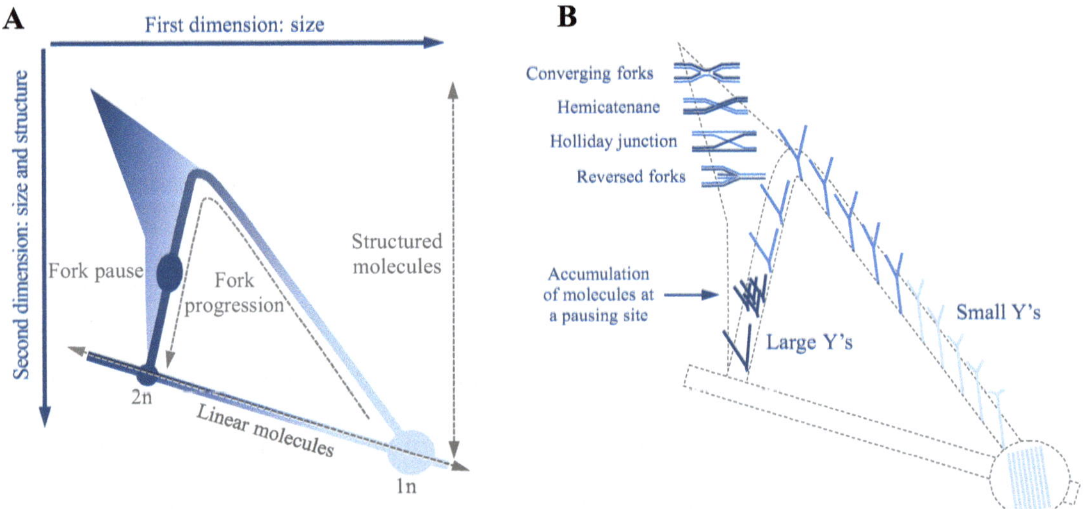

Fig. 1 Different replication and recombination intermediates may be detected by 2D gels. (**a**) Linear molecules migrate relatively to their size only, between *n* and 2*n*, whereas structured molecules migrate according to their size and structure in the second dimension and are therefore detected above the linear ones. The Y arc starts from unreplicated molecules (the *n* spot) to almost completely replicated molecules (the 2*n* spot). A conical shape corresponding to non-Y arc structures is sometimes visible. Fork pausing is detected as a thickening of the Y arc wherever the stalling sequence is located. (**b**) Detailed structured molecules corresponding to Y arc or cone signals. Converging forks, hemicatenanes, Holliday junctions, and reversed forks are hard to discriminate based on their structure and migrate in the same conical area. Note that they are not represented at their expected position in the present figure. Their migration will depend on the time point considered and on the restriction enzyme used to digest genomic DNA. For a comprehensive view of what kind of molecules may be detected and their migration patterns, refer to Schvartzman and colleagues [3]

electrophoresis that it was the case, first in bacteria [13], later on in yeast [14–16]. Secondary structure formation is favored by the presence of extensive single-stranded DNA regions (ssDNA). Therefore, double-strand break repair mechanisms known to generate extensive ssDNA, such as break-induced replication (BIR) [17], single-strand annealing (SSA) [18] or gene conversion should increase trinucleotide repeat instability. Indeed, it was shown in *Saccharomyces cerevisiae* that BIR promotes CAG/CTG repeat expansions [19] and that SSA drives contractions [20], whereas gene conversion induces a high level of both expansions and contractions [21] (reviewed in [22]). In addition, secondary structures may also modify DNA migration in agarose gels, leading to an apparent aberrant mobility [23].

Two-dimensional agarose gel electrophoresis gives a global picture of the replication fork dynamics: replication origin firing, replication fork progression, fork stalling, reversed replication forks, and various replication and recombination intermediates can all be theoretically detected by 2D gels (Fig. 1b) [3, 24, 25]. Variations of this technique were extensively used in *S. cerevisiae* to study replication and recombination intermediates. In order to improve signal quality and signal over background ratio, it is convenient to synchronize yeast cells, either by alpha-factor arrest [18] or by centrifugal elutriation [26]. Cells are subsequently collected at different time points after release into S phase and total genomic DNA is extracted. Different methods can be used to enrich the fraction containing ssDNA, including BND-cellulose columns [27] or extraction in the presence of CTAB (cetyltrimethylammonium bromide), a detergent which stabilizes ssDNA secondary structures [28]. In the present chapter, we describe the 2D gel method on synchronized yeast cells using a simplified CTAB protocol [29] that does not involve a preliminary step of yeast spheroplast preparation. In the following experiments, a $(CAG)_{80}$ or $(CTG)_{80}$ trinucleotide repeat was integrated at the *ARG2* locus on the left arm of yeast chromosome X (strain background BY4741 [30]), 7 kb away from an early replication origin, located in telomeric proximal position as compared to the *ARG2* gene. Maximal replication at this locus occurs 50 min after release from alpha-factor arrest.

2 Materials

Prepare all solutions with deionized water and analytical grade reagents. The quality of the water is crucial in this protocol and changing the water providing source may dramatically alter experimental results. Prepare and store reagents at room temperature, unless otherwise indicated. Follow all waste disposal regulations specific to your institute or country.

2.1 Replication Time Course

1. Alpha-factor (1 mg/mL). Dissolve 10 mg in 10 mL ethanol 100%. Store at 4 °C.
2. Sodium azide. It is kept as a frozen liquid solution at −20 °C, at 100× concentration (10%). It is used as a 0.1% solution to kill yeast cells.
3. 10 mM Tris–HCl, pH 8.0.
4. YPD medium (10 g/L yeast extract, 20 g/L Bacto peptone, 20 g/L dextrose). Autoclave for 20 min at 110 °C. Store at room temperature.
5. 15 mL and 50 mL polypropylene tubes.

2.2 Genomic DNA Extraction

1. Zymolyase 100T (Seikagaku, 30 mg/mL).
2. Extraction solutions.
   Solution I: 2% CTAB (cetyltrimethylammonium bromide), 1.4 M NaCl, 100 mM Tris–HCl pH 7.5, 25 mM EDTA pH 8.0.
   Solution II: 1% CTAB, 50 mM Tris–HCl pH 7.5, 10 mM EDTA.
   Solution III: 1.4 M NaCl, 10 mM Tris–HCl pH 7.5, 1 mM EDTA
3. RNAse A (10 mg/mL).
4. Proteinase K (20 mg/mL).
5. DTT 2 M.
6. Chloroform–isoamyl alcohol 24:1. Order as 250 mL solution, store at 4 °C and use rapidly after opening.

2.3 First Dimension

Use only ultrapure agarose (Lonza Seakem GTG or similar) 0.35% in 300 mL 1× TBE buffer (89 mM Tris–HCl pH 8.0, 89 mM boric acid, 2 mM EDTA pH 8.0). Do *not* add ethidium bromide. Pour the gel in a cold room to quicken polymerization.

2.4 Second Dimension

Use the same agarose. Prepare 300 mL of a 0.9% agarose gel in 1× TBE buffer. Add 9 μL ethidium bromide to the gel *and* 30 μL to 1 L of 1× TBE buffer (0.3 μg/μL final concentration in both gel and buffer).

2.5 Blot

1. Depurination solution, 0.25 N HCl, 1 L.
2. Denaturation solution, 0.5 M NaoH, 1.5 M NaCl, 1 L.
3. Neutralization solution, 0.02 M NaOH, 1 M NH4OAcetetate, 1 L.
4. Six sheets of 3 MM Whatman absorbent paper, cut to the gel dimension.
5. Positively charged nylon membrane cut to the gel dimension (*see* Subheading 3.6).

6. A plastic platform and a plastic tray to set up the transfer (*see* Subheading 3.7).
7. 10× saline sodium citrate (SSC) buffer: 1.5 M NaCl, 150 mM trisodium citrate (adjusted to pH 7.0 with HCl), 1 L.

2.6 Hybridization

1. Hybridization and washes are performed in sodium phosphate buffer ("Church buffer"). Prepare 1 L of 500 mM Na_2HPO_4 adjusted to pH 7.4 with 4 mL orthophosphoric acid.
2. Hybridization: sodium phosphate buffer 250 mM (pH 7.4), SDS 7%, EDTA 1 mM.
3. Washes: 20 mM sodium phosphate buffer (pH 7.4), 1% SDS, 1 mM EDTA.

2.7 Probe Labeling

1. Random Primer (hexadeoxyribonucleotide mix: pd(N)6, 6-mer, 80 nmol), diluted to 120 pmol/μL.
2. 10× Random Priming buffer: 500 mM Tris–HCl pH 7.0, 100 mM $MgSO_4$, 1 mM DTT.
3. [α32P]-dATP, 6000 Ci/mmole.
4. Klenow polymerase 10 U/μL.

3 Methods

3.1 Replication Time Course

Yeast cells respond to the pheromone of the opposite sexual type. Therefore, to perform alpha-factor arrest, cells must be MATa. If working with MATα strains, it is possible to purchase alpha-factor, but its prohibitive price makes this working hypothesis unlikely. If limited amount of alpha-factor are available, it is possible to inactivate the *BAR1* gene, encoding the secreted aspartyl protease that degrades the pheromone, in order to use much lesser amounts of alpha-factor. The amounts indicated here are those recommended for *BAR1* strains, in which the protease is active.

1. Day 1: Grow one colony in 3 mL YDP at 30 °C overnight.
2. Day 2: Transfer in an Erlenmeyer flask, add 200 mL YPD and grow overnight at 23 °C to slow down cell cycle.
3. Day 3: Collect 8×10^9 cells in four 50 mL polypropylene tubes and wash them twice with 20 mL sterile water. Resuspend cells in 800 mL fresh YPD at 9×10^6 cells/mL and incubate 1 h at 23 °C. Add 4 mg alpha-factor (final concentration 5 μg/mL), and incubate cells for 1½ h at 23 °C. Check cell shape under the microscope. They should start to "shmoo" (one end of the cell starts to slightly elongate) in response to the pheromone. If less than 90% of cells are arrested, add an extra 4 mg alpha-factor and incubate cells for an extra 30–45 min. Check cell shape under the microscope. If necessary, an extra 2 mg alpha-

factor may be added to the culture, for a total of 10 mg. When more than 90% of yeast cells are arrested in G1 phase, as shown by microscope observation of "shmoos," centrifuge, wash the culture with 10 mM Tris–HCl (pH 8.0) and resuspend them in fresh YPD at 23 °C. This is the beginning (T_0) of the time course. Progression through cell cycle may be subsequently monitored by microscope observation or followed by FACS, as described in Chapter 5.

4. For each time point, collect 2 × 10^9 cells (i.e., 200 mL) at 40, 50, 60, and 90 min (*see* **Note 1**).
5. Cells are killed by addition of 2 mL 100× sodium azide (0.1% final concentration). Note that Na-azide is a poison for all eukaryotic cells since it by inhibits mitochondrial oxidative phosphorylations. It is therefore recommended to prepare four flasks containing 2 mL of Na-azide, and to leave them on ice for the duration of the experiment, to avoid repeated manipulations of the stock solution. After incubation with sodium azide, leave cells on ice for 10 min (*see* **Note 2**).
6. Centrifuge cells and discard sodium azide-containing YPD in appropriate waste container. Wash once with 50 mL cold sterile water.
7. Resuspend cells in 50 mL cold sterile water, centrifuge, remove water and freeze dried cell pellet at −80 °C until DNA preparation may take place.

3.2 DNA Extraction, Day 1

1. Thaw the four dried pellets on ice. Resuspend each in 2 mL H_2O, 2.5 mL Solution I, 5 μL DTT (2 M) and 167 μL Zymolyase 100T (Seikagaku, 30 mg/mL). Incubate tube at 30 °C for 1 h. The cell lysate must be viscous. Note that zymolyase digestion of yeast cell wall is performed directly in Solution I, in the presence of CTAB. This is an improvement from former protocols in which spheroplasts had first to be prepared, before Solution I was added.
2. Add 200 μL RNAse (10 mg/mL) in each tube for ½ h at 50 °C.
3. Add 200 μL Proteinase K (20 mg/mL) in each tube for 1.5 h at 50 °C.
4. Add 100 μL Proteinase K (20 mg/mL) in each tube and incubate at 37 °C overnight.

3.3 DNA Extraction, Day 2

Centrifuge tubes 15 min at 3200 × *g* (4000 rpm in our centrifuge). In subsequent steps, pellets and supernatants are independently processed.

3.3.1 Supernatants

1. Gently transfer each supernatant in a 15 mL polypropylene tube.
2. Add 2.5 mL 24:1 chloroform–isoamyl alcohol and gently mix by inversion 5–6 times.
3. Centrifuge 15 min at 3200 × *g*.
4. Gently and slowly transfer each supernatant in a 50 mL polypropylene tube.
5. Add 10 mL of Solution II. Wait 2 to 3 h (*see* **Note 3**).
6. Centrifuge 10 min at 4000 rpm. Discard the supernatant.
7. Add 2.5 mL of Solution III and incubate tubes at 37 °C for 10 min to help dissolve DNA.

3.3.2 Pellets

1. Add 1 mL of Solution III to each pellet. Incubate tubes at 50 °C for 1 h.
2. Add one volume of chloroform–isoamyl alcohol and gently mix by inversion 5–6 times.
3. Centrifuge 10 min at 3200 × *g*.
4. Transfer each supernatant in 15 mL polypropylene tubes containing 2.5 mL of Solution III.
5. Add 5 mL of isopropanol and mix by inversion 5–6 times.
6. Centrifuge 10 min at 4000 rpm.
7. Wash each tube with 2 mL of 70% ethanol.
8. Resuspend each pellet in 250 μL 10 mM Tri–HCl pH 8.0 and incubate tubes at 37 °C for 10 min to help dissolve DNA (*see* **Note 4**).
9. Estimate DNA concentration by loading an aliquot on an agarose gel or using a dedicated setup.
10. Keep DNA at 4 °C (*see* **Note 5**).

3.4 Genomic DNA Restriction Digest

1. Quantify DNA recovered at former step by UV absorbance at 260 nm.
2. Digest 10 μg of DNA for each time point, in a final volume of 100 μL, with 20 units of restriction enzyme (ClaI in our experiments) and 2 μL RNAse A (10 mg/mL) during 6 h. Add 20 more units and leave digestion overnight (*see* **Note 6**).

3.5 First Dimension

1. Pour a 0.35% agarose gel in 300 mL 1× TBE buffer, in a cold room to accelerate polymerization. Do *not* add ethidium bromide. After polymerization, handle the gel with much care because it is *very* fragile.
2. Add 20 μL of 6× loading dye to each digestion and load in wells large enough to accommodate 120 μL. Leave one empty well between each sample for convenient cutting at the next step (Fig. 2a).

3. Run gel overnight at 1 V/cm.
4. With a clean scalpel, cut the lane containing the molecular weight ladder and stain it with ethidium bromide. Measure the distance between which you want to study replication intermediates. For example, if your restriction fragment measures 6 kb, you want to cut first dimension pieces of agarose between ~6 kb and ~12 kb (to catch molecules between n and $2n$ in size, *see* **Note 7**).
5. Cut four pieces of similar sizes, one for each time point (Fig. 2b). Watch out at this step because 0.35% agarose is *very* fragile and easily breaks.

3.6 Second Dimension

1. Rotate each piece of DNA by 90° and place them in an empty tray (Fig. 2c).
2. Prepare the volume of agarose 0.9% sufficient to fill the tray up to the height of the four agarose pieces. Add ethidium bromide (0.3 μg/μL final concentration) and let the melted agarose cool down until you may hold the flask (~50 °C).
3. In the meantime, prepare 1× TBE buffer supplemented with ethidium bromide (0.3 μg/μL final concentration) and fill the migration tank in a cold room.
4. Pour the cooled down agarose under a chemical hood, at room temperature and wait for solidification.
5. Take it to the tank in the cold room and migrate the gel at 5 V/cm for ~4.5 h, or until the DNA signal corresponding to linear molecules of n size reaches the bottom of the gel. Take a picture under 260 nm UV lamp (Fig. 2d).

3.7 Transfer

1. Soak the gel in 1 L depurination solution (0.25 N HCl) for 10 min.
2. Soak the gel in denaturation solution (0.5 M NaOH/1.5 M NaCl) for 30 min.
3. Soak the gel in neutralization solution (0.02 M NaOH/1 M NH4 Acetate) for 30 min.
4. Cut a positively charged nylon membrane to the size of the gel and soak it in 10× SSC for 5 min (*see* **Note 8**).
5. Transfer the gel by setting up a classical Southern blot apparatus, in a tray filled with 10× SCC buffer: a plastic platform, 3 MM paper soaked in 10× SSC, the gel, the membrane, three layers of 3 MM paper soaked in 10× SSC, finished by a thick layer (20 cm) of absorbent paper. The bottom 3 MM paper must be larger than the gel and soaks into the SSC-containing tray. Leave the transfer overnight.
6. Crosslink DNA to the membrane in a Stratagene Stratalinker at 0.120 J (or a similar UV cross-linker).

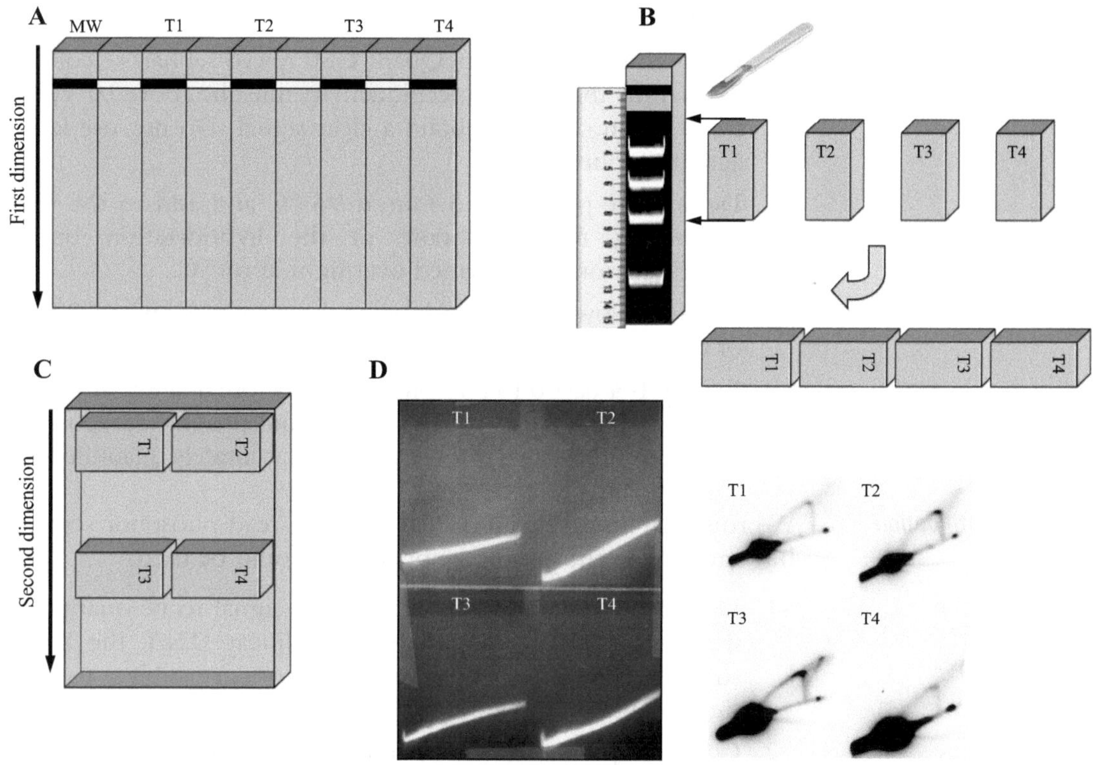

Fig. 2 First and second dimension procedures. (**a**) Each of the four (or more) sample is loaded on an agarose gel, leaving one well free between each sample. Migration is performed at low voltage, in the absence of ethidium bromide. (**b**) The lane containing the molecular weight ladder is cut off and stained to make molecular weight measurements. Each lane containing a DNA sample is subsequently cut between the appropriate molecular weights, as measured on the ladder lane. (**c**) Each cut piece of agarose is turned 90° to be run in the second dimension, at high voltage and in the presence of ethidium bromide. (**d**) Left: Second dimension agarose gel at the end of migration. Linear DNA is stained by ethidium bromide. Structured DNA may sometimes be visible as a weak and fuzzy signal above linear molecules. Right: Hybridization with a radioactive probe specific of the locus studied

3.8 Hybridization

Prehybridization and hybridization are performed at 65 °C in a hybridization oven in a rotating tube.

1. Prehybridize the membrane with 10 mL Church buffer.
2. Prepare the probe by random priming. Use a purified PCR fragment covering the region of interest. Mix 50–60 ng of this PCR product with 120 pmoles hexadeoxyribonucleotide mix (pd(N)6) in 15 μL of 1× random priming buffer (500 mM Tris–HCl (pH 7.0), 100 mM $MgSO_4$, 1 mM DTT).
3. Denaturate DNA for 5 min at 95 °C, then put rapidly on ice.
4. Add 3 μL of α ^{32}P dATP (6000 Ci/mmol), 1 μL of the three remaining dNTP (10 mM each), and 10 units of Klenow polymerase fragment.

5. Incubate at 37 °C for 30–60 min.
6. Purify the probe a ProbeQuant G50 micro sepharose column to quantify the probe. Specific activity must be above 10^8 cpm/μg DNA in order to obtain a clear signal. Do not use lower activity probes.
7. Denaturate probe for 5 min at 95 °C and add to the tube containing the membrane in the hybridization buffer. Hybridization is performed overnight at 65 °C.
8. On the following day, wash twice the membrane with 100 mL of Church washing buffer, for 15 min.
9. Expose 1–4 days on a phosphor screen before quantification. We usually expose 1 day, read the result and possibly reexpose for 2–4 days if the signal is too weak to be accurately quantified.

3.9 Quantification

We routinely use a Fujifilm FLA-9000 to read phosphor screens, but any similar phosphorimaging system could be used.

1. Draw forms surrounding each of the signal to be quantified: the large spot corresponding to *n*, linear DNA, the Y arc, structured molecules migrating as a cone, possibly a pausing signal (Fig. 3 left, *see* **Note 9**).
2. Copy and paste the forms in an area of the membrane containing only background signal (Fig. 3, right).
3. Export data into a spreadsheet. For each signal, subtract the background of the corresponding form.
4. Only signals that are above background by 20% or more were kept for further calculation. Discard other signals.

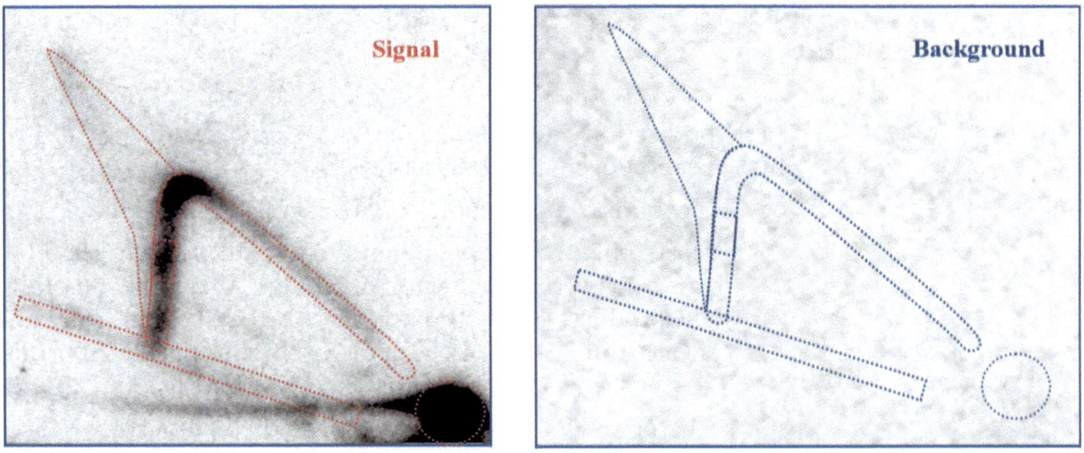

Fig. 3 2D gel quantification. Left: forms of different shapes are drawn around each signal: *n*, linear DNA, Y arc, cone and pausing signal. Right: The same forms are duplicated in another region of the gel in which there is no signal, used as the background to be subtracted from each signal. (Gel originally published by D. Viterbo and G.-F. Richard and reprinted with permission from Elsevier [16])

5. If pausing signals are to be quantified, one may determine a Pausing index (P), as the ratio of pausing signal over Y arc signal, compared to their respective areas. Pausing indexes above one indicate a more intense signal at the pausing locus than on the average of the Y arc [18].

4 Notes

1. In the present experiment, maximum replication timing was known to occur 50 min after alpha-factor release and S phase was finished by 90 min. When working with other yeast strains than S288C (or BY4741) derivatives, or at other genomic loci than *ARG2*, it is advised to experimentally determine the maximum replication timing in preliminary experiments and possibly adjust the above time point values accordingly.
2. Some authors do not use sodium azide, cells are killed by freezing. However, ATP-dependent DNA nucleases may be still active during subsequent steps of DNA isolation, possibly leading to partial DNA degradation, particularly ssDNA. To limit this potential problem, we prefer to shut down ATP metabolism by poisoning the respiratory chain with sodium azide.
3. During this step, the solution must become blurred over time, indicating that DNA is precipitating. If the solution remains crystal clear, it means that the extraction failed or that too little DNA was recovered to form a visible precipitate. If this happens, it is better to stop the experiment at this stage and start over the time course, rather than pursuing through the long and tedious 2D gel protocol with too little DNA to obtain a clear signal at the end.
4. When pipetting DNA use blue tips or yellow tips whose end was cut off with a clean scalpel and slowly pipette to avoid shearing DNA molecules containing single-stranded regions.
5. After extraction, DNA may be kept at 4 °C for weeks. Do not store at −20 °C, to avoid repeated cycles of freezing and thawing, if several experiments are planned.
6. It is very important at this stage that genomic DNA is totally digested. Partial digestion will result in the DNA of interest migrating above its expected size, ending up in missing it when cutting the first dimension gel.
7. Practically, as a security, we recommend cutting agarose a little bit below the n size and a little bit above $2n$ size, to ensure that the entire replication arc will be visible.
8. We used the PerkinElmer charged nylon membrane (NEF1017001PK). However, the experiment may be performed with any other positively charged membrane.

9. Due to the physical properties of a 2D gel, the top of a Y arc always shows more signal than the rest of the arc. Therefore, if planning to study a replication fork pause, choose the restriction enzyme so that the pause will not be exactly in the middle of the restriction fragment, else the pausing signal will be at the top of the Y arc and hard to distinguish from the natural stronger signal at this location (Fig. 3). The enzyme should be chosen so that the pause is in the middle of the ascending or descending Y arc.

Acknowledgments

Work on 2D gels in our lab was generously supported by the Centre National de la Recherche Scientifique (CNRS) and by the Institut Pasteur.

References

1. Bell L, Byers B (1983) Separation of branched from linear DNA by two-dimensional gel electrophoresis. Anal Biochem 130:527–535
2. Brewer BJ, Fangman WL (1987) The localization of replication origins on ARS plasmids in S. cerevisiae. Cell 51:463–471
3. Schvartzman JB, Martinez-Robles ML, Lopez V, Hernandez P, Krimer DB (2012) 2D gels and their third-dimension potential. Methods 57:170–178
4. Schwacha A, Kleckner N (1995) Identification of double Holliday junctions as intermediates in meiotic recombination. Cell 83:783–791
5. Hunter N, Kleckner N (2001) The single-end invasion: an assymetric intermediate at the double-strand break to double-Holliday junction transition of meiotic recombination. Cell 106:59–70
6. Kim JC, Mirkin SM (2013) The balancing act of DNA repeat expansions. Curr Opin Genet Dev 23:280–288
7. Richard G-F, Kerrest A, Dujon B (2008) Comparative genomics and molecular dynamics of DNA repeats in eukaryotes. Microbiol Mol Biol Rev 72:686–727
8. Pearson CE, Edamura KN, Cleary JD (2005) Repeat instability: mechanisms of dynamic mutations. Nat Rev Genet 6:729–742
9. McMurray CT (2010) Mechanisms of trinucleotide repeat instability during human development. Nat Rev Genet 11:786–799
10. Usdin K, House NC, Freudenreich CH (2015) Repeat instability during DNA repair: insights from model systems. Crit Rev Biochem Mol Biol 50(2):142–167. https://doi.org/10.3109/10409238.2014.999192
11. Orr HT, Zoghbi HY (2007) Trinucleotide repeat disorders. Annu Rev Neurosci 30:575–621
12. McMurray CT (1999) DNA secondary structure: a common and causative factor for expansion in human disease. Proc Natl Acad Sci U S A 96:1823–1825
13. Samadashwily G, Raca G, Mirkin SM (1997) Trinucleotide repeats affect DNA replication in vivo. Nat Genet 17:298–304
14. Pelletier R, Krasilnikova MM, Samadashwily GM, Lahue R, Mirkin SM (2003) Replication and expansion of trinucleotide repeats in yeast. Mol Cell Biol 23:1349–1357
15. Anand RP et al (2012) Overcoming natural replication barriers: differential helicase requirements. Nucleic Acids Res 40:1091–1105
16. Viterbo D, Michoud G, Mosbach V, Dujon B, Richard G-F (2016) Replication stalling and heteroduplex formation within CAG/CTG trinucleotide repeats by mismatch repair. DNA Repair 42:94–106
17. Saini N et al (2013) Migrating bubble during break-induced replication drives conservative DNA synthesis. Nature 502:389–392
18. Sugawara N, Haber JE (1992) Characterization of double-strand break-induced recombination: homology requirements and single-stranded DNA formation. Mol Cell Biol 12:563–575

19. Kim JC, Harris ST, Dinter T, Shah KA, Mirkin SM (2017) The role of break-induced replication in large-scale expansions of (CAG)n/(CTG)n repeats. Nat Struct Mol Biol 24:55–60
20. Mosbach V, Poggi L, Viterbo D, Charpentier M, Richard G-F (2018) TALEN-induced double-strand break repair of CTG trinucleotide repeats. Cell Rep 22:2146–2159
21. Richard G-F, Goellner GM, McMurray CT, Haber JE (2000) Recombination-induced CAG trinucleotide repeat expansions in yeast involve the MRE11/RAD50/XRS2 complex. EMBO J 19:2381–2390
22. Mosbach V, Poggi L, Richard G-F (2018) Trinucleotide repeat instability during double-strand break repair: from mechanisms to gene therapy. Curr Genet 65(1):17–28. https://doi.org/10.1007/s00294-018-0865-1
23. Gomes-Pereira M, Monckton DG (2017) Ethidium bromide modifies the agarose electrophoretic mobility of CAG•CTG alternative DNA structures generated by PCR. Front Cell Neurosci 11:153
24. Fierro-Fernandez M, Hernandez P, Krimer DB, Schvartzman JB (2007) Replication fork reversal occurs spontaneously after digestion but is constrained in supercoiled domains. J Biol Chem 282:18190–18196
25. Fierro-Fernandez M, Hernandez P, Krimer DB, Schvartzman JB (2007) Topological locking restrains replication fork reversal. Proc Natl Acad Sci USA 104:1500–1505
26. Marbouty M, Ermont C, Dujon B, Richard G-F, Koszul R (2014) Purification of G1 daughter cells from different Saccharomycetes species through an optimized centrifugal elutriation procedure. Yeast 31:159–166
27. Holmes A et al (2012) Lsd1 and lsd2 control programmed replication fork pauses and imprinting in fission yeast. Cell Rep 2:1513–1520
28. Lopes M, Cotta-Ramusino C, Liberi G, Foiani M (2003) Branch migrating sister chromatid junctions form at replication origins through Rad51/Rad52-independent mechanisms. Mol Cell 12:1499–1510
29. Liberi G et al (2006) Methods to study replication fork collapse in budding yeast. Methods Enzym 409:442–462
30. Brachmann CB et al (1998) Designer deletion strains derived from Saccharomyces cerevisiae S288C: a useful set of strains and plasmids for PCR-mediated gene disruption and other applications. Yeast 14:115–132

Chapter 5

Genetic Assays to Study Repeat Fragility in *Saccharomyces cerevisiae*

Erica J. Polleys and Catherine H. Freudenreich

Abstract

Trinucleotide repeats are common in the human genome and can undergo changes in repeat number and cause length-dependent chromosome fragility. Expanded CAG repeats have been linked to over 14 human diseases and are considered hotspots for breakage and genomic rearrangement. Here we describe two *Saccharomyces cerevisiae* based assays that evaluate the rate of chromosome breakage that occurs within a repeat tract (fragility), with variations that allow the role of transcription to be evaluated. The first fragility assay utilizes end-loss and subsequent telomere addition as the main mode of repair of a yeast artificial chromosome (YAC). The second fragility assay relies on the fact that a chromosomal break stimulates recombination-mediated repair. A PCR-based assay can be used to evaluate instability of the repeat in the same conditions used to measure repeat fragility. These assays have contributed to understanding the genetic mechanisms that cause chromosome breaks and tract-length changes at unstable trinucleotide repeats.

Key words Chromosome breakage, Fragility, Repeat instability, Yeast artificial chromosome (YAC), Direct duplication recombination assay (DDRA)

1 Introduction

Stretches of repetitive DNA sequence are common in eukaryotic genomes and are capable of forming alternative DNA structures, such as hairpin loops. These alternative DNA structures effectively function as a physical barrier, making it difficult for error free DNA replication and repair to occur, and can result in changes in repeat length, chromosomal breakage, and genome instability. One type of repetitive DNA sequence that is common in the human genome are CNG repeats, which when expanded, have been causally associated with over 16 human diseases including Huntington's disease (HD), myotonic dystrophy (DM), spinocerebellar ataxias (SCAs), and fragile X syndrome (FXS) [1, 2].

Long regions of CAG/CTG and CGG/GCC trinucleotide repeats break and undergo aberrant repair at a higher frequency than

Guy-Franck Richard (ed.), *Trinucleotide Repeats: Methods and Protocols*, Methods in Molecular Biology, vol. 2056, https://doi.org/10.1007/978-1-4939-9784-8_5,

nonrepetitive DNA, which can result in mutation and changes in repeat copy number. Breakage of the DNA strands (referred to herein as "fragility") and changes in repeat copy number (referred to herein as "instability") are two sides of the same coin. For example, if normal replication or repair is impaired when encountering a repeat tract, a stalled fork, nick, gap, or double-strand break (DSB) can occur. If the fork is restarted or if there is healing within the nick, gap or break, repeat units can be lost or gained. Alternatively, the DNA lesion may be repaired by a less conservative form of repair that leads to deletion of flanking sequence, loss of a chromosome arm, or other chromosome rearrangements. This dramatic loss of genetic material can be easily monitored in *S. cerevisiae* by loss of a neighboring genetic marker, and is indicative that a break in the chromosome occurred. Such a marker loss assay is an underestimate of the "true" rate of breakage, as it only measures the incidents that are healed after loss of flanking DNA sequence, and not those that heal within the repeat, or those that fail to repair resulting in cell death. Nonetheless, such genetic fragility assays are very useful for comparative studies and can be used to determine if a gene or condition is involved in replication or repair of repetitive DNA.

Repeat fragility rates are generally dependent on repeat length, since longer repeats are more likely to interfere with DNA replication or repair. Therefore it is important to start any fragility assay with cells containing a known repeat size, ideally a pure population of the length of interest. This is best done using a physical PCR assay for trinucleotide repeat instability that captures all (or most) of the repeat sizes present in the starting colony. Therefore a description of PCR size analysis for CAG repeats is included in these methods (Method 3.1), which can be adapted for other types of repeats. A more detailed description of PCR analysis of CAG repeat instability frequencies is available in a previous issue [3]. There are also genetic assay systems that can be used to select for repeat expansion or contraction events [3–5]. Such selection systems differ from the PCR-based instability assay as they capture only the events that yield a phenotype in the selective system, thus they allow for the study of rare repeat length changes. However they are not appropriate for the purpose of identifying starting colonies for a fragility assay.

To determine the rate at which breakage occurs within a repeat tract, two unique yeast systems have been developed. The first is a yeast artificial chromosome (YAC) system wherein the YAC VS5 is modified such that the potential fragile sequence is integrated between a telomere seed sequence $(G_4T_4)_{13}$ and a *URA3* marker gene [6, 7] (Fig. 1) (Method 3.2). The version of this YAC with an

Fig. 1 (continued) logarithmically growing cultures. (**d**) Wild-type fragility data of *S. cerevisiae* strain BY4705 where the fragile sequence integrated between the G_4T_4 and *URA3* marker are different tract lengths of CAG repeats. Assays done with this (CAG)n-*URA3* YAC show that 5-FOA resistance increases with increasing number of CAG repeats. (Data sourced from [8–12])

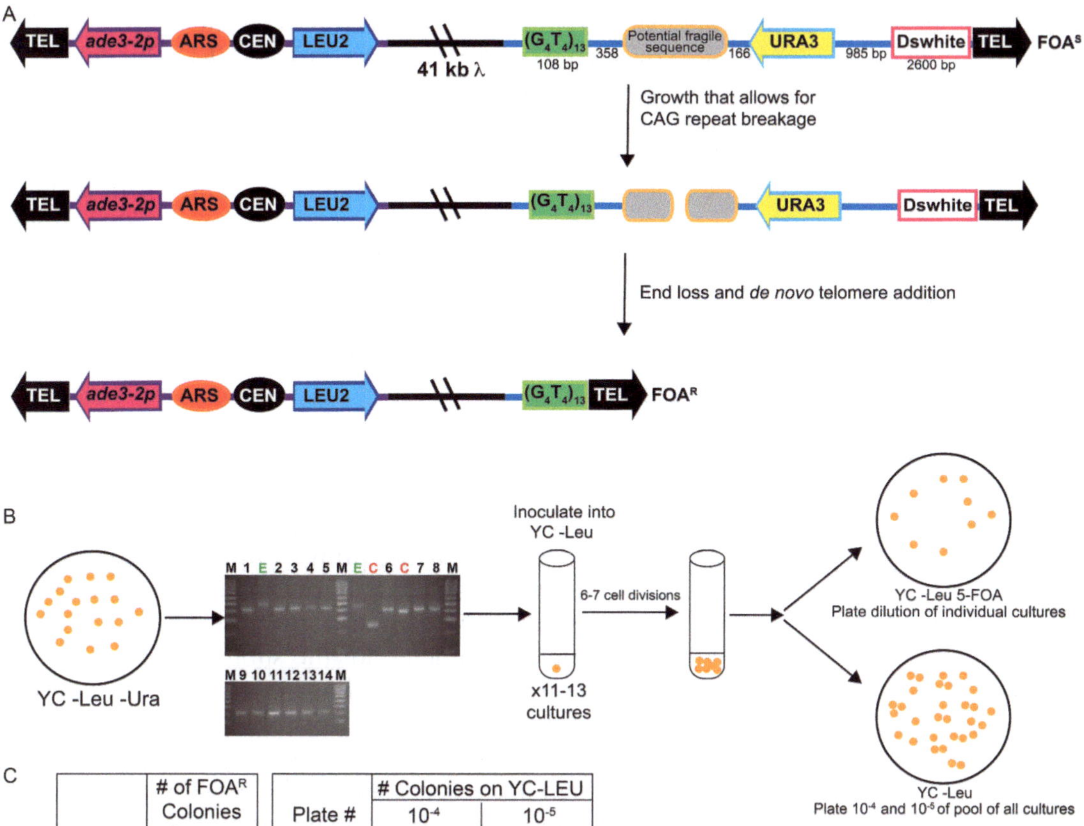

C

Plate #	# of FOA^R Colonies *(in 100ul)
1	**184**
2	**246**
3	**250**
4	**338**
5	**302**
6	**318**
7	**190**
8	**274**
9	**284**
10	**274**

Plate #	# Colonies on YC-LEU 10^{-4}	10^{-5}
1	**240**	**25**
2	**215**	**20**
Average	**227.5**	**22.5**
Total cell count *(in 100ul)	**2,275,000**	**2,250,000**

Method	**Rate**
Median	**23.1 x 10^{-6}**
Maximum Likelihood	**25.3 x 10^{-6}**

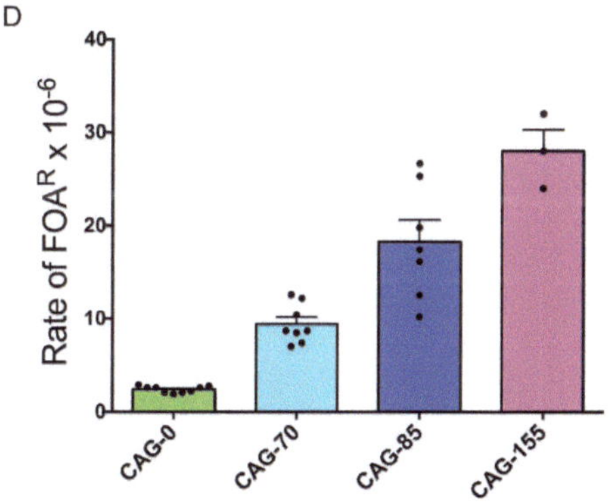

Fig. 1 Schematic of the YAC breakage assay. (**a**) In this system, a potential fragile sequence (such as an expanded CAG repeat tract) is integrated onto a yeast artificial chromosome between a telomere seed sequence $(G_4T_4)_{13}$ and the *URA3* gene. Breaks that occur within the fragile sequence are subject to resection and telomere addition, which results in loss of the *URA3* gene and renders cells 5-FOA^R. The YAC additionally contains a *LEU2* marker gene, which allows for maintenance of the YAC, a centromere (CEN4) and an origin of replication (ARS1). The blue line indicates the pYIP5 plasmid backbone, the black line indicates lambda DNA, and the purple line corresponds to pUC18 plasmid backbone. (**b**) In the YAC end loss assay, strains are plated for single colonies on YC –Leu –Ura plates and 10 individual colonies of the correct tract length (should be verified if testing an unstable repeat sequence) are grown in YC –Leu for 6–7 cell divisions. A portion of each individual culture is plated onto YC –Leu +5-FOA plates, and a portion of the culture is pooled and serially diluted to obtain single colonies on YC –Leu, which serves as the total viable cell count. (**c**) Example of the calculation of fragility rate for a 10-colony YAC CF1 CAG-85 fragility assay. Colony counts are used to determine the number of mutants and the number of viable cells in 100 μL of

integrated CAG repeat tract has been termed the (CAG)n-*URA3* YAC, also referred to in the literature as YAC CF1. One feature of this YAC system is that other modifications are easily made by replacing the right end of the YAC with the desired sequence (Method 3.3). We have used this technique to add additional genetic markers, promoters, and terminators (Fig. 2). In addition the type of potential fragile element can be changed. For example, other derivatives of this YAC have been made that contain the CAG repeat in the opposite orientation (CTG)n [8], AT repeats that are present in the FRA16D common fragile site [15] (Fig. 2), the expanded ATTCT repeat present in SCA10 [16], and inverted repeats [17].

1.1 The YAC Assay

An important feature of the YAC is that it contains little homology to any of the natural yeast chromosomes. This feature, together with the telomere seed sequence placed proximal to the potential fragile sequence, ensures that the primary mode of healing is by telomere addition rather than recombination. Healing via telomere addition is ideal as relatively few genes affect the efficiency of telomere addition. Known examples are the subunits of the enzyme telomerase, which are needed for telomere addition, and the Pif1 helicase, which inhibits promiscuous telomere addition [6]. Thus, in most cases an increase in YAC end loss is caused by increased breakage rather than decreased healing. The position of the potential fragile sequence on the YAC is such that on the proximal side of the sequence there is a 108 bp $(G_4T_4)_{13}$ telomeric seed sequence from *Oxytrica,* which serves as an efficient substrate for *S. cerevisiae* telomerase, but does not recombine with the natural yeast telomere sequence [18]. Therefore, if breakage within the fragile sequence occurs, resection and degradation of the broken end exposes the G_4T_4 sequence as a template for telomerase (Fig. 1). The G_4T_4 seed provides an efficient pathway for healing of breakage events, which is different from another commonly used assay for end loss of chromosome V [19], where healing can occur by a variety of mechanisms including telomere addition onto short naturally occurring GT sequences or recombination with other chromosomes.

In the YAC fragility assay, breakage that results in loss of the right arm of the YAC renders cells *ura3-* and resistant to 5-fluoroorotic acid (5-FOA). The number of cells that are 5-FOA resistant serves as a measure of the rate of breakage, and the effect of a potential fragile sequence can be compared to a control sequence of the same length and base composition, or a YAC that does not contain the fragile sequence. One additional design consideration of the YAC is the distance between the *URA3* gene and the telomere, such that the placement of the *URA3* gene promoter is far enough away from the telomere not to be subject to telomere position effect; this is the reason for the presence of filler sequence

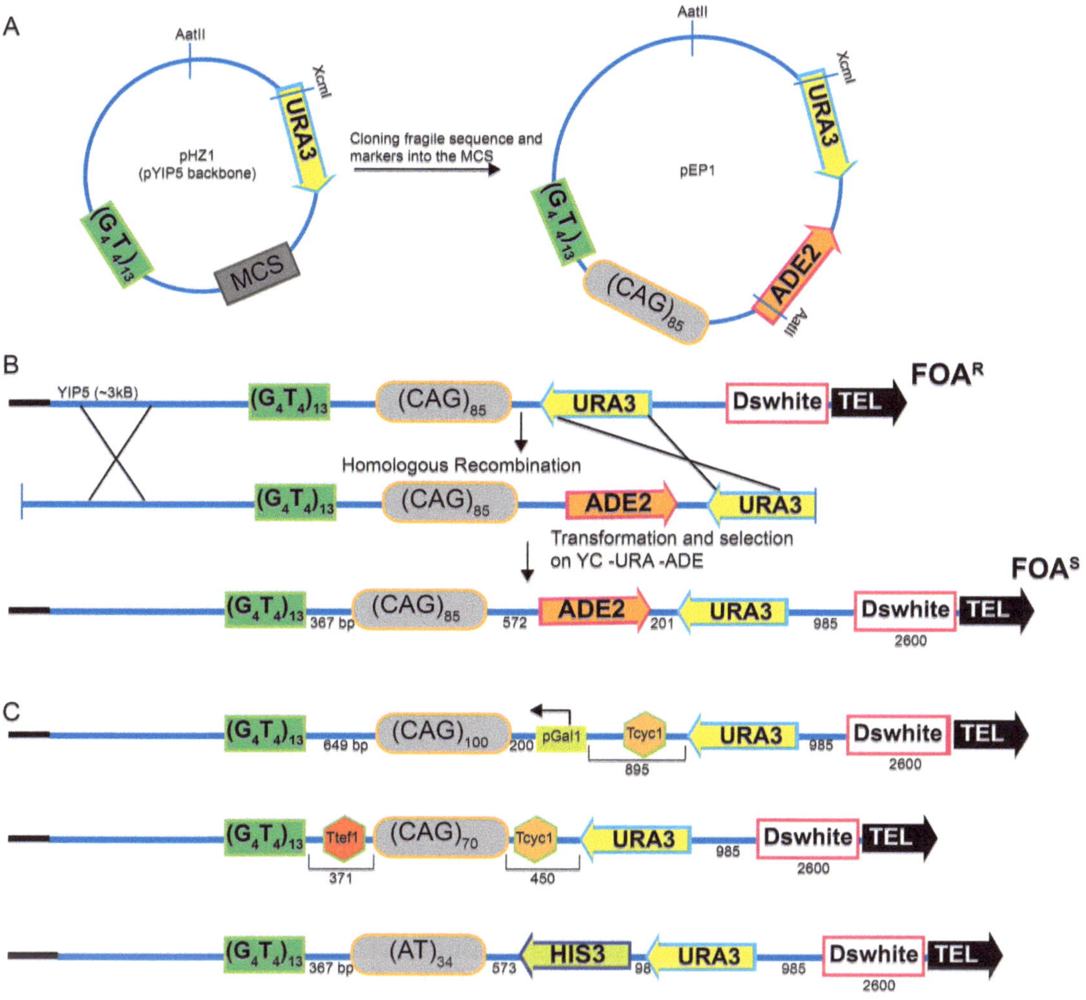

Fig. 2 Schematic of YAC modification. (**a**) Schematic of pHZ1 wherein a telomere seed sequence $(G_4T_4)_{13}$ has been inserted into the pYIP5 plasmid backbone such that G_4T_4 and the *URA3* gene are on either side of the multiple cloning site (MCS). The AatII site has been previously used to linearize the plasmid for transformation into YAC containing strains. If AatII is not a unique restriction site after cloning (as shown for pEP1), XcmI can also be used. (**b**) Schematic detailing integration of a triplet repeat and a second selectable marker into the YAC construct. Transformation of the linear fragment and homologous recombination should result in a novel YAC that incorporates the *ADE2* selectable marker as well as the repeat. Correct transformants can be selected for on YC −Leu −Ura −Ade plates. The resultant YAC contains the *ADE2* marker gene such that transcription of *ADE2* is away from the CAG repeat. Colonies that lose the ADE2 gene will be red on media that contains a limiting amount of adenine [13]. Adding a second selectable marker provides an easy selection for end loss, however other schemes are also possible. Selecting for *URA3* revertants from a YAC that contains a *ura3* mutation is one way to insert markerless modifications to the YAC; CRISPR-Cas9-based integration strategies could also be used. (**c**). Examples of published CF1 YAC derivatives. In the top construct, to determine the role of transcription on CAG repeat fragility, an inducible *GAL1* promoter was added adjacent to the repeat tract [13]. In the middle construct, to determine the role of readthrough transcription from *URA3* on CAG repeat fragility, two terminator sequences were added such that the Tcyc1 terminator sequence was added between the *URA3* marker gene and the CAG repeat and the *TEF1* terminator sequence was added between the G_4T_4 and repeat tract [13, 14]. In the bottom construct, an AT_{34} repeat tract from the common fragile site *FRA16D* was integrated with the addition of the *HIS3* gene (the *Schizosaccharomyces pombe HIS5* gene) [15]

(the *Drosophila* white gene) next to the telomere (Fig. 1). Elsewhere on the YAC, on the left arm there is a *LEU2* marker gene, which allows for maintenance of the YAC, a yeast origin of replication (ARS1), and a centromere (CEN4). Finally, an *ade3-2p* allele can be used to screen for cells that have obtained two YACs by colony color (which occurs occasionally by nondisjunction) in strains with an *ade3* background, but it is not necessary to use this feature for most applications.

For the original (CAG)n-*URA3* YAC, the CAG repeat tract is integrated such that the CAG repeat is on the lagging strand template, which has been shown to be the orientation less prone to repeat tract contractions [20]. For the CAG repeat, it has been established that there is a length dependent increase in breakage as measured by 5-FOA resistance [7] (Fig. 1d). This YAC system can also be used to study CAG repeat stability using similar conditions used for measuring breakage [3]. These instability assays revealed a length dependent increase in contractions and expansions, though contractions occur with greater frequency than expansions in a replicating yeast population [7]. The CAG instability frequency measured on this YAC is similar to that measured at the chromosome II *LYS2* locus for the same orientation with respect to replication [20, 21], though it is known that factors such as distance from an origin, transcription level, and chromatin structure can alter instability frequencies (*see* [1] for review). A useful feature of both fragility assays described herein is that both fragility and instability can be monitored under the same conditions (genomic location, strain background, transcriptional status, etc.).

1.2 The Direct Duplication Recombination Assay

The second system for measuring repeat fragility is a direct duplication recombination assay (DDRA) (Method 3.4). In the original version of this assay, a potential fragile sequence was integrated adjacent to a *URA3* reporter and between a full length *LYS2* gene and a duplication of the 3′ end of *LYS2* on chromosome II [22, 23] (Fig. 3a). If breaks occur within the integrated sequence, resection occurs and repair results from single strand annealing of the duplicated regions of the *LYS2* gene. This results in the loss of the *URA3* gene and resistance to the drug 5-FOA. In this system, it was noted that there is a length dependent increase in 5-FOA

Fig. 3 (continued) subject to resection and recombination, which renders cells Lys + and 5-FOA^R. (**b**) In the *ADE2* DDRA, a potential fragile sequence and the *URA3* gene are integrated between 5′ and 3′ portions of the *ADE2* gene, rendering cells Ade- and 5-FOA^S. Breaks that occur within the repeat are subject to resection and repair via single strand annealing between the 968 bp duplicated region of *ADE2*, thus rendering cells Ade + and 5-FOA^R. (**c**) Schematic of DDRA protocol. Cells are initially plated on YC –Ura media and then plated for single colonies on YEPD (or other nonselective media) to allow loss of *URA3*. Ten individual colonies are selected and each resuspended in water. A portion of each colony suspension is then plated onto ten separate 5-FOA plates (–Lys or –Ade, depending on the assay) and 100 μL of each colony suspension is pooled, diluted and plated for single colonies onto YC plates for a total cell count

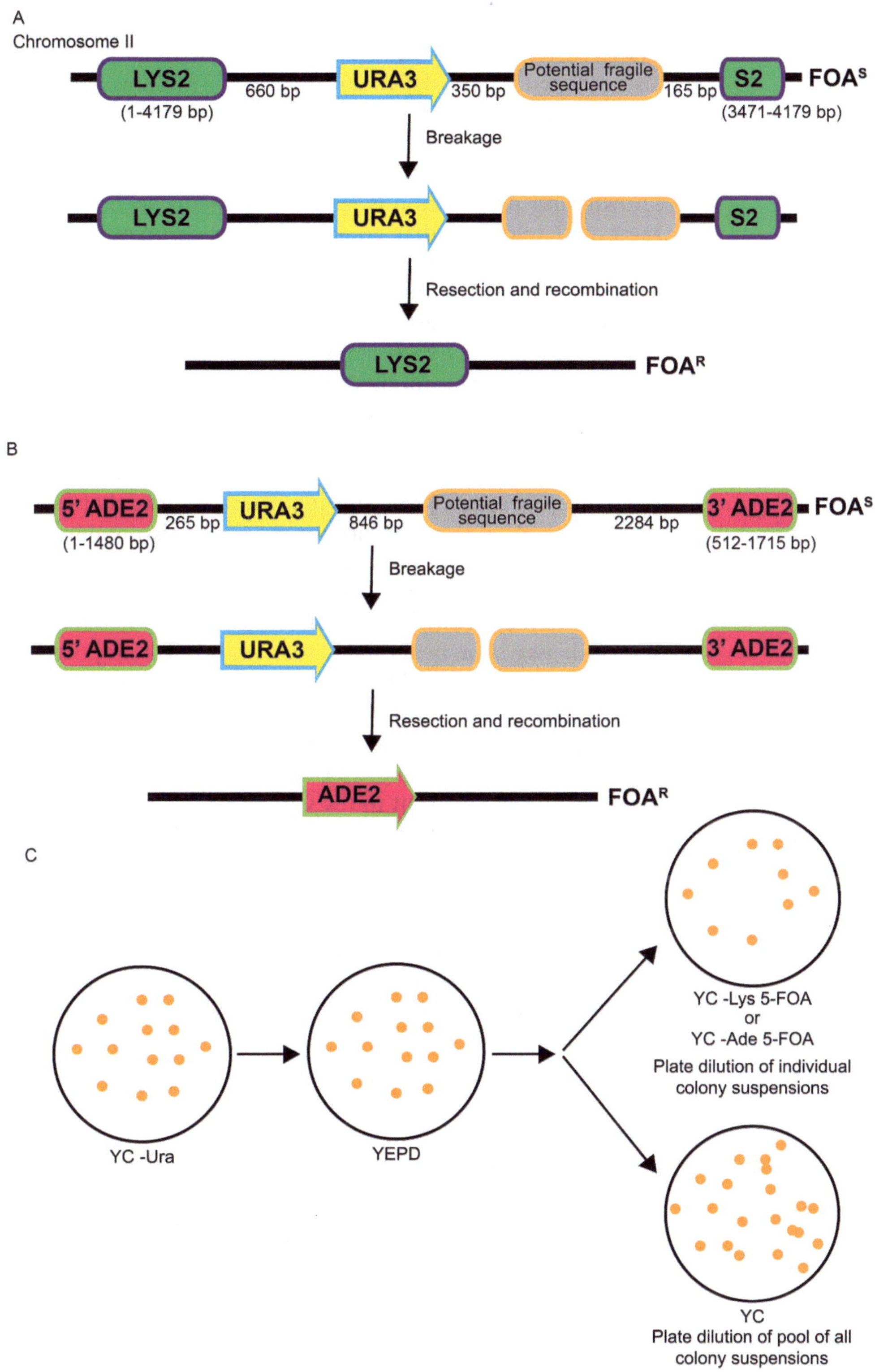

Fig. 3 Schematic of the direct duplication recombination assay (DDRA). (**a**) In this chromosomal system, a potential fragile sequence and the *URA3* gene are integrated between a direct duplication of 708 bp of the 3′ end of the *LYS2* gene; these cells are Lys + and 5-FOA^S. Breaks that occur within the fragile sequence are

resistance which was due to breaks within or very close to an integrated CAG repeat tract [22], and expanded CGG/CCG repeats also induced length-dependent fragility [23]. This system is ideal for understanding the role that recombination plays in the repair of breaks that occur within a repeat tract. Also, as it is located in the middle of a natural yeast chromosome, the replication program is known, and the location is far from elements such as the centromere and telomere that could influence chromatin structure or nuclear positioning. A modification of the DDRA utilizes the same principle, but with a duplication of the *ADE2* gene, designed such that the starting strain is Ade- and recombination products will become Ade + 5-FOA^R (Brian A. Lenzmeier and Virginia A. Zakian; [24]) (Fig. 3b). This modification allows for selection of recombinants, eliminating other events that can generate 5-FOA^R, and the cassette can be integrated anywhere in the genome. It has been used to study increased recombination rates induced by G4 motifs [24] and AT repeats [25]. It is important to note that many genes that are involved in replication or repair are also required for efficient recombination, which makes it more difficult to determine whether a gene is required to prevent fragility or facilitate healing in this system, as compared to the YAC end loss system.

Both assays can be modified to contain different potential fragile sequences or to modify other parameters, such as transcription level. For the YAC assay, we have made modifications to reduce transcription by flanking the CAG tract with transcriptional terminators [14] or increasing transcription by adding the inducible *GAL1* promoter adjacent to the CAG tract [13] (Fig. 2c). We have also added a second marker distal to the CAG tract, either *ADE2* or *HIS3*, which allows end loss events to be verified by loss of the second marker, rather than PCR (Fig. 2). For example, addition of the *ADE2* marker allows identification of YAC end loss events (in an *ade2* strain background) by observation of red color development of 5-FOA^R colonies [13]. Note that in the original (CAG) n-*URA3* YAC, the lack of an efficient transcription terminator in the adjacent *URA3* gene leads to read-through transcription through the CAG tract, and this is significantly reduced by introduction of either a transcription terminator or the *ADE2* gene between *URA3* and the CAG tract, which can effect repeat fragility and instability levels in some backgrounds [13, 14].

Taken together, both assays, the YAC end loss system and the chromosomal direct duplication recombination assay, have provided novel insight into the mechanisms of fragility and instability of repetitive DNA sequences and can be utilized to understand the breakage and repair of any sequence of interest.

2 Materials

2.1 Colony PCR to Determine CAG Repeat Tract Length

1. Taq polymerase.
2. 10× Taq polymerase buffer.
3. 20 mM magnesium sulfate ($MgSO_4$).
4. 5× CG buffer (*see* **Note 1**).
5. 10 mM dNTPs.
6. Primers that span the CAG repeat (*see* Table 1, **Note 2**).
7. P20 or P200 micropipette tips.
8. 2% Metaphor agarose or other high-resolution gel system.
9. Electrophoretic gel box, running buffer (1× TBE or TAE), and power supply.
10. 10 mg/mL ethidium bromide or other DNA detection chemical.
11. Microtubes.

Table 1
Primers that are used for PCR amplification the CAG repeat tract

Direction	Primer name	Sequence	Distance to repeat tract
Forward	CTGrev2	5′ CCC AGG CCT CCA GTT TGC 3′	74 bp
	NewCAGFor	5′ CCT CAG CCT GGC CGA AAG AAA GAA A 3′	42 bp
Reverse	T720	5′ TAA TAC GAC TCA CTA TAG GG 3′	80 bp
	T720b	5′ GAA TTC GAG CTC CAC CGC GG 3′	60 bp
	NewCAGrev	5′ CAG TCA CGA CGT TGT AAA ACG ACG G 3′	117 bp

These primers work for the CAG tract cloned into the YAC and DDRA constructs described herein. The forward primers anneal to sequence from the human DM1 sequence that flanks the CAG tract. The reverse primers anneal to sequence in or near the MCS that the repeat was cloned into. Primers can be used in a variety of combinations depending on the construct and repeat length

2.2 Determination of Chromosome Fragility by a YAC End Loss Assay

1. Starting colonies that have been checked for repeat tract length by colony PCR (*see* Subheading 3.1 for CAG repeats).
2. Spectrophotometer and cuvettes for measuring optical density (OD).
3. 5 mL glass test tubes with caps.
4. P20 or P200 micropipette tips.
5. Roller drum or shaker at 30 °C.
6. YC –Leu liquid medium; *see* ref. 26 for yeast media recipes; YC stands for yeast complete media, missing amino acids noted as "–".
7. YC –Leu –Ura plates.
8. YC –Leu plates.
9. YC –Leu +5-FOA plates (standard 5-FOA concentration is 1.0 g/L).
10. Sterile glass beads or sterile spreaders.

2.3 Modification of the YAC

1. YIP5-based plasmid with desired components added (potential fragile sequence, markers, promoters, terminators, etc.).
2. Luria broth (LB) + 50 μg/mL ampicillin liquid media.
3. LB + 50 μg/mL ampicillin plates.
4. Restriction enzyme: AatII or XcmI.
5. Water bath at 37 °C.
6. Transformation reagents:
   (a) 1 M lithium acetate pH 7.5.
   (b) 100 mM Tris–HCl, pH 7.5.
   (c) 50% polyethylene glycol (PEG) 3350; (*see* [27] for solution recipes).
   (d) High molecular weight single-stranded DNA (e.g., deoxyribonucleic acid sodium salt type III from salmon testes), denatured at 100 °C and cooled on ice.
   (e) Water bath at 42 °C.
7. YC–Ura–Leu yeast medium (other amino acids dropped out according to the desired marker selection; *see* ref. 26 for recipes).
8. Toothpicks or sterile loops.

2.4 Direct Duplication Recombination Assay (DDRA)

1. YC –Ura plates (*see* ref. [26] for yeast media recipes).
2. YEPD plates (rich media containing yeast extract, peptone, and dextrose).
3. YC –Lys +5-FOA plates (*LYS2* assay) or YC –Ade 5-FOA plates (*ADE2* assay).
4. YC plates.

3 Methods

3.1 Colony PCR to Determine CAG Repeat Tract Length

1. Plate or streak for single colonies on YC–Ura, which will select against breakage events, from a master patch (it may be appropriate to drop out additional amino acids according to the fragility assay markers) (*see* **Note 3**).
2. Select individual colonies and clearly mark which PCR reactions will correspond to which colony.
3. Combine a bulk PCR reaction mix on ice and aliquot 12.5 μL per PCR tube. The volume can be adjusted if desired. The 1× PCR reaction is:

Sterile diH_2O	5.8 μL
10× buffer (w/o $MgCl_2$):	1.25 μL
20 mM $MgSO_4$:	1.25 μL
6.25 pmol primer 1:	0.625 μL (of 10 pmol/μL stock)
6.25 pmol primer 2:	0.625 μL (of 10 pmol/μL stock)
10 mM dNTPs:	0.25 μL
Mix thoroughly, then add,	
Taq polymerase:	0.2 μL
5× CG-rich buffer:	2.5 μL (*see* **Note 4**)
Total reaction mix is	12.5 μL

Using a pipette tip, add a small amount of yeast cells from the center of the colony into the PCR reaction mix. When mixing the cells with reaction mix, either place a gloved finger on the wider end of pipette tip or use a pipetteman and push the plunger completely to ensure all liquid entering the tip by surface tension is expelled (*see* **Note 5**).

4. PCR cycle profile

95 °C	4′	
95 °C	30″	
	←	35×
54 °C	1′	
68 °C	3′	
68 °C	7′	
4 °C	Hold	

5. Once the PCR protocol is complete, add an appropriate amount of loading dye to the 12.5 μL reaction and run out the entire PCR reaction on a 2% Metaphor gel or other gel sizing system (*see* **Notes 6** and 7). Load markers on both ends of the gel; a third marker in a middle lane is helpful for gel systems that do not run evenly across the gel box (*see* **Notes 8** and **9**). Run the gel in 1× TAE at 70 V for 90 min.
6. Post-stain with ethidium bromide or other DNA detection dye for 30 min. Transfer gel tray to diH_2O and photograph the gel using a UV transilluminator (*see* **Note 10**).

3.2 Determination of Chromosomal Fragility by a YAC End Loss Assay

1. Plate for single colonies on YC –Leu –Ura, which will select against breakage events, from a master patch.
2. If the potential fragile sequence is an unstable repeat able to be sized via PCR, do colony PCR on 10–20 colonies to check for the appropriate repeat tract length (*see* Method 1; **Note 9**).
3. Inoculate colonies of correct tract length for the fluctuation assay. Colonies should be as fresh as possible; ideally less than 2 weeks old. Select starting colonies that have the appropriate size of repeat tract length with no visible contractions or expansions. Two methods of inoculation may be used, but whenever possible use preferentially method 1.
   (a) Inoculation method 1: 10 colony protocol (preferred):
   (b) For this methodology there will be 10 unique colonies that are inoculated into 10 separate cultures.
      - Pipet 1 mL of YC –Leu into each of ten 5 mL test tubes.
      - Inoculate 1 to 3 tubes with a small number of cells and take the OD_{600} (using the entire 1 mL culture; these are referred to as the "OD_{600} cultures"). The starting OD_{600} should be ~0.02–0.06. Once the OD_{600} has been taken, return the 1 mL culture to the initial test tube. Always work under sterile conditions (*see* **Note 11**).
      - Inoculate the remaining tubes with approximately the same amount of cells by eye, so that they will also have a starting OD_{600} of ~0.02–0.06 (*see* **Note 12**).
   (c) Inoculation method 2: 1 colony protocol (*see* **Note 13**):
   (d) For this methodology there will be 1 colony that is divided into 10 cultures.
      - Suspend one entire colony with the correct tract length in 1.3 mL of YC-Leu media.
      - Take 100 μL of the resuspended mix and inoculate into 0.9 mL of YC-Leu media in a 5 mL test tube. Repeat for each of the 10 cultures.

- Take 1 mL of one of the cultures out of the test tube and measure the OD_{600}. The OD_{600} should be between ~0.02 and 0.06. Return the 1 mL culture to the initial test tube.

4. Allow the cultures to grow with constant agitation or in a spinning roller drum for 6–7 doublings at 30 °C. This step allows the breakage and healing to occur (*see* **Notes 12**, **14**, and **15**).
5. In order to determine the number of doublings, take 100 μL of the OD_{600} culture(s) and resuspend into 900 μL of YC –Leu media and measure the final OD. Multiply this reading by 10. If the ideal starting OD_{600} was ~0.02, the appropriate final OD_{600} range is 1.25–2.5 (*see* **Notes 11** and **12**).
6. Spread 100 μL from each of the 10 tubes onto 10 YC –Leu 5-FOA plates using a consistent number of sterile glass beads or a sterile glass spreader. The amount plated can be adjusted up or down for strains with a higher or lower rate of 5-FOA^R; just remember to adjust the number of colonies counted to the number of mutants per 100 μL in the rate calculations (*see* **Notes 16** and **17**).
7. To determine the viable total cell count, combine 100 μL from each of the 10 undiluted cell cultures and mix together. Serially dilute the mixed cultures in sterile water (usually to 10^{-4} and 10^{-5}) and plate 100 μL on of each dilution onto YC –Leu plates. Total cell count plates should be plated in duplicate.
8. Incubate the plates at 30 °C for 4 days.
9. Count colonies on the YC –Leu 5-FOA plates.
10. Order the plate counts from low to high to determine the median number of colonies for each set (i.e., each 10 plate assay). If necessary, adjust the number to obtain the median number of mutants in 100 μL. Average the number of colonies on the 2 "total cell count" plates to determine the number of viable cells in 100 μL. Determine the rate of 5-FOA^R by using a fluctuation rate calculator such as FALCOR (http://www.keshavsingh.org/protocols/FALCOR.html) [28] or FluCalc ([29]; http://flucalc.ase.tufts.edu/) using either the Maximum Likelihood Method (preferred, if the spread is not too great; this method uses the number of mutants obtained on all selective plates) or the Method of the Median (using the median number of mutants in 100 μL, as described above). *See* [30] for an excellent discussion of calculating fluctuation rates (*see* **Notes 18–22**).
11. The assay should be repeated at least three times per strain, and standard error and confidence intervals calculated.

3.3 Modification of the YAC

1. Using pHZ1, a YIP5 derivative which contains the *URA3* gene and the $(G_4T_4)_{13}$ telomeric seed sequence, clone in genetic elements and fragile sequences as desired. The MCS is between the G_4T_4 and *URA3* marker gene. If a new fragile element is being added, it should be added between the G_4T_4 and *URA3* marker gene (Fig. 2a).
2. Once all new genetic elements have been added and confirmed, linearize the plasmid such that the *URA3* marker and G_4T_4 are on either end of the linear fragment. Previously we have used AatII or XcmI to linearize the modified pHZ1 plasmid.
3. Using a standard *S. cerevisiae* transformation protocol [31], transform the fragment into cells that contain the YAC.
4. Selection for proper transformants will depend on the nature of the DNA elements that are being inserted. If nonselectable elements are being added (such as a promoter or terminator sequence), transformation will need to occur in a strain that contains a *URA3* point mutation so that transformation selection can occur on YC –Ura. CRISPR-Cas9 gene editing strategies can also be employed to make markerless modifications to the YAC.
5. Confirmation of integration into the YAC can be done via PCR between a new element added (e.g., *ADE2* in the example) and an element not included in the integrating fragment, such as the Drosophila white gene. YAC structure can also be confirmed via Southern blot using a lambda probe to the YAC and digest with BstEII [7], or digests and probes specific to the modified area.

3.4 Direct Duplication Recombination Assay: A Recombination Based Method to Assess Chromosome Breakage

1. Patch strain to test onto a YC –Ura plate and allow to grow for 2 days at 30 °C.
2. Plate for single colonies on YEPD at 30 °C for 3 days such that there are 50 ± 10 colonies per plate (this step allows recombination events to occur).
3. Randomly select 10 colonies and resuspend half of each colony in 300 μL diH_2O (*see* **Note 23**).
4. Plate a portion of the suspension on a 5-FOA plate with the goal being to get ~100 colonies per plate to count after 4–5 days of growth at 30 °C. For the *LYS2* assay (Fig. 3a), this should be a YC –Lys +5-FOA plate (Lysine dropout optional); For the *ADE2* assay, (Fig. 3b), this should be a YC –Ade +5-FOA plate (*see* **Notes 24** and **25**).
5. To determine the viable cell count combine 100 μL of each of the 10 colony suspensions. Plate 100 μL of a 10^{-4} dilution onto 2 YC plates. Plate a dilution that will yield ~30–300 colo-

nies single colonies per YC plate. Total cell count plates should be plated in duplicate (*see* **Note 26**).

6. Count the number of colonies on the 5-FOA plates. To obtain the number of mutants and the total number of cells per 100 μL, multiply the number of colonies growing on 5-FOA and the average of the 2 total cell count plates by the dilution factors used. To determine the rate of recombination, use the method of maximum likelihood or the method of the median and a fluctuation analysis calculator (e.g., FALCOR [28] or FluCalc [29]; *see* Subheading 3.2).
7. The assay should be repeated at least three times per strain, and standard error and confidence intervals calculated.

4 Notes

1. A 5× GC rich buffer may aid in amplification across the repetitive tract. One 5× GC rich buffer that has been used in amplification of the CAG repeat tract is Phusion GC Buffer (New England Biolabs, B0519S).
2. In order to obtain robust tract lengths PCR, primers should be designed such that there is a region of nonrepetitive flanking sequence included on both sides of the repeat. Generally, we recommend between 40 and 80 bp of nonrepetitive sequence be included on each side of the repeat. For examples of primers that span the CAG repeat for both the (CAG)n-*URA3* YAC and the (CAG)n *LYS2* DDRA constructs *see* Table 1.
3. This protocol is written for a CAG tract on the CF1 YAC, but can be adapted to other locations or repeats.
4. Taq polymerase & CG buffer should be added last to the master mix after everything else and mixed gently.
5. The amount of cells added to the PCR reaction should be no larger than the tip of the p200 or p20 pipette tip. Too few cells will result in a very faint PCR product, too many will result in a background smear in the lane.
6. The 2% Metaphor agarose gels should be made according to the manufacturer's instructions.
7. Instead of using 2% Metaphor gels for separation of fragments, PCR reactions can be run on a denaturing PAGE gel or other high resolution gel system for size analysis, with appropriate DNA detection. Alternatively an appropriate concentration of DNA-grade agarose may be used.
8. The ideal molecular weight marker used should have bands that change in size every 100 bp or less. Adding an additional marker in the middle of the gel helps with sizing the CAG repeat.

9. If the PCR is of poor quality, then expansions may have not amplified well and could be underestimated, therefore only use good quality PCR reactions to decide on starting colonies. A 2% Metaphor gel can resolve fragments that differ by 2%, that is, 8 bp for a fragment size of 400 bp or about 3 (CAG) repeats added or subtracted for a (CAG)85 repeat tract.
10. Ethidium bromide can be added directly to Metaphor gel if preferred. The ideal concentration is 0.5 μg/mL (e.g., 15 μL 10 mg/mL stock in 300 mL 1× TAE).
11. There is a risk of contamination during the process of taking the OD_{600}. If this is an issue, extra "OD_{600} cultures" can be started that are only used for taking the OD_{600} throughout the experiment and discarded before plating.
12. The method is designed to test for fragility occurring during log phase growth. Ensuring cells grow through several divisions in logarithmic phase is important as this growth step allows the breakage and healing to occur. The OD_{600} range could be altered according to the purpose of the experiment.
13. The 1 colony method is less preferred, but can be used when finding 10 starting colonies of the same repeat tract length is technically difficult.
14. For mutant strains that affect growth, discard any cultures that do not grow or grow especially poorly, and do not include them in the mix for the total cell count. For such strains, more than 10 cultures can be started to allow for this.
15. For wild type, 6–7 divisions will take approximately ~16–18 h. For strains with poor division potential, the total number of divisions can be altered to fewer divisions (e.g., 3–5 divisions). Wild-type strains done as a comparison should be grown for the same number of divisions as mutant strains.
16. The amount of cells plated on 5-FOA can be adjusted for strains or YACs with higher or lower rates of breakage. For example, less than 100 μL may need to be plated for mutants showing increased end loss of the (CAG)n-*URA3* YAC, and 1 mL should be plated for the (CAG)n-*ADE2*-*URA3* YAC.
17. It is best to adjust the amount of cells plated on 5-FOA such that the median number of colonies is between 50 and 250.
18. Make sure you enter the number of mutants and total cells for the *same volume*—usually per 100 μL (per 1 mL can be used for very low rates).
19. For experiments with zeros or a large spread between low and high numbers of mutants (happens with lower rate assays), use the Method of the Median to calculate the rate.
20. Certain mutants could alter *URA3* gene function or 5-FOA^R by increasing the mutation rate of *URA3*, altering *URA3*

expression, or affecting the toxicity of 5-FOA, resulting in increased 5-FOA^R that is not due to chromosome breakage. To confirm that there is loss of the right arm of the YAC, PCR amplify the *URA3* gene (or a portion of it) from 1 colony off of each YC –Leu +5-FOA plate (10 colonies total) to confirm there is loss of the right arm of the YAC. This should be done for 3 assays (a total of 30 independent colonies checked). The expected end loss frequency for wild type is 90–100%. Make sure to also PCR amplify from your starting strain as a positive control.

21. Verify the structure of the YAC in 20 independent 5-FOA^R colonies (plated from independent cultures) by Southern blot, using a lambda probe to the YAC and digest with BstEII digest (*see* [7]).
22. The fragility assay can be combined with an instability assay by analyzing the repeat tract length of the daughter colonies plated for the total cell count [3]. Even though these plates do not select for the presence of the repeat (e.g., the YC –Leu plates for the YAC assay), usually the rate of breakage is low enough that most colonies tested will have retained a repeat tract. One disadvantage to this method is that the starting parent colony and the daughter colonies are no longer correlated, reducing the ability to detect jackpot events.
23. Establish a standard size of colony to use to allow equal generations of growth between colonies and strains.
24. Generally, for rates in the 10^{-5} range, approximately 1/ninth of a colony is plated, though a pilot experiment can determine the best amount to plate. Keep in mind that the more fragile the sequence, the less should be plated.
25. For plating onto 5-FOA, use about a 10^{-2} dilution of cells for strains with low recombination rates, a 10^{-3} dilution of cells for strains with high recombination rates.
26. The dilution plated for the viable cell count may depend on the size of the colonies that were picked for the assay. For initial assays it's best to plate a series of dilutions, such as 10^{-3}, 10^{-4}, and 10^{-5}.

Acknowledgments

Work in our laboratory is currently supported by grants from the National Institute of Health (GM105473, GM122880) and National Science Foundation (MCB 1817499). We would like to thank past and present members of the C. H. Freudenreich and V.A. Zakian labs for their contributions to the development of these assays.

References

1. Usdin K, House NC, Freudenreich CH (2015) Repeat instability during DNA repair: insights from model systems. Crit Rev Biochem Mol Biol 50(2):142–167. https://doi.org/10.3109/10409238.2014.999192
2. McMurray CT (2010) Mechanisms of trinucleotide repeat instability during human development. Nat Rev Genet 11(11):786–799. https://doi.org/10.1038/nrg2828
3. Polleys EJ, Freudenreich CH (2018) Methods to study repeat fragility and instability in *Saccharomyces cerevisiae*. Methods Mol Biol 1672:403–419. https://doi.org/10.1007/978-1-4939-7306-4_28
4. Shishkin AA, Voineagu I, Matera R, Cherng N, Chernet BT, Krasilnikova MM, Narayanan V, Lobachev KS, Mirkin SM (2009) Large-scale expansions of Friedreich's ataxia GAA repeats in yeast. Mol Cell 35(1):82–92. https://doi.org/10.1016/j.molcel.2009.06.017
5. Dixon MJ, Bhattacharyya S, Lahue RS (2004) Genetic assays for triplet repeat instability in yeast. Methods Mol Biol 277:29–45. https://doi.org/10.1385/1-59259-804-8:029
6. Schulz VP, Zakian VA (1994) The saccharomyces PIF1 DNA helicase inhibits telomere elongation and de novo telomere formation. Cell 76(1):145–155
7. Callahan JL, Andrews KJ, Zakian VA, Freudenreich CH (2003) Mutations in yeast replication proteins that increase CAG/CTG expansions also increase repeat fragility. Mol Cell Biol 23(21):7849–7860
8. Kerrest A, Anand RP, Sundararajan R, Bermejo R, Liberi G, Dujon B, Freudenreich CH, Richard GF (2009) SRS2 and SGS1 prevent chromosomal breaks and stabilize triplet repeats by restraining recombination. Nat Struct Mol Biol 16(2):159–167. https://doi.org/10.1038/nsmb.1544
9. Sundararajan R, Gellon L, Zunder RM, Freudenreich CH (2010) Double-strand break repair pathways protect against CAG/CTG repeat expansions, contractions and repeat-mediated chromosomal fragility in Saccharomyces cerevisiae. Genetics 184(1):65–77. https://doi.org/10.1534/genetics.109.111039
10. House NC, Yang JH, Walsh SC, Moy JM, Freudenreich CH (2014) NuA4 initiates dynamic histone H4 acetylation to promote high-Fidelity sister chromatid recombination at postreplication gaps. Mol Cell 55(6):818–828. https://doi.org/10.1016/j.molcel.2014.07.007
11. Nguyen JH, Viterbo D, Anand RP, Verra L, Sloan L, Richard GF, Freudenreich CH (2017) Differential requirement of Srs2 helicase and Rad51 displacement activities in replication of hairpin-forming CAG/CTG repeats. Nucleic Acids Res 45(8):4519–4531. https://doi.org/10.1093/nar/gkx088
12. Yang JH, Freudenreich CH (2010) The Rtt109 histone acetyltransferase facilitates error-free replication to prevent CAG/CTG repeat contractions. DNA Repair 9(4):414–420. https://doi.org/10.1016/j.dnarep.2009.12.022
13. Koch MR, House NCM, Cosetta CM, Jong RM, Salomon CG, Joyce CE, Philips EA, Su XA, Freudenreich CH (2018) The chromatin remodeler Isw1 prevents CAG repeat expansions during transcription in Saccharomyces cerevisiae. Genetics 208(3):963–976. https://doi.org/10.1534/genetics.117.300529
14. Su XA, Freudenreich CH (2017) Cytosine deamination and base excision repair cause R-loop-induced CAG repeat fragility and instability in Saccharomyces cerevisiae. Proc Natl Acad Sci U S A 114(40):E8392–EE401. https://doi.org/10.1073/pnas.1711283114
15. Zhang H, Freudenreich CH (2007) An AT-rich sequence in human common fragile site FRA16D causes fork stalling and chromosome breakage in S. cerevisiae. Mol Cell 27(3):367–379. https://doi.org/10.1016/j.molcel.2007.06.012
16. Cherng N, Shishkin AA, Schlager LI, Tuck RH, Sloan L, Matera R, Sarkar PS, Ashizawa T, Freudenreich CH, Mirkin SM (2011) Expansions, contractions, and fragility of the spinocerebellar ataxia type 10 pentanucleotide repeat in yeast. Proc Natl Acad Sci U S A 108(7):2843–2848. https://doi.org/10.1073/pnas.1009409108
17. Lu S, Wang G, Bacolla A, Zhao J, Spitser S, Vasquez KM (2015) Short inverted repeats are hotspots for genetic instability: relevance to cancer genomes. Cell Rep 10(10):1674–1680. https://doi.org/10.1016/j.celrep.2015.02.039
18. Pluta AF, Zakian VA (1989) Recombination occurs during telomere formation in yeast. Nature 337(6206):429–433. https://doi.org/10.1038/337429a0
19. Chen C, Kolodner RD (1999) Gross chromosomal rearrangements in Saccharomyces cerevisiae replication and recombination defective mutants. Nat Genet 23(1):81–85. https://doi.org/10.1038/12687

20. Freudenreich CH, Stavenhagen JB, Zakian VA (1997) Stability of a CTG/CAG trinucleotide repeat in yeast is dependent on its orientation in the genome. Mol Cell Biol 17(4): 2090–2098
21. Su XA, Dion V, Gasser SM, Freudenreich CH (2015) Regulation of recombination at yeast nuclear pores controls repair and triplet repeat stability. Genes Dev 29(10):1006–1017. https://doi.org/10.1101/gad.256404.114
22. Freudenreich CH, Kantrow SM, Zakian VA (1998) Expansion and length-dependent fragility of CTG repeats in yeast. Science 279(5352):853–856
23. Balakumaran BS, Freudenreich CH, Zakian VA (2000) CGG/CCG repeats exhibit orientation-dependent instability and orientation-independent fragility in Saccharomyces cerevisiae. Hum Mol Genet 9(1):93–100
24. Paeschke K, Capra JA, Zakian VA (2011) DNA replication through G-quadruplex motifs is promoted by the Saccharomyces cerevisiae Pif1 DNA helicase. Cell 145(5):678–691. https://doi.org/10.1016/j.cell.2011.04.015
25. Kaushal S, Wollmuth CE, Das K, Hile SE, Regan SB, Barnes RP, Haouzi A, Lee SM, House NCM, Guyumdzhyan M, Eckert KA, Freudenreich CH. Sequence and Nuclease Requirements for Breakage and Healing of a Structure-Forming (AT)n Sequence within Fragile Site FRA16D. Cell Rep. 2019 Apr 23;27(4):1151-1164.e5. https://doi.org/10.1016/j.celrep.2019.03.103
26. Dunham MJ, Dunham MJ, Gartenberg MR, Brown GW (2015) Methods in yeast genetics and genomics: a Cold Spring Harbor Laboratory course manual, Maitreya J. Dunham, University of Washington, Marc R. Gartenberg, Robert Wood Johnson Medical School, Rutgers, The State University of New Jersey, Grant W. Brown, University of Toronto. Cold Spring Harbor, New York: Cold Spring Harbor Laboratory Press; xvii, p 233. ISBN 978-1-621821-34-2
27. Amberg DC, Burke D, Strathern JN, Burke D (2005) Cold Spring Harbor laboratory. Methods in yeast genetics: a Cold Spring Harbor laboratory course manual, vol xvii. Cold Spring Harbor Laboratory Press, Cold Spring Harbor, NY, p 230
28. Hall BM, Ma CX, Liang P, Singh KK (2009) Fluctuation analysis CalculatOR: a web tool for the determination of mutation rate using Luria-Delbruck fluctuation analysis. Bioinformatics 25(12):1564–1565. https://doi.org/10.1093/bioinformatics/btp253
29. Radchenko EA, McGinty RJ, Aksenova AY, Neil AJ, Mirkin SM (2018) Quantitative analysis of the rates for repeat-mediated genome instability in a yeast experimental system. Methods Mol Biol 1672:421–438. https://doi.org/10.1007/978-1-4939-7306-4_29
30. Rosche WA, Foster PL (2000) Determining mutation rates in bacterial populations. Methods 20(1):4–17. https://doi.org/10.1006/meth.1999.0901
31. Amberg DC, Burke DJ, Strathern JN (2006) High-efficiency transformation of yeast. CSH protocols 2006(1). https://doi.org/10.1101/pdb.prot4145

Chapter 6

Genetic Screens to Study GAA/TTC and Inverted Repeat Instability in *Saccharomyces cerevisiae*

Wenying Guo and Kirill S. Lobachev

Abstract

Instability of trinucleotide and inverted repeats is a causative factor in the development of a number of neurological diseases, hereditary syndromes, and cancer. To understand the mechanisms that lead to repeat-induced genome destabilization it is important to identify factors that affect repeat metabolism. Here we present an approach that utilizes systematic and unbiased genome-wide screen in yeast *Saccharomyces cerevisiae* aimed to find genes that govern GAA/TTC and inverted repeat instability. These screens allowed for the identification of more than 30 mutants with increased fragility of both repeat motifs.

Key words Trinucleotide repeats, Inverted repeats, Genome instability, Double-strand breaks, Gross chromosomal rearrangements, Genome-wide screen

1 Introduction

DNA sequences that can adopt noncanonical secondary structures cause double-strand breaks (DSBs) and chromosomal rearrangements in humans and model organisms [1]. We have demonstrated that triplex-forming GAA/TTC repeats and long inverted repeats that form hairpin and cruciform structures induce chromosomal breakage in baker yeast *S. cerevisiae* [2–5]. One of the consequences of repeat-induced breaks is gross chromosomal rearrangements (GCRs). In the GCR reporters, initially developed in Dr. Kolodner's laboratory [6], the repeats are inserted next to the counterselectable marker *CAN1* on the left arm of chromosome V. DSBs at the fragile motifs lead to loss of the 40 kb telomere-proximal fragment and subsequent repair events restoring the telomere at the broken chromosome. These GCRs cause loss of *CAN1* and give rise to the growth of canavanine-resistant colonies. Depending on the nature and length of the repeats, the GCR levels are increased from 100- to 1000-fold due to the presence of the fragile motifs [3, 5, 7].

Guy-Franck Richard (ed.), *Trinucleotide Repeats: Methods and Protocols*, Methods in Molecular Biology, vol. 2056, https://doi.org/10.1007/978-1-4939-9784-8_6,

The GCR assay is also a convenient tool to monitor changes in the level of instability of the trinucleotide and inverted repeats. To systematically identify genes that control repeat metabolism we combined the repeat carrying GCR cassette marked with *hphMX* with mutant alleles marked with *kanMX*. We utilized three Open Biosystem mutant collections and employed a modified genome-wide approach developed by C. Boone and colleagues [8]. This analysis allowed us to test a complete set of 4786 deletion mutations (YKO collection) and ~800 essential genes, for which expression is either regulated by doxycycline (yTHC collection) or compromised due to mRNA perturbation (DAmP collection). As a result, we have identified 33 mutants with augmented GAA/TTC fragility [4, 5]. Upon further examination, we found that the same mutants exhibited an increase in the large-scale expansions in the *URA3*-artifical intron assay [9] indicating the existence of common intermediates that can drive both types of instability. Moreover, the identity of mutants led us to discover the replication-dependent mechanism of GAA/TTC instability operating during S-phase and transcription-dependent breakage in nondividing cells. In the case of inverted repeats, genome-wide screen revealed that depletion or lack of components of the DNA replication machinery, the replication-pausing checkpoint pathway, proteins involved in Fe-S cluster biogenesis, the telomere maintenance complex or the Sgs1-Top3-Rmi1 dissolvasome augment fragility at the *Alu*-quasi-palindrome [4].

Below, we describe in details how we combined a GCR-based genome-wide screen approach for systematic identification of genes responsible for maintenance of repeat stability. Potentially, similar approach can be utilized (1) to identify not only hyperfragility but also hypofragility mutants; (2) to study instability of other secondary structure-forming motifs (e.g., CTG/CAG and CGG/CCG repeats); (3) to use other developed libraries based on the BY4730/BY4741 background (e.g., a collection of temperature-sensitive mutants [10].

2 Materials

2.1 Media and Solutions

1. YPD: dissolve 10 g yeast extract, 20 g peptone and 20 g glucose in 950 mL water in a 2–3 L flask, adjust to 1 liter, add 17 g agar. Autoclave for 30 min, at 120 °C and pour ~35 plates after cooling media to 55 °C.
2. YPD + G418 and Hygromycin B: Autoclave 1 L of YPD medium, cool down to 55 °C, add 3 mL of G418 solution (100 mg/mL stock solution in water made from the powder) and 6 mL of Hygromycin B solution (50 mg/mL stock solution in PBS).

3. YPD + doxycycline: Autoclave 1 L of YPD medium, cool down to 55 °C, add 1 mL of doxycycline (2 mg/mL stock solution in water). Cover plates with foil to prevent exposure of plates to the light.
4. Sporulation medium: dissolve 20 g potassium acetate, 2.5 g Bacto yeast extract, 1 g glucose, 20 mg adenine sulfate, 20 mg L-arginine–HCl, 100 mg L-aspartic acid, 20 mg L-histidine–HCl, 100 mg L-glutamic acid, 30 mg L-isoleucine, 100 mg L-leucine, 30 mg L-lysine–HCl, 20 mg L-methionine, 400 mg L-serine, 50 mg L-phenylalanine, 200 mg L-threonine, 20 mg L-tryptophan, 30 mg L-tyrosine, 20 mg uracil, 150 mg L-valine in 950 mL water in a 2–3 L flask. Adjust pH to 7.0 with KOH and add water to 1 L. Add 17 g agar, autoclave for 30 min, at 121 °C and pour plates after cooling media to 55 °C.
5. SD –his, SD –arg, SD –trp, or SD –ura dropout: Prepare each of them as a mix of the following 16 compounds, omitting one required amino acid or base (e.g., SD –his is prepared by mixing 15 out of the 16 compounds, omitting histidine): 20 mg adenine sulfate, 20 mg L-arginine–HCl, 100 mg L-aspartic acid, 20 mg L-histidine–HCl,100 mg L-glutamic acid, 30 mg L-isoleucine, 100 mg L-leucine, 30 mg L-lysine–HCl, 20 mg L-methionine, 400 mg L-serine, 50 mg L-phenylalanine, 200 mg L-threonine, 20 mg L-tryptophan, 30 mg L-tyrosine, 20 mg uracil, 150 mg L-valine.
6. SD –his + cycloheximide: SD –his dropout, 6.7 g yeast nitrogen base with ammonium sulfate and without amino acids, 20 g glucose, 17 g agar. Autoclave for 30 min, at 120 °C, cool down to 55 °C, add 0.5 mL of cycloheximide solution (10 mg/mL stock solution in DMSO) and pour plates.
7. Canavanine: SD –arg dropout, 6.7 g yeast nitrogen base with ammonium sulfate and without amino acids, 20 g glucose, 17 g agar. Autoclave for 30 min, at 120 °C, cool down to 55 °C, add 3 mL/L (20 mg/mL canavanine stock solution in water) and pour plates.
8. 5-FOA: Filter-sterilize 7 g yeast nitrogen base with ammonium sulfate and amino acids, 1 g 5-fluoroorotic acid, 50 mg uracil, 20 g glucose dissolved in 500 mL water. Warm up solution to 50 °C. Autoclave 500 mL of 4% agar, cool down to ~60 °C and mix with prewarmed 5-FOA solution. Pour plates.
9. Galactose medium: Filter-sterilize 2% galactose, 1% yeast extract, 2% Bacto peptone.

2.2 Accessories

1. We used a simple template for patching yeast cells depicted in Fig. 1. For the best results in visual identification of the GCR-caused papillae on the plate, we suggest crossing the query strains with the mutant strains from the libraries by making 6

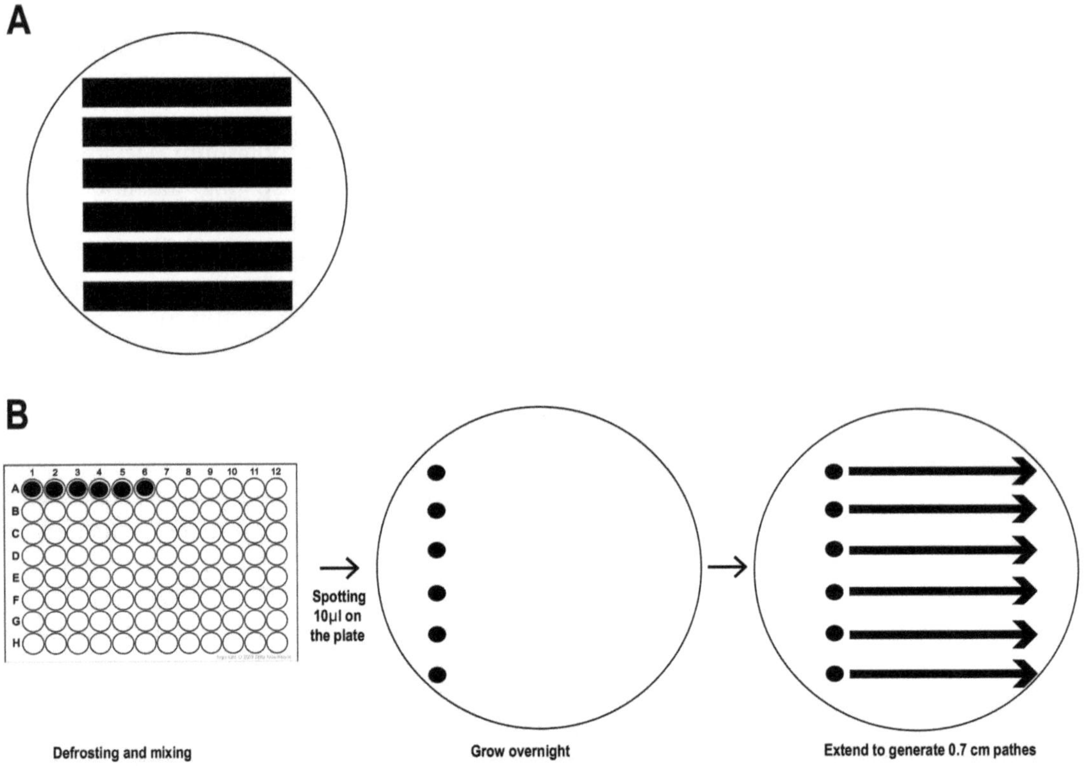

Fig. 1 Preparation of the query and tester strains for the screen. (**a**) Template for making plates with six patches of 0.7 cm wide. (**b**) Diagram for the recovery of the tester strains from collections and making streaks for crosses

patches of the control and experimental strains (*see* below), per plate. Each patch should be approximately 0.7 cm wide.

2. To reduce the cost of the replica-plating experiments, we custom made 6″ velveteen squares by cutting several yards of velvet fabric.

2.3 Yeast Strains and Plasmids

1. Query strains are derivatives of BY4742 from Open Biosystems (MATα, *ura3-Δ*, *leu2-Δ*, *his3-Δ*, *lys2-Δ*). The genotype of the query strain, used in the screens is: MATα, *ura3-Δ*, *leu2-Δ*, *his3-Δ*, *lys2-Δ*, *rpl28-Q38K*, *mfa1Δ::MFA1pr-HIS3*, *V29617::hphMX*, *V34205::lys2::Fragile motif*. Fragile motifs inserted into *LYS2* were (GAA/TTC)$_{230}$, or the 100% and 94% homologous inverted *Alus*. For query strain construction, *see* Subheading 3.
2. The three collections of tester strains: yTHC (~860 strains), DAmP (~860 strains), YKO (4786 strains), were purchased from Open Biosystems (currently they are available from Dharmacon (https://dharmacon.horizondiscovery.com). The yTHC collection is a set of strains where the expression of essential genes is under control of the doxycycline-regulatable

TET promoter. The DAmP collection is a library of strains where the expression of essential genes is reduced by four to tenfold due to destabilization of their mRNA. The YKO collection is a set of gene-disruption mutants. In all three cases, mutant alleles are labeled with the *kanMX* cassette.

3. *MAT*a and *MAT*α lys5 mating type tester strains.

3 Methods

1. Query strain construction.
   (a) The *LYS2* fragment from the pFL39*LYS2* plasmid [11] was PCR amplified with primers canlys5 and canlys3 that carry homology to the *V34205* region (Table 1). The PCR product was transformed into the BY4742 strain to insert *LYS2* on the left arm of chromosome V telomere distal to *CAN1* (*see* **Note 1**).
   (b) The mating type of this strain was switched to MATa using the pJH132 plasmid (gift from Dr. James Haber) carrying the HO gene under control of the GAL1-GAL10 promoter. Transformants were selected on the SD –trp medium. Then, they were inoculated into 5 mL of galactose medium and shook for 2–4 h to induce HO expression and plated on YPD to get individual colonies. Colonies were patched on YPD and crossed with α- and a-specific *ade5* testers to identify MATa isolates. MATa clones that lost pJH132 were selected on 5-FOA media.
   (c) The *MFA1pr-HIS3* cassette was PCR amplified from y2454 [12] (gift from Dr. Kyungjae Myung) using primers mfa1-amp5 and mfa1-amp3 (Table 1) and inserted into the *MFA1* locus. Transformants were selected on SD –his medium.
   (d) The mating type was switched back to MATα using pJH132 as described in 1.2.
   (e) The *hphMX* cassette was PCR amplified from the pAG32 plasmid [13] and inserted telomere proximal from *CAN1* on chromosome V at the position V29617 using km-5v and km-3v primers (Table 1).
   (f) We obtained spontaneous resistant colonies to the cycloheximide (YPD media supplemented with 5 mg/L cycloheximide). Selected clones were sequenced and found to contain the *rpl28-Q38K* mutation, identified in another study where cycloheximide was used as a selection drug [14].
   (g) The $(GAA)_{230}$ tract was moved to the *Bam*HI site of *LYS2* via *delitto perfetto* [15]. First, the CORE cassette (*URA3*cl*kanMX*) was PCR amplified from the pCORE

Table 1
Primers used

Name	Sequence
canlys5	5′ **GTTCTTGTTCTAATTAATTGTAACTATTTTT**ATGCATGCGGCCGC*CCACTTGCAATTACATAAAAAATTCCGGCGG* 3′[a]
canlys3	5′ **GATACGATTACTCCAGTTCCTCTTACAAGAA**GGCGCGCCCATATTTAATTATTGTA*CATGGACATATCATACGTAATGC* 3′[a]
mfa1-amp5	5′ GCACCTACTGCTACGGTTGG 3′
mfa1-amp3	5′ GTCGAAGCCGATGAAACGAC 3′
Km-5v	5′ **CAAATAATTTCATACATGCACATATAGCTACTACATAGTCAAGAACATATCATAACATTT***ATCGATGAATTCGAGCTCG* 3′[b]
Km-3v	5′ **TCGGTAGAGCCAGCATCAGATGCAAAGCCATGCAAAGACTGATATAAAGACTGTTATACC***CGTACGCTGCAGGTCGAC* 3′[b]
lys2-core5	5′ **TGATATAATTATCCATAATGGTGCGTTAGTTCACTGGGTTTATCCATATGCCAAATTGAG***GAGCTCGTTTTCGACACTGG* 3′[c]
lys2-core3	5′ **AAGAACTTTGGCTTGCCGACGGCGGCTAAGCTCATAACATTGATAGTTGAAATAACATTT***TCCTTACCATTAAGTTGATC* 3′[c]
230PF	5′ **GGTGCGTTAGTTCACTGGGTTTATCCATATGCCAAATTGAGGATC**GCCCGGGCGATCGCGAGGA*GCTCGAGTGCAGACCTCAAATTCGAT* 3′[d]
230PR	5′ **CGGCTAAGCTCATAACATTGATAGTTGAAATAACATTTGGATC**GGCGCG*CGATGTGCAGAACCTGAAGCTTGATC* 3′[d]
cpcr3	5′ CGACGGCGGCTAAGCTCATAAC 3′
s3393	5′ GTCAGGGCCAAGGATGAAG 3′

[a]Bold: homology to Chromosome V, italics: sequence annealing to *LYS2*
[b]Bold: homology to the Chromosome V, italics: sequence annealing to *hphMX*
[c]Bold: homology to *LYS2*, italics: sequence annealing to pCORE
[d]Bold: homology to *LYS2*, italics: sequence specific to the flanking regions of the $(GAA)_{230}$ tract

plasmid using primers lys2-core5 and lys2-core3. $G418^R Ura^+ Lys^-$ transformants were used to verify insertion of CORE into *LYS2*. Second, $(GAA)_{230}$ tract was PCR amplified from the pYES-GAA228 plasmid [16] using primers 230PF and 230PR (Table 1). The resulting PCR fragment was used to replace CORE in *LYS2*. The correct replacements were verified in 5-FOA^R and $G418^S$ clones by PCR using *LYS2*-specific primers: cpcr3 and s3393.

(h) The 100% or 94% homologous inverted *Alus* were integrated into the chromosomal *LYS2* gene using plasmids pHS-I and p36-I via pop-in and pop-out method as previously described [11].

2. Preparation of query and tester strains for the experiment. Patch MATα query strains marked with hphMX (containing 100% or 94% homologous inverted *Alus* and $(GAA)_{230}$ tract) and 6 MATa tester strains carrying *kanMX* on YPD plates overnight in the following way. Streak out query strains for single-colonies and verify the presence of the unchanged $(GAA)_{230}$ tracts using colony PCR (this step is unnecessary in the case of strains with inverted repeats). Patch cells from single colonies in duplicates using template depicted on Fig. 1a. Defrost cells from the collections frozen in glycerol in 96 well plates on the bench, mix by pipetting using a multichannel pipette and spot 10 μL of the cultures from 6 wells containing mutants to one side of the YPD plate as a column. Allow yeast to grow at 30 °C overnight and extend the original 6 spots to 6 rows of long patches by spreading the cells with flat-ended toothpicks (Fig. 1b). The overall scheme for combining mutant alleles marked with *kanMX* cassette and repeat-induced GCR assay is depicted in Fig. 2. Use the following protocol to carry out the screen (*see* **Note 2**).
3. Cross strains by replica-plating and incubate at 30 °C on YPD overnight.
4. Select diploids on medium containing 300 mg/L G418 and 300 mg/L hygromycin B.
5. Replica-plate diploids to sporulation medium and incubate for 5 days at 23 °C.
6. Transfer a mixture of diploids and asci containing MATa/MATα haploid tetrads to SD –his plates supplemented with 5 mg/L cycloheximide. Incubate for 2 days. Since the query strain carries a mating type-specific reporter MFA1pr-*HIS3* and a recessive mutation *rpl28-Q38K* that provides resistance to cycloheximide, this procedure allows selecting only for MATa haploid progeny. The MFA1promoter allows to eliminate MATα haploids, while the presence of *rpl28-Q38K* prevents growth of MATa/MATa diploids that occur due to the

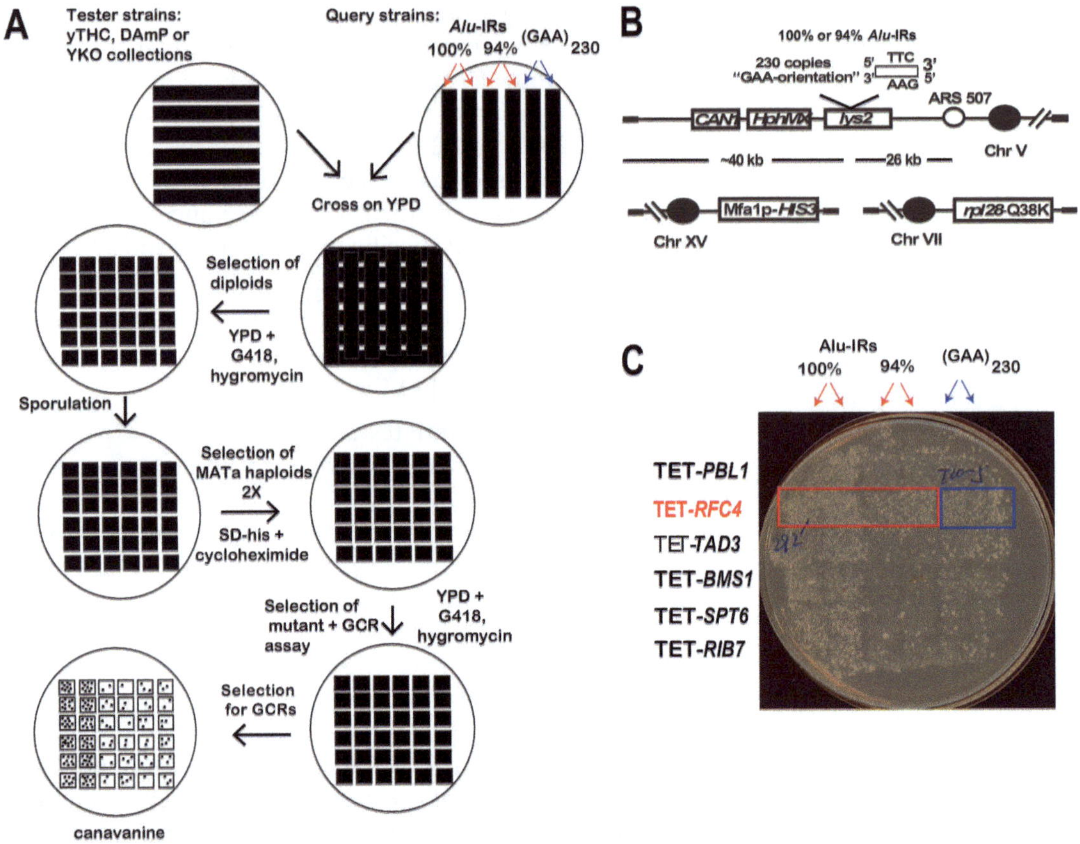

Fig. 2 Methodology for genome-wide screens. (**a**) Flowchart of the screen (*see* detailed description in the Methods). (**b**) Relevant constructs in query strains for the discovery of the genotypes with increased inverted and GAA/TTC repeat fragility. The 100% or 94% homologous inverted *Alus* (*Alu*-IRs) and 230 copies of GAA/TTC repeats ($(GAA)_{230}$) were integrated next to *CAN1* on the left arm of chromosome V. The location of *HIS3* ORF under control of a MATa-specific promoter and *rpl28-Q38K* allele on chromosomes IV and VII, correspondingly, are shown. (**c**) Example of the screening plate. Columns are duplicates of the query strains containing repeats. Each row is one of the tester strains from the collections. The level of arm loss in TET-*PBL1*, TET-*TAD3*, TET-*BMS1*, TET-*SPT6*, is comparable to the GCRs observed in wild-type (not shown). Visible increase in the number of canavanine-resistant colonies on the intersections of the patch of the strain with down-regulated *RFC4* gene and patches of the strains with the GCR assay indicates that disruption of PCNA-loading RFC complex leads to destabilization of inverted *Alus* and GAA/TTC trinucleotide repeats (red and blue boxes, respectively)

gene conversion of mating type locus. To assure the selection of haploids, repeat this step.

7. Select MATa haploids harboring the chromosome V with repeats and mutated genes on medium containing G418 and hygromycin B.
8. In experiments involving YKO and DAmP collections, replica-plate cells to canavanine-containing plates. Strains from the yTHC collection incubate overnight on YPD medium containing 2 μg/mL doxycycline and then replica-plate to canavanine-containing plates.

9. Evaluate the GCR-inducing capacity of tested mutants after incubation of yeast on canavanine media for 5 days. Record the number of revertants on canavanine plates on square patches resulting from the crosses of query strains with mutants and compare this amount with patches coming from the control crosses of repeat-containing strains with wild-type. Since the GCR rate induced by $(GAA)_{230}$ repeats ($\sim 2 \times 10^{-6}$) and 100% *Alu*-IRs ($\sim 2 \times 10^{-5}$) is ~10 and 100 times, correspondingly, higher than the mutation rate ($\sim 3 \times 10^{-7}$) at the *CAN1* locus in wild-type strains, the screen preferentially selects for GCR inducers or strong mutators (*see* **Note 3**).

4 Notes

1. Repeat tracks that can be amplified by PCR, such as GAA/TTC repeats, might be targeted next to *CAN1* directly using *delitto perfetto* approach [15], so insertion of *LYS2* can be omitted. Unlike trinucleotide repeats, inverted repeats cannot be amplified by PCR using currently available thermostable polymerases (K. S. Lobachev, unpublished data). Thus, we had to use already available *lys2::IR* alleles which in turn necessitated *LYS2* integration.
2. Selection of diploids, induction of sporulation, selection of MATa progeny might be done in liquid cultures using robot systems that is utilized for replica pinning procedures (e.g., described in Costanzo and Boone [17]). However, the frequency of the repeat-induced GCRs is too low to readily detect changes in the number of canavanine-resistant papillae when pin-sized prints are replica-plated. Therefore, upon using robotic systems two last steps should be carried out similarly to what is described in this protocol by making approximately 0.7 × 0.7 cm patches of cells.
3. The validity of the effects detected in the identified mutants in the genome-wide screen should be verified by recreating the hyperfragile alleles in strains where the consequences of GCR events can be easily distinguished from mutations in *CAN1*. This step is also required to prevent erroneous annotations, unavoidable in large collections of yeast strains. We reassessed the effect of the identified mutants by recreating the hyperfragile alleles in strains with the *ADE2* gene inserted between *CAN1* and repeats that allows differentiation of GCRs from mutations based on the color of canavanine-resistant clones [4, 5].

Acknowledgments

We thank Dr. N. Degtyareva for critical reading of the manuscript and Dr. Y. Zhang for carrying out the screens. This work was supported by NIH grant R01GM129119 to KSL.

References

1. Saini N, Zhang Y, Usdin K, Lobachev KS (2013) When secondary comes first--the importance of non-canonical DNA structures. Biochimie 95:117–123
2. Lobachev KS, Gordenin DA, Resnick MA (2002) The Mre11 complex is required for repair of hairpin-capped double-strand breaks and prevention of chromosome rearrangements. Cell 108:183–193
3. Kim HM, Narayanan V, Mieczkowski PA, Petes TD, Krasilnikova MM, Mirkin SM, Lobachev KS (2008) Chromosome fragility at GAA tracts in yeast depends on repeat orientation and requires mismatch repair. EMBO J 27:2896–2906
4. Zhang Y, Saini N, Sheng Z, Lobachev KS (2013) Genome-wide screen reveals replication pathway for quasi-palindrome fragility dependent on homologous recombination. PLoS Genet 9:e1003979
5. Zhang Y, Shishkin AA, Nishida Y, Marcinkowski-Desmond D, Saini N, Volkov KV, Mirkin SM, Lobachev KS (2012) Genome-wide screen identifies pathways that govern GAA/TTC repeat fragility and expansions in dividing and nondividing yeast cells. Mol Cell 48:254–265
6. Chen C, Kolodner RD (1999) Gross chromosomal rearrangements in Saccharomyces cerevisiae replication and recombination defective mutants. Nat Genet 23:81–85
7. Narayanan V, Mieczkowski PA, Kim HM, Petes TD, Lobachev KS (2006) The pattern of gene amplification is determined by the chromosomal location of hairpin-capped breaks. Cell 125:1283–1296
8. Tong AHY, Evangelista M, Tyers M, Boone C, Parsons AB, Xu H, Bader GD, Pagé N, Robinson M, Raghibizadeh S, Hogue CW, Bussey H, Andrews B (2001) Systematic genetic analysis with ordered arrays of yeast deletion mutants. Science 294:2364–2368
9. Shishkin AA, Voineagu I, Matera R, Cherng N, Chernet BT, Krasilnikova MM, Narayanan V, Lobachev KS, Mirkin SM (2009) Large-scale expansions of Friedreich's ataxia GAA repeats in yeast. Mol Cell 35:82–92
10. Li Z, Vizeacoumar FJ, Bahr S, Li J, Warringer J, Vizeacoumar FS, Min R, VanderSluis B, Bellay J, DeVit M, Fleming JA (2011) Systematic exploration of essential yeast gene function with temperature-sensitive mutants. Nat Biotechnol 29:361–367
11. Lobachev KS, Stenger JE, Kozyreva OG, Jurka J, Gordenin DA, Resnick MA (2000) Inverted Alu repeats unstable in yeast are excluded from the human genome. EMBO J 19:3822–3830
12. Smith S, Hwang JY, Banerjee S, Majeed A, Gupta A, Myung K (2004) Mutator genes for suppression of gross chromosomal rearrangements identified by a genome-wide screening in Saccharomyces cerevisiae. Proc Natl Acad Sci 101:9039–9044
13. Goldstein AL, McCusker JH (1999) Three new dominant drug resistance cassettes for gene disruption in Saccharomyces cerevisiae. Yeast 15:1541–1553
14. Kaufer NF, Fried HM, Schwindinger WF, Jasin M, Warner JR (1983) Cycloheximide resistance in yeast: the gene and its protein. Nucleic Acids Res 11:3123–3135
15. Storici F, Lewis LK, Resnick MA (2001) In vivo site-directed mutagenesis using oligonucleotides. Nat Biotechnol 19:773–776
16. Krasilnikova MM, Mirkin SM (2004) Replication stalling at Friedreich's ataxia (GAA)n repeats in vivo. Mol Cell Biol 24:2286–2295
17. Costanzo M, Boone C (2009) SGAM: an array-based approach for high-resolution genetic mapping in Saccharomyces cerevisiae. Methods Mol Biol 548:37–53

Chapter 7

Monitoring Double-Strand Break Repair of Trinucleotide Repeats Using a Yeast Fluorescent Reporter Assay

Lucie Poggi, Bruno Dumas, and Guy-Franck Richard

Abstract

Cells can repair a double-strand break (DSB) by homologous recombination if a homologous sequence is provided as a template. This can be achieved by classical gene conversion (with or without crossover) or by single-strand annealing (SSA) between two direct repeat sequences flanking the DSB. To initiate SSA, single-stranded regions are needed adjacent to the break, extending up to the direct repeats in such a way that complementary strands can anneal to each other to repair the DSB. In the present protocol, we describe a GFP reporter assay in *Saccharomyces cerevisiae* allowing for the quantification of nuclease efficacy at inducing a DSB, by monitoring the reconstitution of a functional GFP gene whose expression can be rapidly quantified by flow cytometry.

Key words Endonuclease, CRISPR-Cas9, Flow cytometry, GFP-based reporter assay, Yeast, Homologous recombination

1 Introduction

Double-strand DNA endonucleases have been used for decades as biotechnological tools to engineer DNA sequences, first on plasmids, later on in whole genomes. Their activities were determined mainly using biochemical approaches. Among the four large families of highly specific DNA endonucleases [1], meganucleases were the first to have been used to engineer mammalian genomes [2] The first meganuclease to be characterized was I-*Sce* I which was isolated from a mitochondrial intron in *S. cerevisiae* [3] and its activity was assessed in vitro on a plasmid carrying its recognition site [4]. The development of new target specificities for meganucleases also relied on in vitro assays to assess cleavage efficiencies of synthetic meganucleases [5]. Zinc-finger nucleases (ZFN) were engineered from Zinc-finger transcription activators fused to the FokI endonuclease domain, and in vitro assays were carried out on λ DNA to test cleavage efficacy, sequence recognition specificity and time course of cleavage [6]. Fifteen years later, Transcription

Guy-Franck Richard (ed.), *Trinucleotide Repeats: Methods and Protocols*, Methods in Molecular Biology, vol. 2056,
https://doi.org/10.1007/978-1-4939-9784-8_7,

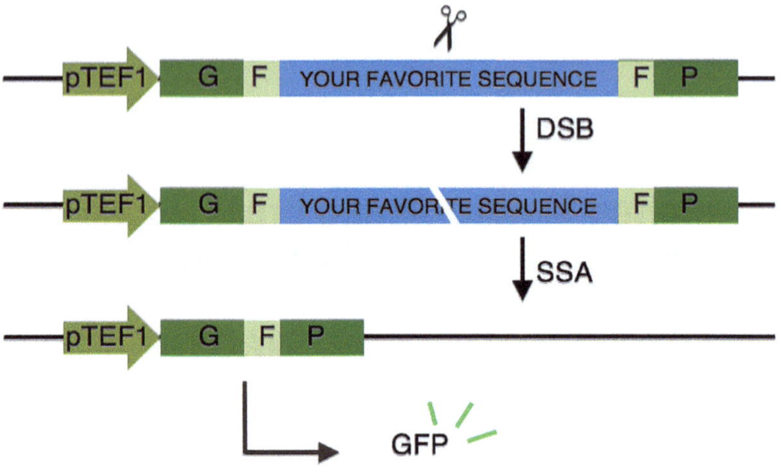

Fig. 1 Cassette integrated into the FYBL1-4D strain. pTEF1 is a strong constitutive promoter driving the expression of the GFP cassette. Upon nuclease induction, a double-strand break is made within the CTG repeat tract, generating recombination intermediates that lead to annealing between the two GFP moieties by Single-Strand Annealing, regenerating a functional protein. Readouts of nuclease efficacy is made by counting GFP-positive cells using flow cytometry

Activator-Like Effectors (TALE) were also fused to FokI to make TALE Nucleases (TALEN). This new family of nucleases was validated as a bona fide DNA double-strand strand endonuclease in vivo, on a yeast plasmid [7]. More recently, *Streptococcus pyogenes* Cas9 (SpCas9) and variants that were engineered to be more specific were characterized using a cutting-edge technology based on FRET experiments to identify off-target sites in vitro [8]. Here, we propose a simple in vivo assay, in the yeast *Saccharomyces cerevisiae* to test cleavage efficacy of any DNA endonuclease on any target sequence. The assay uses homologous recombination as a proxy for nuclease efficacy. Homologous recombination assays have already been used to quantify repair efficacy after the induction of a DSB [9]. Here we introduced in a *S. cerevisiae* S288C derivative strain a reporter gene made of a CTG trinucleotide repeat integrated in a GFP bipartite gene containing 100 bp overlapping homology regions flanking the repeat (Fig. 1). Upon nuclease induction, cells repair the DSB by single-strand annealing (SSA) between the two overlapping GFP moieties, reconstituting a functional gene that can be easily quantified by flow cytometry. This method is adapted to high throughput data acquisition to study DSB repair efficacy at any given target sequence integrated in the GFP cassette, using any endonuclease targeting this region. Here we present the protocol developed to study the efficacy of the *Streptococcus pyogenes* Cas9 nuclease (SpCas9) at repairing a DSB made into CTG trinucleotide repeats, but the nuclease as well as the target sequence may be easily changed, to make it a versatile assay.

2 Materials

Use good laboratory practices to avoid contaminating yeast cultures. Always manipulate cells in a sterile environment.

2.1 Yeast Media

1. YPD medium: 20 g Bacto peptone, 10 g yeast extract, 20 g glucose, H_2O to 1 L, autoclave for 20 min at 120 °C. For solid medium, add 20 g agar before autoclaving and pour 25 mL in each plate.
2. SC –Ura –Leu medium: 6.7 g yeast nitrogen base without amino acids, 20 g glucose, 2 g –Ura –Leu dropout mix, H_2O to 1 L, autoclave for 20 min at 120 °C. For solid medium, add 20 g agar before autoclaving and pour 25 mL in each plate. –Ura –Leu dropout mix contains 1 g adenine, 2 g alanine, 2 g arginine, 2 g aspartic acid, 2 g asparagine, 2 g cysteine, 2 g glutamic acid, 2 g glutamine, 2 g glycine, 2 g histidine, 2 g isoleucine, 2 g lysine, 2 g methionine, 2 g phenylalanine, 5 g proline, 2 g serine, 2 g threonine, 2 g tryptophan, 2 g tyrosine, and 2 g valine.
3. GAL –Ura –Leu medium: 6.7 g yeast nitrogen base without amino acids, 20 g galactose, 2 g –Ura –Leu dropout mix, H_2O to 1 L, autoclave for 20 min at 120 °C.

2.2 Yeast Transformation

1. FYBL1-4D strain (or another S288C derivative) into which the bipartite GFP-CTG cassette was integrated.
2. Sterile toothpicks.
3. Sterile 1.5 mL microtubes.
4. Sterile micropipette blue and yellow tips.
5. Sterile 2 and 25 mL disposable pipettes.
6. Sterile glass beads (or a sterile spreader).
7. TE/LiAc solution: 10 mM Tris–HCl pH 7.5, 1 mM EDTA pH 8.0, 100 mM lithium acetate pH 7.5. Sterilize the solution on a 0.22 μm filter unit.
8. PEG/TE/LiAc solution: 10 mM Tris–HCl pH 7.5, 1 mM EDTA, 100 mM Lithium acetate pH 7.5, 40% PEG3350. Sterilize on a 0.22 μm filter unit.
9. Carrier DNA: 10 mg/mL salmon sperm DNA denatured at 100 °C for 5 min then put on ice (*see* **Note 1**).
10. Water bath set at 42 °C.

2.3 Flow Cytometry

1. 1.3 mL sterile 96 deep-well plates.
2. Breathable sealing membrane.
3. 96 well plates.
4. Incubator with a 25 mm shaking diameter (*see* **Note 2**).

5. PBS buffer: 137 mM NaCl, 2.7 mM KCl, 10 mM Na_2HPO_4, 1.8 mM KH_2PO_4.
6. Flow cytometer buffers (storage, running, washing).
7. Flow cytometer (*see* **Note 3**). It must be turned on 30 min before starting experiments, in order to allow lasers to warm up. Calibration should be carried out every day.

2.4 Vectors

1. pGAL-Cas9 [10]: This centromeric plasmid contains a *GAL1* promoter driving the expression of *Streptococcus pyogenes* Cas9 and *LEU2* as a selectable marker.
2. pRS416-CTG: This plasmid was constructed by integrating a synthetic cassette containing the *SNR52* promoter, the guide RNA target sequence TGCTGCTGCTGCTGCTGCTG, the guide RNA scaffold and the *SUP4* terminator into the pRS416 plasmid [11]. The sequence of the full cassette can be found at the end this chapter. This centromeric plasmid carries *URA3* as a selectable marker.

3 Methods

3.1 Transformation of FYBL1-4D Containing the Bipartite GFP-CTG Cassette

1. Thaw cells from −80 °C freezer, plate on YPD plate and let them grow for 48 h.
2. Pick a single colony using a sterile toothpick and start an overnight culture in 3 mL YPD. Incubate at 30 °C, 160 rpm.
3. Dilute saturated culture 1:50 in YPD and incubate at 30 °C, 160 rpm until cell density reaches 1×10^7–3×10^7 cells/mL.
4. Preheat water bath at 42 °C.
5. Wash cells with 20 mL TE/LiAc solution.
6. Resuspend pellet in TE/LiAc so that 50 μL contain 10^8 cells. Example: 50 mL at 1×10^7 cells/mL is resuspended after wash in 250 μL TE/LiAc.
7. Incubate cells for 15 min at 30 °C without shaking.
8. Prepare a 1.5 mL sterile microtube containing 300 μL PEG/TE/LiAc solution, 100 ng pGAL-Cas9 plasmid, 100 ng pRS416-CTG, 50 μg boiled carrier DNA. Vortex.
9. Add 50 μL of cells and gently mix using micropipette and a sterile yellow tip.
10. Incubate at 30 °C for 30 min without shaking.
11. Heat-shock at 42 °C for 20 min without shaking.
12. Centrifuge for 3 min at 3220 × *g*. Resuspend cells in sterile H_2O.
13. Plate cells on GLU −Ura −Leu plate.
14. Incubate at 30 °C for 40 h.

3.2 Flow Cytometry Assay

Each test should be carried out in triplicate, both in GLU −Ura −Leu and GAL −Ura −Leu media.

1. Fill one 96 deep-well plate with 300 μL of liquid GLU −Ura −Leu or GAL −Ura −Leu medium.
2. Using a toothpick seed one colony into each well. Be careful not to pick untransformed cells close to the colony (*see* **Note 4**). Gently agitate the toothpick so that the cells are transferred into the liquid medium.
3. Prepare another 96 well plate and add 100 μL of PBS in each well.
4. Transfer 100 μL of each well from the culture plate using a multichannel pipette to the 96-well plate containing the PBS.
5. Seal deep-well plate with breathable sealing membrane and incubate in a rotating incubator at 300 rpm, 30 °C.
6. On the flow cytometer, use the appropriate parameters for 96 well plates.
7. Select channels FSC, SSC both Area and Height. Voltages set up are as follows: 316 V (linear) for FSC, 350 V (linear) for SSC. To read FITC use channel B1 from the 488 nm laser with 525/50 nm filter. Use 390 V (log3) in voltage settings for this channel.
8. Select population on the FSC-A/SSC-A window to eliminate cellular debris (*see* **Notes 5** and **6**) then eliminate doublets on the SSC-A/SSC-H window. Quantify number of GFP-positive cells on the FITC-A histogram (Fig. 2).
9. After 12 h, prepare a new 96 well plate in which 100 μL of PBS is added. Harvest 30 μL of each well in the 96 deep-well culture plate and add them to the PBS plate.
10. Proceed from **step 6** to **8**, as above.
11. Repeat from **step 9** at 24 and 36 h (*see* **Note 7**) (Fig. 3).
12. At the end of the experiment, export all data to FCS files for subsequent analysis using FlowJo (or any appropriate software).

3.3 Data Analysis

Quantify the number of GFP-positive cells over time, using your favorite software (we use FlowJo 10.0). Use the following guidelines:

1. Select a homogeneous population on FSC-A/SSC-A graph to remove cell debris. Debris are usually only visible at T0 and most probably correspond to cell mortality due to the transformation process (Fig. 2a).
2. Select single cells on SSC-H/SSC-A graph (Fig. 2b).
3. On a glucose control population, select GFP- cells. Use this gate to define the same GFP- population in other samples. Cells exhibiting fluorescence above this limit are considered GFP+ (Fig. 2c).

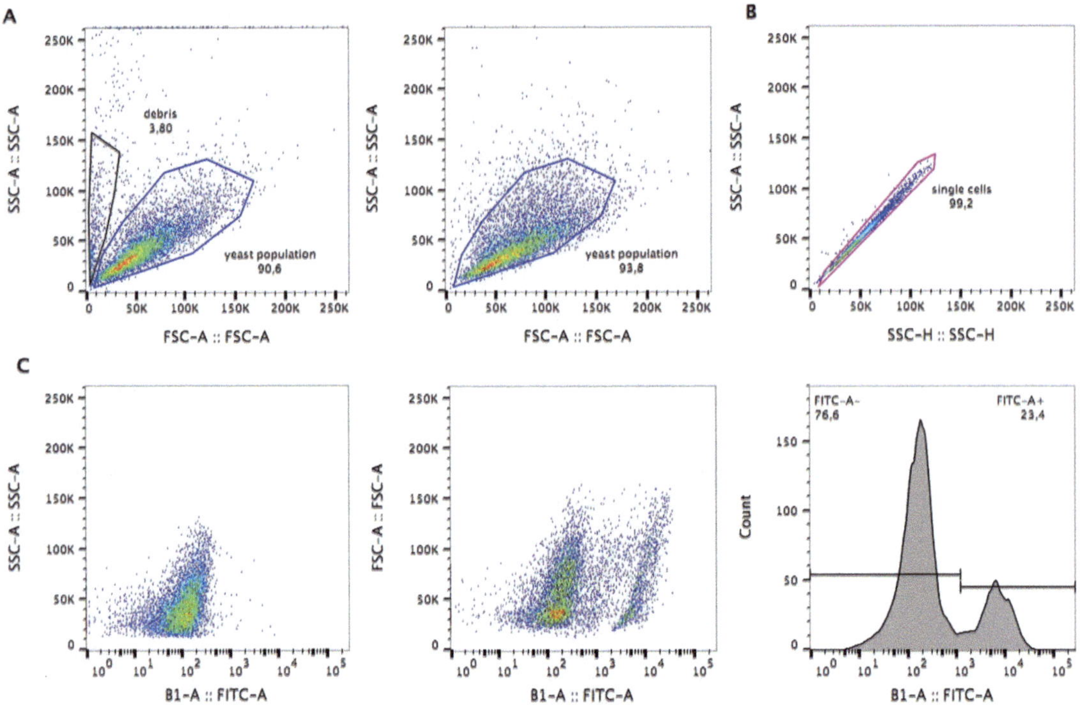

Fig. 2 Flow cytometry (**a**) Yeast total population analysis. Left: The FYBL1-4D-CTG strain was transformed with pGAL-Cas9 and pRS416-CTG plasmids, freshly picked from GLU –Ura –Leu plate 40 h after transformation. Yeast population is selected in a gate on the FSC-A/SSC-A graph and circled in blue. Debris are circled in black and not considered for subsequent analyses. Right: The same strain analyzed 12 h later. Note that cell debris are not visible anymore (**b**) Single cells are selected on the SSC-H/SSC-A graph (circled in pink on the figure) (**c**) Analysis of GFP expression. Single cells are now analyzed for GFP fluorescence. Left: Yeast cells at T0. Middle: Cells after 36 h in galactose medium. Note the shift of fluorescence corresponding to GFP-expressing cells. Right: GFP-positive cells are counted in the selected population: 23.4% of cells are GFP+ and have therefore repaired the DSB by Single-Strand Annealing

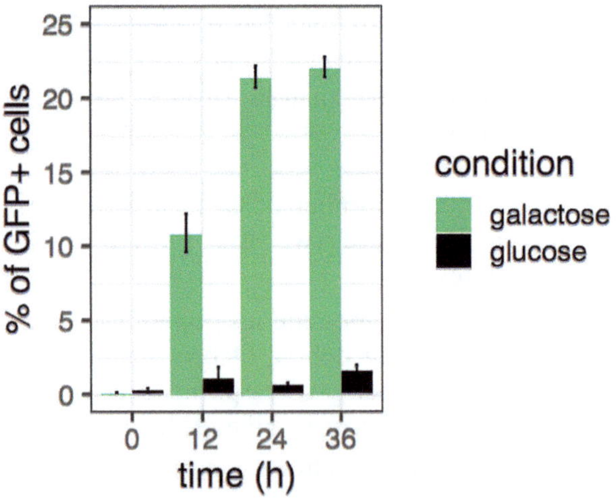

Fig. 3 GFP positive cells in glucose and galactose media during a 36 h time course. A low level of GFP+ cells is detected in glucose medium due to the *GAL1* promoter leakiness

4. Apply the same gating rules to all samples.
5. Export data collection to a spreadsheet.

3.4 Conclusion

In the present protocol, each time course was performed at only four time points (0, 12, 24 and 36 h), but additional points may be added. Note that the limiting step will be the time taken by the flow cytometer to process each sample. In addition, this assay is easily scalable. Here, the repair following a DSB made into a CTG repeat tract by SpCas9 was assessed, but it can be used to test a wide variety of nucleases [1] on many different target sequences. However, the experimenter should keep in mind the technical issue due to frequent leakiness of the *GAL1* promoter, resulting in an elevated background level of GFP+ cells in glucose medium. This is why we recommend carrying the experiment right after plasmid transformation, and as soon as small colonies can be picked.

Sequence of the *SNR52*-CTG-*SUP4* cassette for SpCas9:

TCTTTGAAAAGATAATGTATGATTATGCTTT CACTCATATTTATACAGAAACTTGATGTTTTCTTTC GAGTATATACAAGGTGATTACATGTACGTTT GAAGTACAACTCTAGATTTTGTAGTGCC CTCTTGGGCTAGCGGTAAAGGTGCGCATTTTTT CACACCCTACAATGTTCTGTTCAAAAGATTTTGGTC AAACGCTGTAGAAGTGAAAGTTGGTGCGCA TGTTTCGGCGTTCGAAACTTCTCCGCAGTGA AAGATAAATGATCTGCTGCTGCTGCTGCTGCTG GTTTTAGAGCTAGAAATAGCAAGTTAAAATAAGGCTAG TCCGTTATCAACTTGAAAAAGTGGCACCGAGTC GGTGC*TTTTTTTGTTTTTTATGTCT*.

Bold: SNR52 promoter.
Plain: CTG guideRNA.
Underlined: Scaffold RNA.
Italics: SUP4 terminator.

4 Notes

1. Denaturation step is necessary to ensure that carrier DNA is single stranded and will bind to the cell wall and be degraded by DNases in the cytosol instead of the transformed plasmid. It greatly enhances transformation efficiency.
2. We use an incubator with a 25 mm shaking diameter to provide some oxygenation to yeast cells in 96 deep-well plates.
3. We work with a MACSQuant Analyzer (Miltenyi Biotec), but other cytometers may be used.
4. Very important: we recommend picking colonies right after they start being visible on a plate, 40 h after transformation and without preliminary subcloning. The *GAL1* promoter is

slightly leaky and waiting for a longer time will increase background noise as some cells will start expressing Cas9 and undergoing DSB-repair. This would result in an unwanted high proportion of GFP+ cells at the start of the experiment. Therefore, picking yeast colonies as early as 40 h after transformation is crucial.

5. At $t = 0$ h there can be cell debris due to mortality rate during transformation. These debris will be outnumbered by growing cells in future time points.
6. It is also possible to do a viability staining, using propidium iodide or a commercial viability dye like viability dye from Miltenyi 405/452. Be careful to choose a fluorophore that does not overlap with FITC signal.
7. We do not proceed after 36 h, since the cell culture is are saturated and cells stop dividing and expressing the GFP.

Acknowledgments

L.P. was supported by a CIFRE PhD fellowship from SANOFI. Work in G.-F. Richard laboratory was generously supported by the Institut Pasteur and the Centre National de la Recherche Scientifique (CNRS).

References

1. Richard G-F (2015) Shortening trinucleotide repeats using highly specific endonucleases: a possible approach to gene therapy? Trends Genet 31(4):177–186
2. Choulika A, Perrin A, Dujon B, Nicolas JF (1995) Induction of homologous recombination in mammalian chromosomes by using the I-SceI system of Saccharomyces cerevisiae. Mol Cell Biol 15(4):1968–1973
3. Colleaux L et al (1986) Universal code equivalent of a yeast mitochondrial intron reading frame is expressed into E. Coli as a specific double strand break endonuclease. Cell 44:521–533
4. Colleaux L, D'Auriol L, Galibert F, Dujon B (1988) Recognition and cleavage site of the intron-encoded omega transposase. Proc Natl Acad Sci U S A 85(16):6022–6026
5. Arnould S et al (2006) Engineering of large numbers of highly specific homing endonucleases that induce recombination on novel DNA targets. J Mol Biol 355(3):443–458
6. Kim YG, Cha J, Chandrasegaran S (1996) Hybrid restriction enzymes: zinc finger fusions to Fok I cleavage domain. Proc Natl Acad Sci U S A 93:1156–1160
7. Christian M et al (2010) Targeting DNA double-strand breaks with TAL effector nucleases. Genetics 186(2):757–761
8. Chen JS, Dagdas YS, Kleinstiver BP, Welch MM, Sousa AA, Harrington LB, Sternberg SH, Joung JK, Yildiz A, Doudna JA (2017) Enhanced proofreading governs CRISPR-Cas9 targeting accuracy. Nature 550:407–410
9. Moynahan ME, Pierce AJ, Jasin M (2001) BRCA2 is required for homology-directed repair of chromosomal breaks. Molecular Cell 7:263–272
10. DiCarlo JE et al (2013) Genome engineering in Saccharomyces cerevisiae using CRISPR-Cas systems. Nucleic Acids Res 41(7):4336–4343
11. Sikorski RS, Hieter P (1989) A system of shuttle vectors and yeast host strains designed for efficient manipulation of DNA in Saccharomyces cerevisiae. Genetics 122:19–27

Chapter 8

Analysis of Trinucleotide Repeat Stability by Integration at a Chromosomal Ectopic Site

Rujuta Yashodhan Gadgil, S. Dean Rider Jr., Todd Lewis, Joanna Barthelemy, and Michael Leffak

Abstract

Expansions of CNG microsatellite tracts are responsible for several neurodegenerative diseases, including myotonic dystrophy type 1, Huntington disease, and spinocerebellar ataxia type 8. Here we show that expanded $(CNG)_n$ repeats are susceptible not only to expansions and contractions, but are prone to DNA double strand breaks following replication stress. We describe a general strategy for the construction of clonal cell lines containing CNG repeats of various lengths, in which the microsatellites are integrated using the yeast FLP recombinase at a single ectopic recombination acceptor site in the HeLa genome. We illustrate two types of (CTG/CAG) cell lines, one of which contains dual fluorescent marker genes flanking the (CTG/CAG) repeat, and one which does not. We show that long CNG repeats are prone to DNA double strand breaks (DSBs) upon exposure of these cell lines to prolonged replication stress.

Key words Microsatellite, Trinucleotide repeat, FLP recombinase, Chromosome ectopic site, Ganciclovir, Polymerase chain reaction (PCR), Small-pool PCR, DNA double strand break, Flow cytometry

1 Introduction

Microsatellite sequences, also known as short tandem repeats (STRs) or simple sequence repeats (SSRs), are tandemly repeated tracts of 1–6 bp. These repeats comprise approximately 3% of the human genome [1], with high mutability making them informative genetic markers. Trinucleotide repeats (TNRs) represent a small subfamily of microsatellites which are of special interest because they are prone to length instability, which is attributed to their tendency to form non-B DNA structures during DNA replication and repair [2–4]. Although TNRs (≥6 units) represent only ~0.0005% of the genome [5], TNR expansion has been linked to more than 35 neuromuscular or neurodegenerative diseases [6–8].

TNR instability has been studied extensively in plasmid and chromosomal model systems of bacteria, yeast, and metazoans [9–18].

Guy-Franck Richard (ed.), *Trinucleotide Repeats: Methods and Protocols*, Methods in Molecular Biology, vol. 2056,
https://doi.org/10.1007/978-1-4939-9784-8_8,

In yeast, TNR sequences not only undergo length instability (expansions and contractions), but also induce chromosome fragility (DNA double strand breaks, DSBs) [19–22]. In general, increasing the length of trinucleotide repeats increases replication stalling [17, 23–25], however, the relationship between fork stalling and chromosome breakage is complex. Thus, the fragility of unstable repeats may be mitigated by multiple factors including replication fork remodeling, helicase unwinding, and postreplication repair [13, 26–29].

In humans, complex genome rearrangements (CGRs) have been postulated to arise from replication-dependent DNA double strand breaks. Based on the proximity of breakpoint junction sequences to repetitive elements, the diversity of nonrecurrent copy number variations (CNVs), and multiple iterative template switch signatures of replicative repair-based mechanisms such as Fork Stalling and Template Switching (FoSTeS) and Microhomology-Mediated Break-Induced Replication (MMBIR), replication-dependent mechanisms have been implicated in the complex genome rearrangements characteristic of human tumors and several developmental defects termed chromoanagenesis [30–33].

The coding strand of the dystrophia myotonica protein kinase gene (DMPK, chr19q13.32, NCBI Gene ID 1760) contains a CTG repeat in its 3′ untranslated region. Expansion of the CTG tract to greater than 37 repeats is associated with the appearance of symptoms of myotonic dystrophy 1 (DM1, MIM#160900), while the most severely affected patients can have expansions of >1000 repeats. The length instability of CTG repeats has been related to their tendency to form hairpin or slipped strand structures [3, 34–36]; however, the susceptibility of expanded CTG repeats to DSBs during replication or repair has received limited attention in human cells [29].

We have used the FLP recombinase system to integrate a donor DNA construct stably into a single-copy acceptor locus at a specific location in the human (HeLa) genome. Our laboratory previously constructed the HeLa/406 acceptor line that contains a single integrated ectopic FLP Recombinase Target (FRT) site (Fig. 1). The acceptor cell line was verified by Southern blot for single insertion of the FRT site [37, 38]. RPE1 [39] and HEK293 [40–42] FRT acceptor cell lines are available commercially.

In HeLa/406 cells, FLP recombinase specifically targets the ectopic 48 bp FRT acceptor site in the genome and in a donor plasmid to integrate the plasmid into that location (chromosome 18p11.22 [37, 38]. FLP recombination leads to duplication of the FRT sequence (Fig. 1). In the current systems, $(CTG)_n$ microsatellites were integrated at the ectopic FRT site in HeLa/406 cells and were bordered by the c-myc replication origin core [3, 37, 43]. To aid in the selection of site-specific recombinants, the chromosomal FRT is flanked by bacterial hygromycin phosphotransferase (Hyg) and herpes simplex virus (HSV) thymidine kinase (TK) genes.

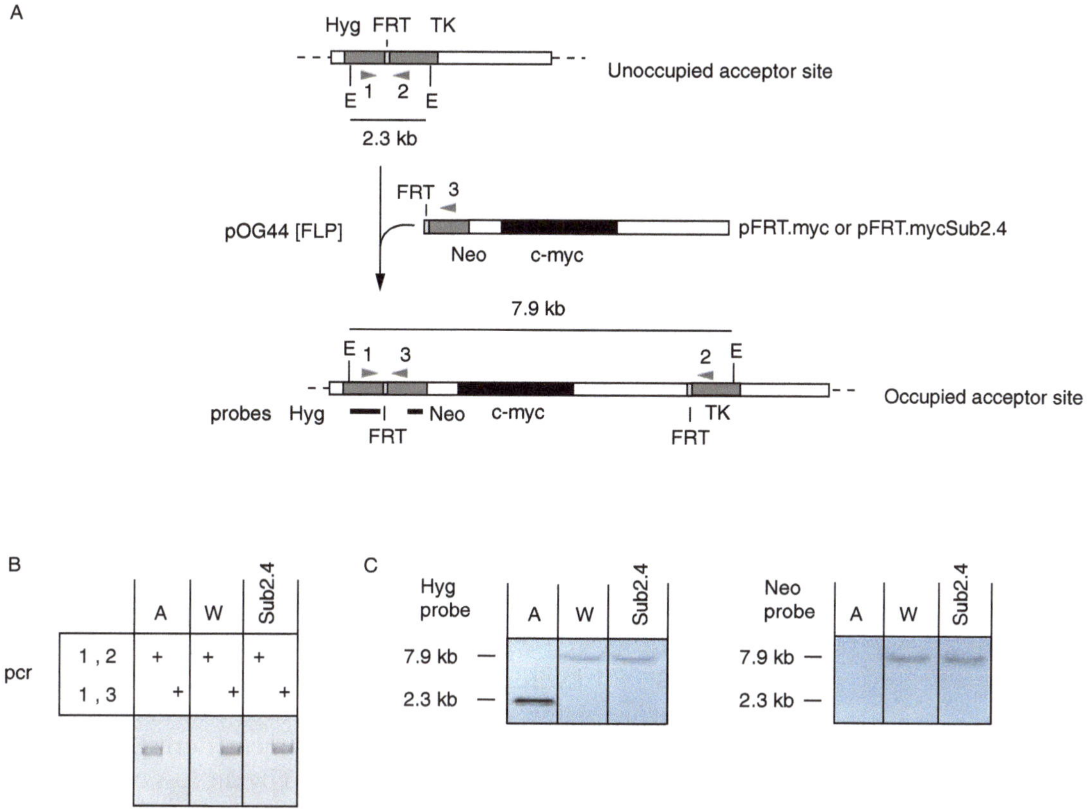

Fig. 1 Ectopic site integration by FLP recombinase (**a**) The acceptor site plasmid pHyg.FRT.TK [38] was transfected into HeLa cells, and clonal cell lines were screened for single copy integration. 406 cells are the HeLa acceptor cell subline containing a single chromosomal copy of the plasmid pHyg.FRT.TK (shown linearized at its *Bgl*II sites) at chromosome 18p11.22 [2–5], representing an unoccupied chromosomal acceptor site. HeLa/406 cells were transfected with the FLP recombinase expression vector p0G44 [9] and the donor plasmids pFRT.myc(CTG)$_{23}$ or pFRT.myc(CTG)$_{100}$. Integrants were selected for resistance to G418 and ganciclovir (GCV). Hyg, hygromycin resistance gene; FRT, FLP recombinase target site; TK, herpes simplex virus thymidine kinase gene. Unfilled rectangles are vector sequences. pFRT.myc (shown linearized) contains the 2.4-kb *Hin*dIII/*Xho*I fragment of the c-*myc* origin. pFRT.myc.Sub2.4 contains the non-origin *Xho*I/*Eco*RV fragment of c-*myc* DNA in place of the *Hin*dIII/*Not*I fragment; the 3′ 46-bp *Not*I/*Xho*I segment of the 2.4-kb *Hin*dIII/*Xho*I fragment is retained in pFRT.myc.Sub2.4. Neo, G418 resistance gene with promoter replaced by FRT. Plasmids are described in detail in [37]. The positions of restriction sites (E, *Eco*RI) and probes (solid bars; Hyg, 756-bp *Eco*RI/*Xba*I fragment of pHyg.FRT.TK; Neo, 405-bp *Nco*I/*Sma*I fragment of pFRT.myc) relevant to Southern analyses are shown. Unrearranged, single copy recombination of the donor plasmids was confirmed by PCR and Southern blotting (**b**) Diagnostic PCR using primers 1 and 2 or 1 and 3 (Table 1) with DNA from 406 acceptor cells (A) with an unoccupied FRT acceptor site and DNA from cells containing the wild type c-*myc* origin fragment (pFRT.myc) (W) or pFRT.myc.Sub2.4 c-myc DNA (Sub2.4) at the acceptor site. PCR primers 1 and 2 give products diagnostic for the unoccupied acceptor site and primers 1 and 3 for the occupied acceptor site (**c**) Hybridization with the Hyg or Neo probe to *Eco*RI-digested DNA from 406 acceptor cells (A) or from 406 cells containing the wild-type c-*myc* origin fragment (W) or pFRT.myc.Sub2.4 (Sub2.4) at the acceptor site

Before insertion of donor DNA at the FRT site, the HeLa/406 acceptor cells are resistant to hygromycin and sensitive to the nucleoside analog ganciclovir (GCV). Once a derivative of the pFRT.myc donor plasmid is integrated into the FRT site, the TK open reading frame is replaced by the promoterless neomycin phosphotransferase (Neo) gene in the donor plasmid. Expression of the Hyg/Neo fusion protein renders the cells resistant to hygromycin and neomycin (G418). Integration of the donor plasmid disrupts the Hyg/TK gene and makes the cells resistant to ganciclovir [38, 44, 45]. Commercially available FLP cells utilize other selectable drug markers (hygromycin, Zeocin).

The clonal cell lines pFRT.myc$(CTG)_{102}$ and pFRT.myc$(CAG)_{102}$ each contain a single ectopic integrant of the human 2.4 kb c-myc core replication origin flanked by a $(CTG/CAG)_{102}$ microsatellite tract (Fig. 2) [29]. When replicated from the flanking c-myc origin, pFRT.myc$(CTG)_{102}$ cells or pFRT.myc$(CAG)_{102}$ cells, respectively, have the CTG repeat or the CAG repeat in the lagging strand template. To assess fragility at (CTG/CAG) microsatellites in pFRT.myc$(CTG)_{102}$ and pFRT.myc$(CAG)_{102}$ cells during prolonged replication stress, FANCJ was knocked down using siRNA in the presence of 0.3 mM hydroxyurea. The FANCJ helicase is one of the Fanconi anemia pathway proteins required to stabilize processive DNA synthesis and replication fork movement during replication stress [46–52]. DNA DSBs were monitored by the loss of small pool PCR signal across the ectopic (CTG/CAG) microsatellite.

A second type of ectopic microsatellite cell lines containing dual fluorescent (DF) reporter genes was also engineered to examine microsatellite fragility via flow cytometry. In DF.myc$(CTG)_{100}$ cells and DF.myc$(CTG)_{23}$ cells the microsatellites are flanked by Tomato and eGFP reporter genes (Fig. 3). DNA double strand breaks induced by replication stress could be evidenced by loss of one or both fluorescent reporter genes (Fig. 4).

2 Materials

Prepare all solutions using ultrapure water (prepared by purifying deionized water to 18 MΩ·cm at 25 °C) and analytical grade reagents. Reagents that cannot be autoclaved are sterilized by ultrafiltration.

2.1 Cell Line Construction

1. Dulbecco's Modified Eagle Medium 1× (DMEM): +4.5 g/l glucose, +L-glutamine, −pyruvate.
2. Fetal bovine serum (FBS). Added to DMEM to 10% (v/v) of final volume.
3. Newborn calf serum (NCS). Added to DMEM to 10% (v/v) of final volume.

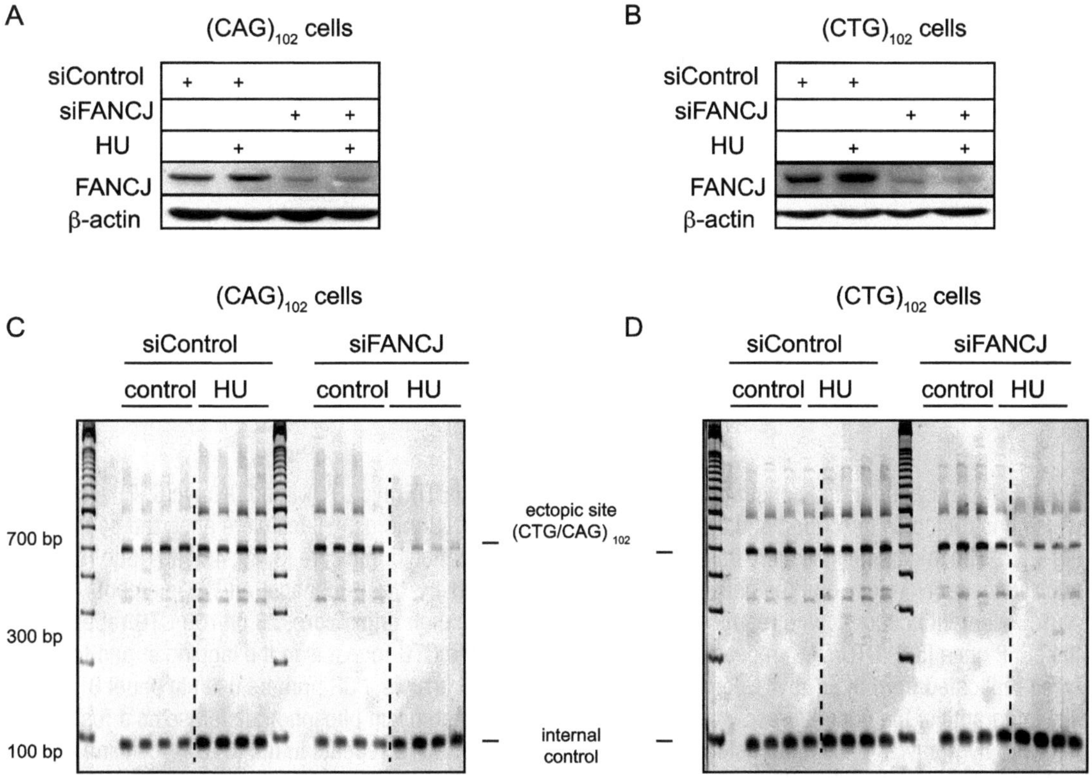

Fig. 2 FANCJ knockdown leads to loss of ectopic CTG/CAG microsatellite signals in $(CTG)_{102}$ and $(CAG)_{102}$ cells under replication stress (**a**, **b**) Western blots. Whole cell extracts were isolated after treatment of cells with siControl or siFANCJ for a total of five transfections, and 0.3 mM hydroxyurea, or parallel untreated cultures, and immunoblotted for FANCJ (**c**, **d**) Duplex small pool PCR with primers spanning the ectopic $(CAG/CTG)_{102}$ repeats and primers for a nonrepeat internal PCR control site. DNA was amplified by small pool PCR (spPCR) using primers within 85 bp 5′ and 3′ to the ectopic $(CTG/CAG)_{102}$ repeats, in the presence of an internal PCR control primer set. In contrast to repeat expansions and contractions observed after repeated cycles of replication inhibition and restart [3, 36, 56], the spPCR signal of the ectopic $(CTG/CAG)_{102}$ repeats was dramatically decreased in DNA from cells depleted of FANCJ and treated continuously with HU (Fig. 2). The polarity of DNA replication relative to the c-myc origin did not affect the sensitivity of the microsatellite to replication stress. These results are consistent with double strand DNA breaks occurring within 85 bp of the $(CTG/CAG)_{102}$ tract that separates the flanking PCR primers. (Reproduced with permission of the publisher, Oxford University Press [29])

4. Cloning rings/cylinders.
5. PCR primers (Table 1).
6. 10× PCR buffer: 100 mM Tris–HCl (pH 8.0), 500 mM KCl, 15 mM $MgCl_2$
7. Geneticin/G418 (*see* **Note 1**).
8. Ganciclovir/GCV.
9. HeLa/406 cells containing a single FRT integration [38] were derived from HeLa cells (ATCC CCL-2). There are also multiple commercially available cell lines containing single copy FRT integrations from Thermo-Fisher (Flp-In™-CV-1,

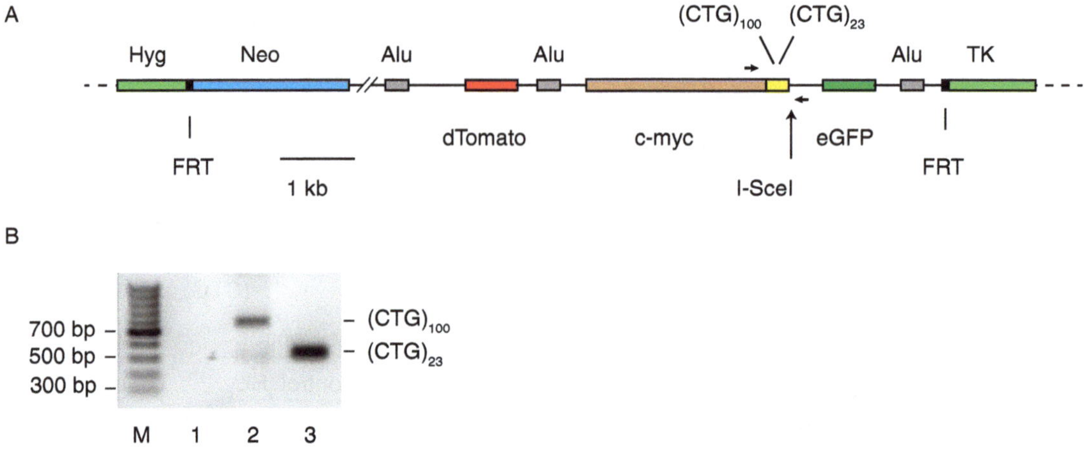

Fig. 3 Ectopically Integrated constructs in DF.myc(CTG)$_n$ cell lines. DF.myc(CTG)$_{23}$ and DF.myc(CTG)$_{100}$ cell lines were constructed as described and the lengths of the ectopic CTG microsatellites were analyzed by PCR (*see* Fig. 2) (**a**) The microsatellites were bordered by the c-myc replication origin core [3, 37, 43], an I-Sce I site, and two fluorescent protein marker genes (Tomato, eGFP) flanked by three identical AluYa5 elements. A third AluYa5 element occurs downstream of the 2.4 kb c-myc replication origin core, 23 or 100 CTG repeats, and the eGFP gene [57] (CTG/CAG) repeats are positioned so that the CTG repeat is in the lagging strand template when replicated from the c-myc origin. Leftward and rightward arrows, PCR primers used in panel B. Ectopic site integrants in the dual fluorescence (DF) cell lines express neomycin phosphotransferase as a fusion protein with hygromycin phosphotransferase (**b**) PCR analysis of the CTG repeats in the (CTG)$_{100}$ cell line (lane 2) and the (CTG)$_{23}$ cell line (lane 3)

Flp-In™-293, Flp-In™-BHK, Flp-In™-Jurkat, Flp-In™-3 T3, Flp-In™-CHO, Flp-In™ T-REx™-293) and Ximbio (RPE1 FRT/TR).

10. Hygromycin/Hyg.
11. Lipofectamine 2000 (Used according to manufacturer's instructions, *see* **Note 2**).
12. Opti-MEM reduced serum medium.
13. Plasmid pOG44 (Invitrogen Life Technologies) (*see* **Note 3**).
14. Penicillin/streptomycin solution (10,000 units/ml penicillin and 10 mg/ml streptomycin in 0.9% (w/v) NaCl diluted 1:100 into DMEM to give 100 mg/ml of streptomycin and 100 units/ml of penicillin).
15. Tissue culture dishes.
16. TrypLE™ Express (Thermo-Fisher Invitrogen).
17. Tris-EDTA (TE) buffer: 10 mM Tris–HCl pH 8.0, 1 mM EDTA pH 8.0. Prepare as a 10× stock solution.

2.2 Small Pool PCR (spPCR)

1. E.Z.N.A. Tissue DNA Kit (Omega BioTek/VWR).
2. Gel Red gel stain or equivalent DNA staining solution.
3. HotStarTaq DNA polymerase Master Mix.

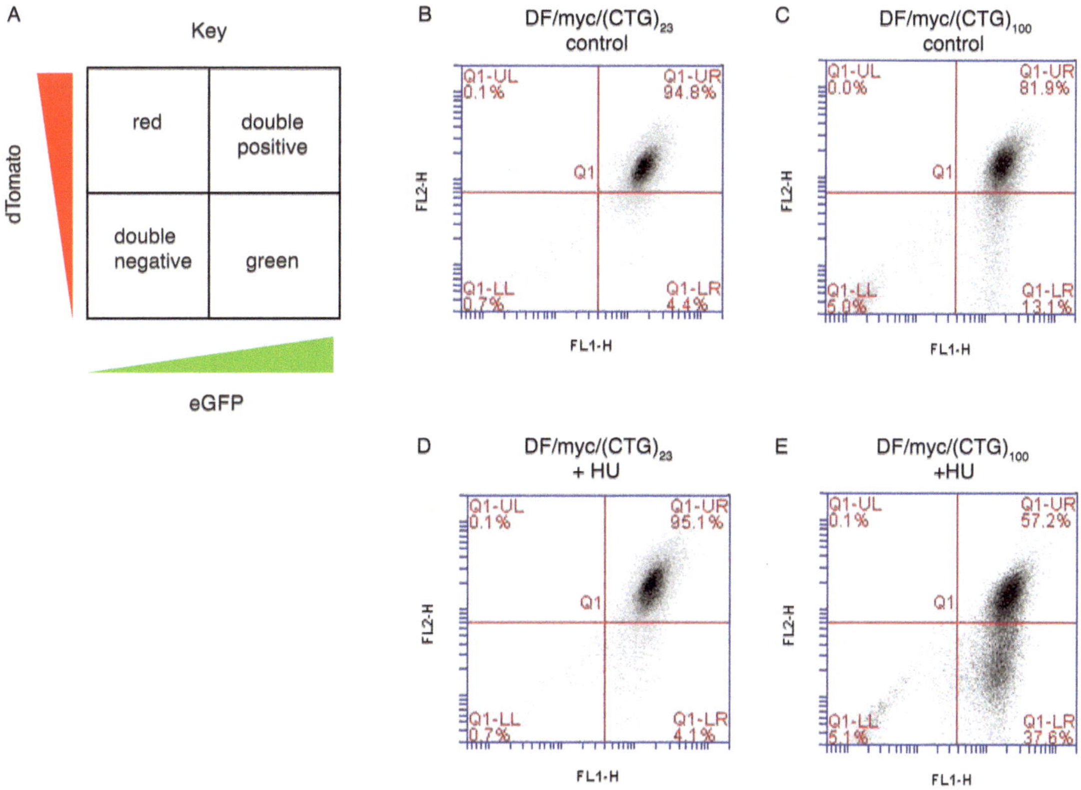

Fig. 4 $(CTG)_n$ length-dependent DNA double strand breaks induced by replication stress. Representative flow cytometry profiles of dual fluorescence cell lines (**a**) key to interpretation of flow cytometry profiles (**b–e**) flow cytometry analysis (**b**) DF/myc$(CTG)_{23}$ cells grown under unperturbed conditions (**c**) DF/myc$(CTG)_{100}$ cells grown under unperturbed conditions (**d**) DF/myc$(CTG)_{23}$ cells treated with hydroxyurea (0.3 mM, 4 days, followed by 8 day recovery in drug-free medium (**e**) DF/myc$(CTG)_{100}$ cells treated with hydroxyurea (0.3 mM, 4 days, followed by 8 day recovery in drug-free medium. The DF.myc$(CTG)_{100}$ cell line and the DF.myc$(CTG)_{23}$ cells express both the dTomato and eGFP reporter genes, appeared in the upper right quadrant (yellow, double positive) when analyzed by flow cytometry. In the DF.myc$(CTG)_{100}$ cells, approximately 13% of cells had spontaneously lost the red reporter (lower right quadrant, green) and 5–6% of cells had lost both reporters (lower left quadrant, double negative). This result suggests that the expanded $(CTG)_{100}$ repeat shows a significant basal level of instability during unperturbed growth. When DF.myc$(CTG)_{23}$ and DF.myc$(CTG)_{100}$ cells were treated with low dose hydroxyurea an increase in the percentage of green (lower right quadrant) DF.myc$(CTG)_{100}$ cells was seen which was not evident in the HU treated DF.myc$(CTG)_{23}$ cells

4. FANCJ siRNA (siGENOME SMARTpool M-010587).
5. Negative control nontargeting siRNA.
6. siPort NeoFX transfection reagent (*see* **Note 4**).
7. PCR primers (Table 1, *see* **Note 5**).
8. Hydroxyurea.
9. Tris–Acetate–EDTA buffer 1×: 40 mM Tris–acetate,1 mM EDTA, pH 8.3.
10. 8% polyacrylamide gel (37.5:1 acrylamide–bisacrylamide).

Table 1
PCR primers used

Diagnostic PCR primers (Subheading 3.1)	
1 (Forward)	5′ TGACTGGAGCGAGGCGAT
2 (reverse)	5′ GCAGTAGCGTGGGCATTT
3 (reverse)	5′ TCAGAGCAGCCGATTGTCT
spPCR primers (Subheading 3.2)	
Ectopic site (forward) (CTG PCR forward primer)	5′ AAAAAAGATCCTCTCTCGCTAATCTCCG
Ectopic site (reverse) (CTG PCR reverse primer)	5′ GGAAGGAGCTGACTGGGTTGAAGG
Internal control (forward) (chromosome 19q13.3)	5′ CTCACTGGTCACTGGTTTCTT
Internal control (reverse) (chromosome 19q13.3)	5′ CCAACCCAACTTCATCCTCTAC

2.3 Flow Cytometry

1. Phosphate-buffered saline (PBS): 120 mM NaCl, 25 mM KCl, 10 mM Na_2HPO4, 3 mM KH_2PO4, pH 7.4. This solution can be made up at 10× concentration, but pH should be checked on dilution.
2. Flow cytometer.

3 Methods

Transfect the acceptor cell line HeLa/406 [37] with the FLP recombinase expression vector pOG44, and one of the experimental donor plasmid constructs (pFRT.myc$(CTG)_n$) at a molar ratio of 8:1 pOG44:donor construct. Within the donor construct is a promoterless neomycin resistance gene (G418^r) that forms a Hyg-Neo fusion gene after successful insertion into the acceptor cell line. Accurate integration inactivates the HSV thymidine kinase (HSV TK) gene making the successfully recombined cells resistant to ganciclovir. Twenty-four hours after transfection, select transfected cells with 600 μg/ml G418 for 14–21 days. For the following 8 days, select integrant cells with 20 μM ganciclovir for 48 h and then switch back to G418 for 48 h.

3.1 pFRT.Myc(CTG/CAG)n Cell Line Construction

1. Plate 1–3 × 10^5 cells in DMEM/10% newborn calf serum (NCS) in each well of a 24-well plate so that the wells are ~90% confluent on the day of transfection.
2. For each well in the dish that is to be transfected, a total of 2.5 μg of supercoiled plasmid is used for transfection (*see* **Note 3**). Add DNA to 250 μl of Opti-MEM serum free medium.

Add this solution to 250 μl of Opti-MEM containing 12 μl of Lipofectamine 2000 and incubate for 20 min at room temperature (*see* **Note 2**). Add the 500 μl of medium containing the DNA–lipid complex to one well of cells (refer to the Lipofectamine 2000 protocol for further details of the transfection). The ratio of the donor plasmid (pFRT.myc or its derivatives) to the FLP recombinase expression plasmid pOG44 [53] should be optimized (the insert sequence and size of the donor plasmid can affect integration efficiency). The lowest molar ratio is 8:1, that is, 8 mol pOG44:1 mol pFRT.myc donor plasmid.

3. Trypsinize cells 24 h after transfection, and transfer all of the cells from one well to one 15 cm diameter plate.
4. Add DMEM/NCS medium with G418 (600 μg/ml active component (*see* **Note 1**), 1.5 times as concentrated as that cited in ref. [37]).
5. Change the growth medium every fourth day, keeping 600 μg/ml G418 (*see* **Note 6**).
6. Monitor cells daily. After 14–21 days cells can be visualized from below the plate to have formed colonies; these mother colonies should be circled accurately from below (*see* **Notes 7–9**).
7. Change the medium to DMEM/NCS + 20 μM GCV for 2 days, then DMEM/NCS + G418 medium (400 μg/ml active component) for 2 days, then DMEM/NCS + 20 μM GCV medium for 2 days. GCV selects for cells that do not express HSV thymidine kinase, since the HSV TK gene is interrupted if there is a successful integration (*see* **Notes 7–9**).
8. Pick single surviving mother colonies with cloning discs or micropipette tips (*see* **Note 10**).
9. Transfer colonies into individual wells of a 24-well plate. To be certain that each well contains cells from an independent colony, harvest only one colony from each 15 cm plate. Maintain colonies in DMEM supplemented with 10% fetal bovine serum/FBS or 10% newborn calf serum/NCS, 1% penicillin/streptomycin and 5% CO_2 at 37 °C.
10. Do not apply drug selection until the colonies have expanded (*see* **Note 11**).
11. Transfer each colony to a 10 cm diameter plate in DMEM/NCS + GCV (20 μM) for 2 days. Add fresh medium including 400 μg/ml G418 (with 500 μg/ml Hyg, if there is a concern that there may be contaminating HeLa cells) (*see* **Notes 12** and **13**).
12. Expand colonies until there are enough to freeze approximately half of them (liquid N_2). Process remaining cells for PCR, qPCR, or Southern blotting.

13. To verify correct integration as determined by the presence of PCR product and PCR product size [8], perform PCR with a primer complementary to the acceptor site and a second primer complementary to the donor plasmid [37] so that the PCR product will cross the insertion junction. Use 50 nanograms of genomic DNA for PCR with diagnostic primer sets for either the unoccupied chromosomal acceptor site (primers 1 + 2, Table 1 and Fig. 1) or the acceptor site after integration of the donor plasmid (primers 1 + 3, Table 1 and Fig. 1).
14. Run PCR reactions in 1× buffer containing 0.2 mM each of dGTP, dCTP, dATP, and dTTP, 1.25 U of HotStar Taq DNA polymerase, and 25 pmol of each primer for the following amplification regimen after an initial dwell at 94 °C for 15 min: 94 °C for 30 s, 55 °C for 30 s, and 72 °C for 30 s, for a total of 30 cycles.
15. Perform Southern blotting with Hyg and Neo probes to verify accurate (Hyg probe), and single copy (Neo probe) integrations or qPCR (donor plasmid PCR) to verify single copy insertion (Fig. 1) using standard methods with 10 μg of genomic DNA and either the 756-bp EcoRI/XbaI fragment of the Hyg gene from plasmid pFRT.Hyg.TK or the 405-bp NcoI/SmaI fragment of the Neo gene from pFRT.myc [37] as probes.

3.2 Detection of DSBs by Small-Pool PCR (spPCR)

1. Grow cell lines in Dulbecco's modified Eagle's medium (DMEM) supplemented with 10% fetal bovine serum/FBS at 37 °C and 5% CO_2.
2. Treat $(CTG/CAG)_n$ cells with 0.3 mM HU for a total of 10 days. Harvest cells on the tenth day of treatment using TrypLE™ Express, a trypsin alternative.
3. Transfect $(CTG/CAG)_n$ cells at a confluency of 60% with siPort NeoFX transfection reagent and 100 nM (final concentration) of pooled small interfering RNAs (siRNAs) (an equal molar mixture of four different siRNAs targeting FANCJ), in a 6-well plate every 48 h, for a total of five transfections, in the presence of hydroxyurea.
4. Harvest cells using TrypLE™ Express 48 h after the fifth transfection. Carry out control experiments in parallel using negative control nontargeting siRNA.
5. After treatment with siRNA and HU, isolate DNA using an E.Z.N.A ® Tissue DNA Kit. Perform PCR on a small amount (10–20 haploid genome equivalents) of DNA template (~50 pg of genomic DNA) per reaction. Perform four small-pool PCR (spPCR) reactions on DNA from each experimental condition (Table 1), in the presence of HotStar Taq polymerase. Amplification conditions are 95 °C (15 min); 35 cycles

of 94 °C (1 min), 54 °C (45 s), 72 °C (1 min); and final extension at 72 °C (7 min), although amplification conditions should be optimized for each primer set. Resolve PCR products in nondenaturing 8% polyacrylamide/Tris-Acetate-EDTA gels. Stained gels are imaged using a Fuji LAS-3000 and ImageReader software (Fig. 2).

3.3 Detection of DSBs by Flow Cytometry

The dual fluorescence cell lines DF.myc$(CTG)_{23}$ and DF.myc$(CTG)_{100}$ (Fig. 3) are constructed and characterized for targeted integration as described above. In addition to the microsatellite repeats, these cell lines contain the c-myc replication origin core [3, 37, 43], an I-Sce I site, and two fluorescent protein marker genes (Tomato, eGFP) flanked by three identical AluYa5 elements, which are potential targets for homology directed DSB repair.

1. Treat cells with a low dose of hydroxyurea (0.3 mM) added to the medium 24 h after plating. Cells are treated with HU for 4 days and allowed to recover in drug-free medium for 8 days. The half-lives of eGFP and Tomato reporter proteins are approximately 24 h [54, 55], therefore 4–8 days are allowed after HU treatment for degradation of the preexisting reporter proteins.
2. Harvest cells and collect them in 1.5 ml Eppendorf tubes and centrifuge at 300 × *g* for 3 min. Aspirate growth medium, wash cells with cold PBS and spin down at 300 × *g* for 3 min. After a final wash with PBS, analyze cells directly using a flow cytometer. The fluorescent proteins are excited using a 488 nm laser and detected with emission filters of 530 nm (eGFP) and 585 nm (dTomato) (Fig. 4).

4 Notes

1. Geneticin/G418 concentrations are given as the concentration of the active component (often ~70% of total G418).
2. Lipofectamine 2000 can be toxic to some cell types. Transfection time may require optimization. Reasonable results can be obtained in some cell types with as little as 90 min exposure to the Lipofectamine/DNA complex.
3. Amplified plasmid should be purified using an endotoxin-free kit (e.g., IBI Scientific Maxi Fast-Ion Plasmid Kit or Qiagen Endofree Plasmid Maxi kit).
4. Used according to manufacturer's instructions for reverse transfection.
5. Primers are at 100 μM in Tris-EDTA (TE) buffer.

6. 600 μg/ml G418 will speed up the screening and clean the plate.
7. Two days of GCV treatment are sufficient to induce DNA damage in most TK^+ cells, however GCV treatment can be extended to 10–12 days. TK^+ cells will continue to die once the GCV is removed due to the DNA damage incurred during the drug treatment.
8. Drug-resistant colonies that are small, healthy, and dividing will contain 2^N cells.
9. In addition to variation in the efficiency of transfection, the FLP recombinase-mediated integration is a rare event. Typically, between 5 and 20 foci should be expected within 10 days of transfection. Mother colonies can be very low in number, and their detection can be painstaking work. Carefully monitoring and marking the mother colonies are key steps that will reduce your subsequent work. If no colonies are visible after 15–20 days, all media, reagents, plasmids, and cells should be re-verified.
10. To pick individual foci, we use either a sterile pipette tip to scrape cells from a single, well-separated colony, or autoclaved cloning rings. To use a cloning ring, mark the position of the colony on the bottom of the plate and remove the medium. Wash the plate carefully with warmed PBS. Spread a very thin layer of vacuum grease on the ring and place over the colony. Avoid any overlapping colonies. If desired, add 50 μl of trypsin to aid in cell detachment. Add 100 μl of medium into the ring and carefully pipette up and down to separate the cells from the plate.
11. Do not use drug in the 24-well step (**step 10**), in order to let the cells grow faster.
12. If there is a concern that the mother colony may contain a mixture of GCV-resistant cells protecting GCV-sensitive cells, cells may be replated at limiting dilution (0.5 cell/well) in a 96-well plate and the drug selection repeated. Although TK^+ HeLa cells are reported to transfer GCV phosphate to TK^- bystander cells, they do not display bystander cytotoxicity [44].
13. If a mixture of integrant and nonintegrant cells is suspected, cells may be replated at limiting dilution (0.5 cell/well) in a 96-well plate and the drug selection repeated.

Acknowledgments

This work was supported by NIH/NIGMS grant GM122976 to M.L., and by the WSU BMS Ph.D. program (T.L., J.B.). We thank David Hitch and French Damewood IV for comments on the manuscript.

References

1. Lander ES, Linton LM, Birren B, Nusbaum C, Zody MC, Baldwin J, Devon K, Dewar K, Doyle M, FitzHugh W, Funke R, Gage D, Harris K, Heaford A, Howland J, Kann L, Lehoczky J, LeVine R, McEwan P, McKernan K, Meldrim J, Mesirov JP, Miranda C, Morris W, Naylor J, Raymond C, Rosetti M, Santos R, Sheridan A, Sougnez C, Stange-Thomann Y, Stojanovic N, Subramanian A, Wyman D, Rogers J, Sulston J, Ainscough R, Beck S, Bentley D, Burton J, Clee C, Carter N, Coulson A, Deadman R, Deloukas P, Dunham A, Dunham I, Durbin R, French L, Grafham D, Gregory S, Hubbard T, Humphray S, Hunt A, Jones M, Lloyd C, McMurray A, Matthews L, Mercer S, Milne S, Mullikin JC, Mungall A, Plumb R, Ross M, Shownkeen R, Sims S, Waterston RH, Wilson RK, Hillier LW, McPherson JD, Marra MA, Mardis ER, Fulton LA, Chinwalla AT, Pepin KH, Gish WR, Chissoe SL, Wendl MC, Delehaunty KD, Miner TL, Delehaunty A, Kramer JB, Cook LL, Fulton RS, Johnson DL, Minx PJ, Clifton SW, Hawkins T, Branscomb E, Predki P, Richardson P, Wenning S, Slezak T, Doggett N, Cheng JF, Olsen A, Lucas S, Elkin C, Uberbacher E, Frazier M, Gibbs RA, Muzny DM, Scherer SE, Bouck JB, Sodergren EJ, Worley KC, Rives CM, Gorrell JH, Metzker ML, Naylor SL, Kucherlapati RS, Nelson DL, Weinstock GM, Sakaki Y, Fujiyama A, Hattori M, Yada T, Toyoda A, Itoh T, Kawagoe C, Watanabe H, Totoki Y, Taylor T, Weissenbach J, Heilig R, Saurin W, Artiguenave F, Brottier P, Bruls T, Pelletier E, Robert C, Wincker P, Smith DR, Doucette-Stamm L, Rubenfield M, Weinstock K, Lee HM, Dubois J, Rosenthal A, Platzer M, Nyakatura G, Taudien S, Rump A, Yang H, Yu J, Wang J, Huang G, Gu J, Hood L, Rowen L, Madan A, Qin S, Davis RW, Federspiel NA, Abola AP, Proctor MJ, Myers RM, Schmutz J, Dickson M, Grimwood J, Cox DR, Olson MV, Kaul R, Raymond C, Shimizu N, Kawasaki K, Minoshima S, Evans GA, Athanasiou M, Schultz R, Roe BA, Chen F, Pan H, Ramser J, Lehrach H, Reinhardt R, McCombie WR, de la Bastide M, Dedhia N, Blocker H, Hornischer K, Nordsiek G, Agarwala R, Aravind L, Bailey JA, Bateman A, Batzoglou S, Birney E, Bork P, Brown DG, Burge CB, Cerutti L, Chen HC, Church D, Clamp M, Copley RR, Doerks T, Eddy SR, Eichler EE, Furey TS, Galagan J, Gilbert JG, Harmon C, Hayashizaki Y, Haussler D, Hermjakob H, Hokamp K, Jang W, Johnson LS, Jones TA, Kasif S, Kaspryzk A, Kennedy S, Kent WJ, Kitts P, Koonin EV, Korf I, Kulp D, Lancet D, Lowe TM, McLysaght A, Mikkelsen T, Moran JV, Mulder N, Pollara VJ, Ponting CP, Schuler G, Schultz J, Slater G, Smit AF, Stupka E, Szustakowki J, Thierry-Mieg D, Thierry-Mieg J, Wagner L, Wallis J, Wheeler R, Williams A, Wolf YI, Wolfe KH, Yang SP, Yeh RF, Collins F, Guyer MS, Peterson J, Felsenfeld A, Wetterstrand KA, Patrinos A, Morgan MJ, de Jong P, Catanese JJ, Osoegawa K, Shizuya H, Choi S, Chen YJ, Szustakowki J, International Human Genome Sequencing C (2001) Initial sequencing and analysis of the human genome. Nature 409:860–921
2. Mirkin SM, Smirnova EV (2002) Positioned to expand. Nat Genet 31:5–6
3. Liu G, Chen X, Bissler JJ, Sinden RR, Leffak M (2010) Replication-dependent instability at (CTG) x (CAG) repeat hairpins in human cells. Nat Chem Biol 6:652–659
4. Ghosh M, Liu G, Randall G, Bevington J, Leffak M (2004) Transcription factor binding and induced transcription alter chromosomal c-myc replicator activity. Mol Cell Biol 24:10193–10207
5. Kozlowski P, de Mezer M, Krzyzosiak WJ (2010) Trinucleotide repeats in human genome and exome. Nucleic Acids Res 38:4027–4039
6. Mirkin SM (2007) Expandable DNA repeats and human disease. Nature 447:932–940
7. Budworth H, McMurray CT (2013) A brief history of triplet repeat diseases. Methods Mol Biol 1010:3–17
8. Liu G, Bissler JJ, Sinden RR, Leffak M (2007) Unstable spinocerebellar ataxia type 10 (ATTCT)*(AGAAT) repeats are associated with aberrant replication at the ATX10 locus and replication origin-dependent expansion at

an ectopic site in human cells. Mol Cell Biol 27:7828–7838
9. Yang Z, Lau R, Marcadier JL, Chitayat D, Pearson CE (2003) Replication inhibitors modulate instability of an expanded trinucleotide repeat at the myotonic dystrophy type 1 disease locus in human cells. Am J Hum Genet 73:1092–1105
10. Gomes-Pereira M, Hilley JD, Morales F, Adam B, James HE, Monckton DG (2014) Disease-associated CAG.CTG triplet repeats expand rapidly in non-dividing mouse cells, but cell cycle arrest is insufficient to drive expansion. Nucleic Acids Res 42:7047–7056
11. Lia AS, Seznec H, Hofmann-Radvanyi H, Radvanyi F, Duros C, Saquet C, Blanche M, Junien C, Gourdon G (1998) Somatic instability of the CTG repeat in mice transgenic for the myotonic dystrophy region is age dependent but not correlated to the relative intertissue transcription levels and proliferative capacities. Hum Mol Genet 7:1285–1291
12. Jarem DA, Wilson NR, Delaney S (2009) Structure-dependent DNA damage and repair in a trinucleotide repeat sequence. Biochemistry 48:6655–6663
13. Viterbo D, Michoud G, Mosbach V, Dujon B, Richard GF (2016) Replication stalling and heteroduplex formation within CAG/CTG trinucleotide repeats by mismatch repair. DNA Repair (Amst) 42:94–106
14. Frizzell A, Nguyen JH, Petalcorin MI, Turner KD, Boulton SJ, Freudenreich CH, Lahue RS (2014) RTEL1 inhibits trinucleotide repeat expansions and fragility. Cell Rep 6:827–835
15. Kovtun IV, McMurray CT (2008) Features of trinucleotide repeat instability in vivo. Cell Res 18:198–213
16. Jackson SM, Whitworth AJ, Greene JC, Libby RT, Baccam SL, Pallanck LJ, La Spada AR (2005) A SCA7 CAG/CTG repeat expansion is stable in Drosophila melanogaster despite modulation of genomic context and gene dosage. Gene 347:35–41
17. Pelletier R, Krasilnikova MM, Samadashwily GM, Lahue R, Mirkin SM (2003) Replication and expansion of trinucleotide repeats in yeast. Mol Cell Biol 23:1349–1357
18. Wojciechowska M, Bacolla A, Larson JE, Wells RD (2005) The myotonic dystrophy type 1 triplet repeat sequence induces gross deletions and inversions. J Biol Chem 280:941–952
19. Freudenreich CH, Kantrow SM, Zakian VA (1998) Expansion and length-dependent fragility of CTG repeats in yeast. Science 279:853–856
20. Freudenreich CH, Lahiri M (2004) Structure-forming CAG/CTG repeat sequences are sensitive to breakage in the absence of Mrc1 checkpoint function and S-phase checkpoint signaling: implications for trinucleotide repeat expansion diseases. Cell Cycle 3:1370–1374
21. Sundararajan R, Gellon L, Zunder RM, Freudenreich CH (2010) Double-strand break repair pathways protect against CAG/CTG repeat expansions, contractions and repeat-mediated chromosomal fragility in Saccharomyces cerevisiae. Genetics 184:65–77
22. Usdin K, House NC, Freudenreich CH (2015) Repeat instability during DNA repair: insights from model systems. Crit Rev Biochem Mol Biol 50:142–167
23. Follonier C, Oehler J, Herrador R, Lopes M (2013) Friedreich's ataxia-associated GAA repeats induce replication-fork reversal and unusual molecular junctions. Nat Struct Mol Biol 20:486–494
24. Voineagu I, Surka CF, Shishkin AA, Krasilnikova MM, Mirkin SM (2009) Replisome stalling and stabilization at CGG repeats, which are responsible for chromosomal fragility. Nat Struct Mol Biol 16:226–228
25. Liu G, Chen X, Gao Y, Lewis T, Barthelemy J, Leffak M (2012) Altered replication in human cells promotes DMPK (CTG)(n). (CAG)(n) repeat instability. Mol Cell Biol 32:1618–1632
26. Shishkin AA, Voineagu I, Matera R, Cherng N, Chernet BT, Krasilnikova MM, Narayanan V, Lobachev KS, Mirkin SM (2009) Large-scale expansions of Friedreich's ataxia GAA repeats in yeast. Mol Cell 35:82–92
27. Daee DL, Mertz T, Lahue RS (2007) Postreplication repair inhibits CAG.CTG repeat expansions in Saccharomyces cerevisiae. Mol Cell Biol 27:102–110
28. Kerrest A, Anand RP, Sundararajan R, Bermejo R, Liberi G, Dujon B, Freudenreich CH, Richard GF (2009) SRS2 and SGS1 prevent chromosomal breaks and stabilize triplet repeats by restraining recombination. Nat Struct Mol Biol 16:159–167
29. Barthelemy J, Hanenberg H, Leffak M (2016) FANCJ is essential to maintain microsatellite structure genome-wide during replication stress. Nucleic Acids Res 44:6803–6816
30. Gu S, Szafranski P, Akdemir ZC, Yuan B, Cooper ML, Magrina MA, Bacino CA, Lalani SR, Breman AM, Smith JL, Patel A, Song RH, Bi W, Cheung SW, Carvalho CM, Stankiewicz P, Lupski JR (2016) Mechanisms for complex chromosomal insertions. PLoS Genet 12:e1006446

31. Lee JA, Carvalho CM, Lupski JR (2007) A DNA replication mechanism for generating nonrecurrent rearrangements associated with genomic disorders. Cell 131:1235–1247
32. Hastings PJ, Ira G, Lupski JR (2009) A microhomology-mediated break-induced replication model for the origin of human copy number variation. PLoS Genet 5:e1000327
33. Holland AJ, Cleveland DW (2012) Chromoanagenesis and cancer: mechanisms and consequences of localized, complex chromosomal rearrangements. Nat Med 18:1630–1638
34. Axford MM, Wang YH, Nakamori M, Zannis-Hadjopoulos M, Thornton CA, Pearson CE (2013) Detection of slipped-DNAs at the trinucleotide repeats of the myotonic dystrophy type I disease locus in patient tissues. PLoS Genet 9:e1003866
35. Voineagu I, Narayanan V, Lobachev KS, Mirkin SM (2008) Replication stalling at unstable inverted repeats: interplay between DNA hairpins and fork stabilizing proteins. Proc Natl Acad Sci U S A 105:9936–9941
36. Liu G, Chen X, Leffak M (2013) Oligodeoxynucleotide binding to (CTG) {middle dot} (CAG) microsatellite repeats inhibits replication fork stalling, hairpin formation, and genome instability. Mol Cell Biol 33:571–581
37. Liu G, Malott M, Leffak M (2003) Multiple functional elements comprise a mammalian chromosomal replicator. Mol Cell Biol 23:1832–1842
38. Malott M, Leffak M (1999) Activity of the c-myc replicator at an ectopic chromosomal location. Mol Cell Biol 19:5685–5695
39. Mansfeld J, Collin P, Collins MO, Choudhary JS, Pines J (2011) APC15 drives the turnover of MCC-CDC20 to make the spindle assembly checkpoint responsive to kinetochore attachment. Nat Cell Biol 13:1234–1243
40. Thankamony SP, Knudson W (2006) Acylation of CD44 and its association with lipid rafts are required for receptor and hyaluronan endocytosis. J Biol Chem 281:34601–34609
41. Weichart D, Gobom J, Klopfleisch S, Hasler R, Gustavsson N, Billmann S, Lehrach H, Seegert D, Schreiber S, Rosenstiel P (2006) Analysis of NOD2-mediated proteome response to muramyl dipeptide in HEK293 cells. J Biol Chem 281:2380–2389
42. Harris EN, Weigel JA, Weigel PH (2004) Endocytic function, glycosaminoglycan specificity, and antibody sensitivity of the recombinant human 190-kDa hyaluronan receptor for endocytosis (HARE). J Biol Chem 279:36201–36209
43. Chen X, Liu G, Leffak M (2013) Activation of a human chromosomal replication origin by protein tethering. Nucleic Acids Res 41:6460–6474
44. Gentry BG, Im M, Boucher PD, Ruch RJ, Shewach DS (2005) GCV phosphates are transferred between HeLa cells despite lack of bystander cytotoxicity. Gene Ther 12:1033–1041
45. Gentry BG, Boucher PD, Shewach DS (2006) Hydroxyurea induces bystander cytotoxicity in cocultures of herpes simplex virus thymidine kinase-expressing and nonexpressing HeLa cells incubated with ganciclovir. Cancer Res 66:3845–3851
46. Suhasini AN, Rawtani NA, Wu Y, Sommers JA, Sharma S, Mosedale G, North PS, Cantor SB, Hickson ID, Brosh RM Jr (2011) Interaction between the helicases genetically linked to Fanconi anemia group J and bloom's syndrome. EMBO J 30:692–705
47. Gupta R, Sharma S, Sommers JA, Kenny MK, Cantor SB, Brosh RM Jr (2007) FANCJ (BACH1) helicase forms DNA damage inducible foci with replication protein A and interacts physically and functionally with the single-stranded DNA-binding protein. Blood 110:2390–2398
48. Wu Y, Shin-ya K, Brosh RM Jr (2008) FANCJ helicase defective in fanconia anemia and breast cancer unwinds G-quadruplex DNA to defend genomic stability. Mol Cell Biol 28:4116–4128
49. Wu Y, Brosh RM Jr (2009) FANCJ helicase operates in the Fanconi Anemia DNA repair pathway and the response to replicational stress. Curr Mol Med 9:470–482
50. Hiom K (2010) FANCJ: solving problems in DNA replication. DNA Repair (Amst) 9:250–256
51. Suhasini AN, Sommers JA, Yu S, Wu Y, Xu T, Kelman Z, Kaplan DL, Brosh RM Jr (2012) DNA repair and replication fork helicases are differentially affected by alkyl phosphotriester lesion. J Biol Chem 287:19188–19198
52. Raghunandan M, Chaudhury I, Kelich SL, Hanenberg H, Sobeck A (2015) FANCD2, FANCJ and BRCA2 cooperate to promote replication fork recovery independently of the Fanconi Anemia core complex. Cell Cycle 14:342–353
53. O'Gorman S, Fox DT, Wahl GM (1991) Recombinase-mediated gene activation and site-specific integration in mammalian cells. Science 251:1351–1355

54. Li X, Zhao X, Fang Y, Jiang X, Duong T, Fan C, Huang CC, Kain SR (1998) Generation of destabilized green fluorescent protein as a transcription reporter. J Biol Chem 273:34970–34975
55. Snapp EL (2009) Fluorescent proteins: a cell biologist's user guide. Trends Cell Biol 19:649–655
56. Barthelemy J, Hanenberg H, Leffak M (2017) FANCJ is essential to maintain microsatellite structure genome-wide during replication stress. Nucleic Acids Res 45:509–511
57. Cormack BP, Valdivia RH, Falkow S (1996) FACS-optimized mutants of the green fluorescent protein (GFP). Gene 173:33–38

Chapter 9

Experimental System to Study Instability of $(CGG)_n$ Repeats in Cultured Mammalian Cells

Artem V. Kononenko, Thomas Ebersole, and Sergei M. Mirkin

Abstract

Expansions of simple trinucleotide repeats, such as $(CGG)_n$, $(CAG)_n$ or $(GAA)_n$, are responsible for more than 40 hereditary disorders in humans including fragile X syndrome, Huntington's disease, myotonic dystrophy, and Friedreich's ataxia. While the mechanisms of repeat expansions were intensively studied for over two decades, the final picture has yet to emerge. It was important, therefore, to develop a mammalian experimental system for studying repeat instability, which would recapitulate repeat instability observed in human pedigrees. Here, we describe a genetically tractable experimental system to study the instability of $(CGG)_n$ repeats in cultured mammalian cells (Kononenko et al., Nat Struct Mol Biol 25:669–676, 2018). It is based on a selectable cassette carrying the HyTK gene under the control of the FMR1 promoter with carrier-size $(CGG)_n$ repeats in its 5′ UTR, which was integrated into the unique RL5 site in murine erythroid leukemia cells. Expansions of these repeats and/or repeat-induced mutagenesis shut down the reporter, which results in the accumulation of ganciclovir-resistance cells. This system is useful for understanding the genetic controls of repeat instability in mammalian cells. In the long run, it can be adjusted to screen for drugs that either alleviate repeat expansions or reactivate the FMR1 promoter.

Key words Trinucleotide repeats, Repeat expansions, Repeat-induced mutagenesis, Fragile X syndrome, Mammalian cell culture, RNA interference

1 Introduction

More than 40 hereditary diseases in humans, largely neurological or neurodegenerative, are caused by the expansions of simple DNA repeats [1]. Most commonly, these are trinucleotide repeats, but there are instances of tetra-, penta-, hexa- and even dodeca-nucleotide repeat expansions. While repeats differ in their sequence composition and their location within a gene, there is one common characteristic for all repeat expansion diseases: expansion of a repeat beyond a certain threshold shuts down its carrier gene or other genes in *trans*, which ultimately leads to disease development [2]. This threshold length can differ significantly: for trinucleotide repeats located in protein coding parts of the genes it is less than

Guy-Franck Richard (ed.), *Trinucleotide Repeats: Methods and Protocols*, Methods in Molecular Biology, vol. 2056, https://doi.org/10.1007/978-1-4939-9784-8_9,

40 copies, while for repeats in the 5′-UTRs, introns or 3′-UTRs of the genes it is around 200 copies.

Given this characteristic, experimental systems to study repeat expansions in cultured eukaryotic cells ranging from yeast to humans have capitalized on the same general principle: repeat-mediated inactivation of a forward selection marker makes cells resistant to a drug, allowing one to detect these events on a specific selective media [3].

Our mammalian experimental system is based on the mechanism of *FMR1* gene silencing mediated by expanded $(CGG)_n$ repeats, which is well known from studies of fragile X syndrome in humans [4]. An *FMR1* locus spans approximately 40 kb on the X chromosome; it has a relatively short promoter region (~400 bp) followed by 17 exons. The $(CGG)_n$ repeats are located in exon 1, ~135 bp downstream from the transcription start site and 99 bp upstream of the translation start codon [5]. In healthy individuals, the number of $(CGG)_n$ repeats ranges from 6 to 30 copies. Intermediate *FMR1* alleles contain 30-to-50 repeats; they are not associated with a disease, but are prone to further expansions [6]. Premutation *FMR1* alleles contain 51-to-200 $(CGG)_n$ repeats. Individuals with premutation alleles are carriers for fragile X syndrome; they can also develop three late-onset disorders: fragile X–associated tremor/ataxia syndrome (FXTAS) [7], fragile X–associated primary ovarian insufficiency (FXPOI) [8], and fragile X–associated diminished ovarian reserve (FXDOR) [9]. Importantly, at this repeat range, expression of the FMR1 gene is not repressed; in fact, the amount of the FMR1 transcript is even slightly elevated [10–12]. Subsequent repeat expansions beyond ~200 copies lead to the full *FMR1* mutation. Full mutation results in the methylation of the *FMR1* promoter and gene silencing [13]. As the repeat continues to expand during intergenerational transmission (it can reach up to 3500 copies), the DNA and histone methylation spreads beyond the *FMR1* locus, ultimately leading to the formation of a later-replicating, megabase-long constitutive heterochromatin zone [14].

We utilized these features of the *FMR1* gene expression in designing our experimental system [15]. Figure 1 shows a schematic of the selectable cassette. Carrier size $(CGG)_n$ repeats were placed downstream of the *FMR1* promoter, replacing the endogenous $(CGG)_n$ repeat, followed by the *HyTK* reporter. In this reporter, the hygromycin phosphotransferase (*hph*) gene is fused in frame with the herpes simplex virus type 1 (HSV-1) thymidine kinase (TK) gene [16]. Consequently, when the *HyTK* gene in ON, cells are resistant to hygromycin and sensitive to ganciclovir,—a guanosine analogue that, upon phosphorylation by TK (and two more rounds of phosphorylation by cellular kinases), incorporates into a growing chain of DNA, thereby triggering apoptosis.

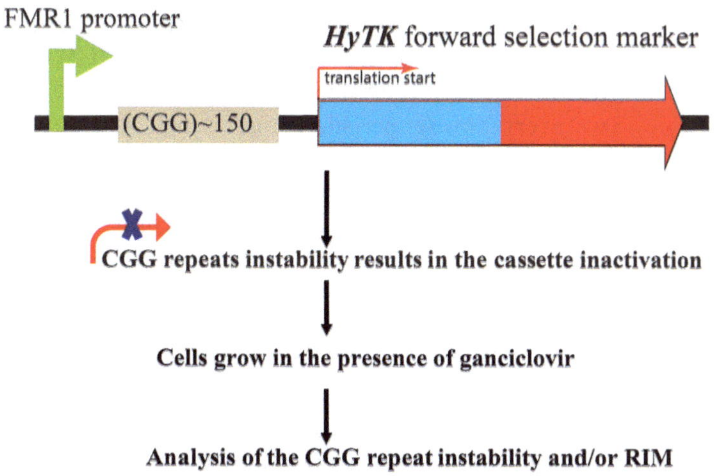

Fig. 1 A selectable cassette to study genome instability caused by $(CGG)_n$ repeats. Large-scale expansions of $(CGG)_n$ repeats and/or repeat-induced mutagenesis lead to the reporter inactivation making cells resistant to ganciclovir. Gc^R clones are then analyzed by PCR and sequencing to detect changes in the repeat length and/or the presence of mutations in the HyTK reporter

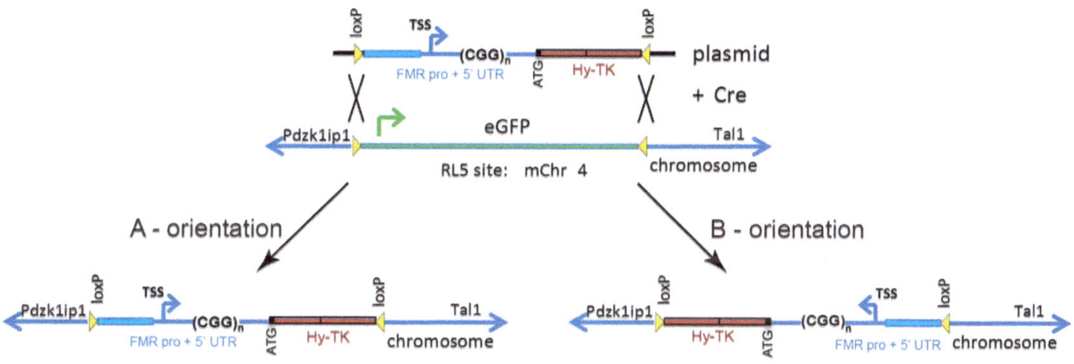

Fig. 2 Integration of a unique copy of the FMR1-CGGn-HyTK cassette into MEL cells. The FMR1-CGG_n-HyTK cassette was integrated into the RL5 locus in MEL cells via Cre-loxP recombination by replacing the eGFP gene. Two orientations of the cassette in this locus are designated as A and B

We reasoned that the reporter inactivation upon repeat expansion or other forms of repeat-mediated instability should make cell resistant to ganciclovir (Fig. 1).

We constructed three FMR-HyTK cassettes with various numbers of repeats: $(CGG)_0$—control, $(CGG)_{53}$—intermediate length, and $(CGG)_{153}$—premutation length. They were then integrated into the RL5 locus located between the Tal1 and Pdzk1ip1 genes on chromosome 4 in murine erythroid leukemia (MEL) cell line [17] (Fig. 2). To this end, we utilized a cell line carrying a eGFP gene flanked by inverted loxP sites at the RL5 site [18]. eGFP was exchanged with loxP-flanked FMR1-$(CGG)_n$-HyTK cassettes via transient Cre-recombinase expression. The RL5 locus was chosen to avert transgene silencing, which commonly happens with transgenes in cultured mammalian cells. The unique feature of this locus is that it is constitutively active transcriptionally, thus, a transgene integrated into it sustains its expression for many months in culture [18]. This feature of the RL5 locus was central to our experimental strategy, since spontaneous silencing of our selectable cassette could create a high background of ganciclovir resistant (Gc^R) clones, which would prevent us from detecting repeat-mediated events.

As our cassettes were flanked by inverted loxP sites, their integration could occur in one of two orientations, which are designated "A" and "B" in Fig. 2. Upon integration of HyTK cassettes with different numbers of CGG repeats, we analyzed individual hygromycin resistant clones to confirm a single copy number for each integrated cassette by qPCR and the integrity of $(CGG)_n$ repeats via PCR and sequencing. This allowed us to create several independent cell lines containing a unique copy of a selectable cassette carrying either 0, 53, or 153 $(CGG)_n$ repeats.

We used the following strategy to detect rare Gc^R clones. Cells carrying various selectable cassettes were first grown without any selection (i.e., in the absence of hygromycin) for 6 days. They were then dispersed into 96-well plates containing 12 μM ganciclovir in the media. After 2–3 weeks of selection the number of ganciclovir resistant subclones was counted for each cell line. Characteristic results are shown in Fig. 3a. One can see that the frequency of Gc^R subclones containing in a cell line with *FMR1*-CGG153-HyTK cassette is ~tenfold higher than in cell lines with either *FMR1*-CGG0-HyTK or *FMR1*-CGG53-HyTK cassettes. Initially we thought that this difference was due to large-scale expansions of the carrier-size $(CGG)_{153}$ repeats leading to the inactivation of the *FMR1* promoter.

Surprisingly, the majority of these Gc^R clones had relatively small-scale expansions or even contractions of the $(CGG)_{153}$ repeat (Fig. 3b). These changes in the repeat length could not be responsible for the promoter silencing, and we confirmed that the reporter is still expressed by qRT-PCR. It appeared that a different mechanism, called RIM (from **r**epeat-**i**nduced **m**utagenesis) [19, 20] could be responsible for the reporter inactivation. We have previously proposed that RIM occurs during the course of break-induced replication (BIR) [19],—a pathway to repair one-ended double-strand breaks in DNA [21, 22]. Several replication and recombination proteins are implicated in BIR in mammals [23, 24]. We have found that the treatment of cells containing the *FMR1*-CGG153-HyTK cassette with siRNAs against those genes,

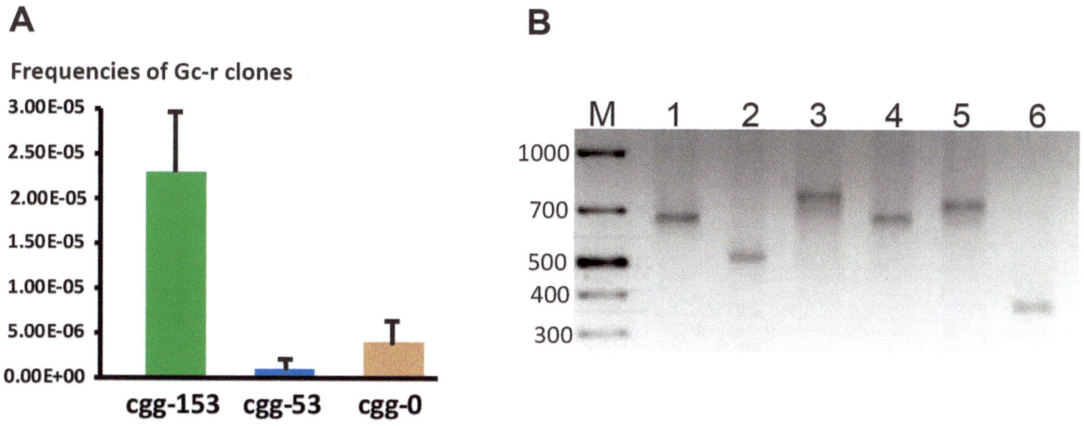

Fig. 3 Analysis of Gc^R subclones obtained in our experimental system. (**a**) Frequencies of Gc^R subclones recovered for cells with CGG153-HyTK, CGG53-HyTK and CGG0-HyTK cassette. (**b**) Sample PCR across the (CGG)153 run showing expanded (lanes 3 and 5), contracted (lanes 2 and 6) and unchanged repeats (lanes 1 and 4). (Adapted from [15] with modifications)

including *POLD3*, *RAD52*, *RAD51* and others, dramatically reduced the number of Gc^R subclones. A hallmark of BIR is the appearance of complex mutations. We have found many complex mutations inactivating the HyTK gene in Gc^R subclones from the cell line with the *FMR1*-CGG153-HyTK cassette. No complex mutations were found in Gc^R subclones in cell lines with the zero-repeat control or *FMR1*-CGG53-HyTK cassettes. Furthermore, sequencing of Gc^R clones recovered upon PolD3 inactivation in *FMR1*-CGG153-HyTK cells revealed the lack of complex mutations [15].

Overall, the majority of Gc^R clones originating in the cell line with the carrier-size $(CGG)_{153}$ repeat in our selectable cassette demonstrate a unique mutational signature: a change in repeat length concurrent with mutagenesis in the reporter gene. Our working model explaining this signature is presented in Fig. 4 [15]. A one-ended DSB results from the replication fork stalling at carrier-size $(CGG)_n$ repeats [25]. Following the end resection, a 3′- repetitive overhang is produced. This repetitive overhang can then invade the sister chromatid using Rad52 and Rad51 proteins to create a single D-loop. Subsequently, this D-loop is extended via conservative DNA synthesis mediated by DNA polymerase delta. Since the 3′-end of the invading strand contains a long repetitive run, the invasion might occur out-of-register, resulting in repeat expansion or contraction. In addition, the conservative nature of DNA synthesis combined with the slipping of DNA polymerase delta can lead to elevated mutagenesis and the appearance of complex mutations [26].

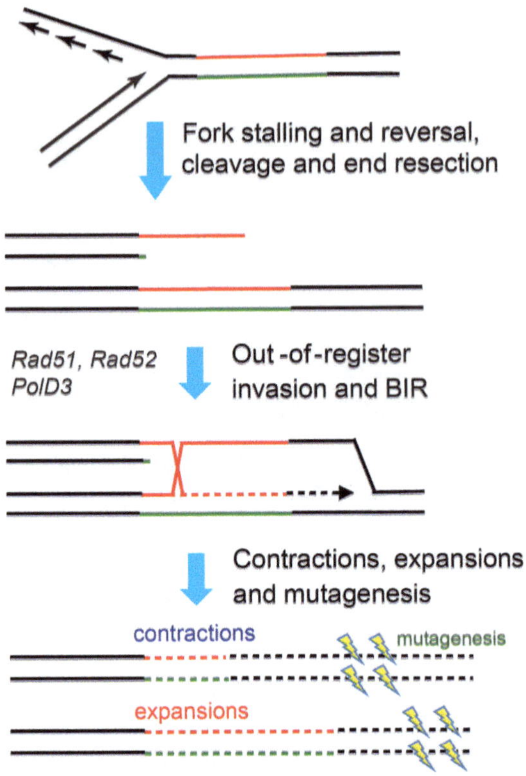

Fig. 4 A working model for mutational events triggered by carrier-size $(CGG)_n$ repeats. The replication fork stalling and reversal can lead to the formation of a one-ended DSB. Repair of this DSB via BIR can result in repeat expansion or contraction concordant with mutagenesis at a distance (*see* text for details). Strands of the repeat are shown in red and green, flanking DNA is in black. Proteins involved in strand invasion are indicated. (Adapted from [15] with modifications)

Could our system can be used to study larger-scale expansions of $(CGG)_n$ repeats that are at heart of fragile X syndrome? We are cautiously optimistic, since we were able to detect the addition of up to 100 repeats to the starting $(CGG)_{153}$ run in ~2% of Gc^R subclones. As one would expect, these expansions partially silenced the *FMR1* promoter resulting in a fivefold drop in the amount of HyTK mRNA as confirmed by qRT-PCR [15]. The low frequency of these large-scale expansions, however, makes their genetic analysis difficult. Our unpublished data indicate that changing a cell line, the location of the repeat in the genome, and/or the selection protocol can shift the repeat instability equilibrium toward large-scale expansions. For example, when our selectable cassette was integrated into a particular genome site in HEK293 cells, the majority of Gc^R subclones contained large-scale repeat expansions. We are currently adjusting our system to perform genetic analysis of large-scale expansions of (CGG)n repeats in mammalian cells.

We are currently tuning up our system up to perform genetic analysis of large-scale expansions of (CGG)n repeats in mammalian cells.

2 Materials

2.1 RL5 Targeting System

1. MEL cells containing the eGFP-Lox511 cassette.
2. pFMR1-CGGn-HyTK targeting plasmid.
3. Cre recombinase vector.
4. DMEM medium.
5. Fetal bovine serum.
6. Penicillin–streptomycin mix.
7. Opti-MEM I Reduced Serum Medium.
8. X-tremeGENE HP DNA Transfection Reagent (Roche).
9. Nontreated tissue culture 6-, 24-, or 96-well plate, flat.
10. Nontreated T25 EasYFlask, Filter Cap.
11. Heracell VIOS 160i CO_2 incubator with copper chamber.
12. Hygromycin B (50 mg/mL).

2.2 Cell Culture

1. CKX41 Inverted Microscope with excitation filter BP460-490C (Olympus).
2. Disposable serological pipets 1, 2, 5, 10, 25, and 50 mL.
3. Disposable aspirating pipets 2 mL.
4. Pipet-Aid.
5. EVOS™ XL Core Imaging System (Thermo Scientific).
6. Cellometer Auto T4 Bright Field Cell Counter (Nexcelom).
7. Ganciclovir.
8. Micropipette (1–10 μL).
9. 10 μL extralong filter/barrier tips
10. Isopropanol-filled cryo 1 °C freezing container,
11. Liquid nitrogen tank,
12. Freezing medium: complete growth medium supplemented with 10% (v/v) DMSO.
13. Phosphate saline buffer (PBS).

2.3 PCR and CGG Repeat Sequencing

1. Taq DNA polymerase.
2. Phusion High-Fidelity DNA Polymerase (Thermo Scientific).
3. 10× Taq Buffer: 750 mM Tris–HCl pH 8.8 at 25 °C, 200 mM $(NH_4)_2SO_4$, 0.1% (v/v) Tween 20, 20 mM $MgCl_2$.

4. 5 M betaine solution.
5. DMSO.
6. Ethidium bromide stock solution: 10 mg/mL.
7. Electrophoresis buffer.

2.4 Mouse Gene Inactivation by Accell siRNAs

1. 5× siRNA Buffer (Dharmacon B-002000-UB-100).
2. RNase-free water.
3. Accell Delivery Media (Dharmacon B-005000).
4. Accell siRNAs against the expression of *POLD3* (Dharmacon E-046305-00-0020), *POLD4* (E-050262-00-0010), *RAD51* (E-062730-00-0010), *RAD52* (E-043751-00-0010), *SMARCAL1* (E-041643-00-0010) gene, or nontargeting control (D-001910-10-20).
5. Centrifuge for cell culture.
6. Cell counter.

3 Methods

3.1 Creating Cell Lines with the FMR1-CGG$_n$-HyTK Cassette in RL5 Locus of MEL Cells

1. Plate 10^6 MEL cells containing the eGFP-Lox511 cassette per 35-mm (6 well) plate and grow overnight in 2 mL of DMEM medium supplemented with 10% FBS at 37 °C under 5% CO_2.
2. Add 1–2 μg of targeting plasmid DNA (pFMR1-CGGn-HyTK) and ~0.3 μg of Cre recombinase expressing vector into 200 μL of Opti-MEM media in a 1.5-mL microcentrifuge tube for each well to be transfected.
3. Add 4 μL of the X-tremeGENE HP DNA Transfection Reagent directly into medium with diluted DNA from **step 2** (*see* **Note 1**). Mix well by gentle pipetting and incubated 30 min at room temperature.
4. Take out the 6-well plate from the incubator. At this step, do not exchange or replace growth media (*see* **Note 2**). DNA/Lipofectamine complex from **step 3** was added to cells in a dropwise manner using tips with a wide orifice. The 6 well plate was then gently shaken.
5. Grow cells overnight in the CO_2 incubator.
6. Next day post transfection, transfer cells into a 15 mL tube and wash with 10 mL of the complete growth media.
7. Dissolve cell pellet in 30 mL of the growth media containing 500 μg/mL of hygromycin B, and distribute a homogenous suspension of cells to 3 × 96 well plates at 100 μL of cells suspension per well.

8. Grow cells for up to 3 weeks. Add 50 μL of fresh growth media supplemented with hygromycin after 1–2 weeks of selection. Pick up hygromycin-resistant clones and analyze for the length of CGG repeats and copy number of the HyTK gene (*see* **Note 3**).
9. Immediately after receiving hygromycin-resistant clones, culture cells in T25 flasks in the presence of 10–15 mL complete growth media.
10. Freeze the seed stock of cells as soon as a surplus of cells became available. Use the isopropanol-filled cryo 1 °C freezing container, freeze cells in freezing medium and store in liquid nitrogen vapor phase. Each experiment was conducted on the cells that have been taken from the fresh seed stocks.
11. Confirm successful cassette exchange in hygromycin resistant colonies by a visual loss of eGFP signal.
12. Confirm the correct integration of a FMR1-CGG_n-HyTK cassette by PCR across the loxP sites using primers loxP "A" upstream and "A" downstream (Table 1) (Tm = 60 °C) for the cassette in "A" orientation, or loxP "B" upstream and "B" downstream (Table 1) (Tm = 60 °C) for the cassette in "B" orientation.
13. Confirm correct locus targeting using PCR with RL5 "A" upstream and downstream primers for "A" orientation (Table 1) (Tm = 68 °C) and RL5 "B" upstream and downstream primers for "B" orientation (Table 1) (Tm = 68 °C) (*see* **Note 4**).
14. Verify single copy insertion by Southern blotting of genomic DNA digested by EcoRV and additionally confirmed by qPCR.

3.2 Repeat Instability Assay

1. Take fresh seed stock of hygromycin-resistant clone of MEL cells containing FMR1-$(CGG)_n$-HyTK cassette stored in liquid nitrogen vapor phase.
2. Warm the cells for 3–5 min at 37 °C water bath and transfer the cell suspension into T25 flask containing 15 mL of prewarmed cell culture media.
3. Grow MEL cells with a selectable cassette in Nunc T25 non-treated cell culture flasks for suspension cells, split the cells on average 1:6. Aspirate most of the media after 2–4 days of culturing to leave 1–3 mL of cell suspension and refill the flask with 10 mL of fresh culturing media. Alternatively, transfer 1–3 mL of MEL suspension to new flask containing 10 mL of complete growth media.
4. Maintain fresh stocks of MEL cells containing FMR-$CGGG_n$-HyTK construct in RL5 locus off selection for 6 days (*see*

Table 1
Primers used in this work

Name	Sequence
loxP "A" upstream	GGAGATGGGGGAGGCTAAC
loxP "A" downstream	ATGACCATGATTACGCCAAG
loxP "B" upstream	TACGCCCTCTCTCACCAGAT
loxP "B" downstream	GGGCAGTGAGCGCAACGCAATTA
RL5 "A" upstream	TGACCCGTAGAGGCAGAAGGTGA
RL5 "A" downstream	TGGAGGCCCCTCTCCACTCA
RL5 "B" upstream	CTGAAGCTTCCCGGGGGTACCGAAT
RL5 "B" downstream	TGGAGGCCCCTCTCCACTCA
CGG upstream	TCAGGCGCTCAGCTCCGTTTCGGTTTCACTTCC
CGG downstream	ACAGACGTCGCGGTGAGTTCAGGCTTTTTCATGG

Note 5). During this time hygromycin B was not added to the culture medium.

5. Disperse ~5 × 10^6 cells into 5 × 96 well plates containing 12 μM ganciclovir in the growth media but without hygromycin B, so finally you get around ~10^6 cells per plate. Place all 96 well plates straight into 37 °C CO_2 incubator.
6. Grow the cells around a week. Add 50 μL of fresh media containing 12 μM of ganciclovir after 7–10 days of selection. Place the cells back in CO_2 incubator and incubate another 10–14 days.
7. Examine every well of the plate with a microscope for signs of colony formation, and mark those that have a clone.
8. Clean up all parts of EVOS™ XL Core Imaging System with wipes soaked in 70% ethanol and place it inside of cell culture hood. Turn on UV light at least for 1 h.
9. Place clean micropipette (1–10 μL) and sterile 10 μL extralong filter/barrier tips into the culture hood. Slightly heat the tip in cigarette lighter flame and bend it to ~90°. Work under aseptic conditions to ensure the tips and the pipet remain sterile.

10. Examine the plate containing marked Gc^R subclones from **step** 7 with EVOS™ XL Core Imaging System. Pick up all Gc^R subclones using the pipet and self-made 90° bent 10 μL barrier tips (*see* **Note 6**).
11. Transfer each Gc^R subclone into 24-well plate containing 0.5 mL of complete growth media with ganciclovir and grow for another 5–6 days.
12. Collect Gc^R cells from each well into 1.5 mL microcentrifuge tube, spin down by centrifugation 376 × *g* for 3 min and wash by PBS one time. Isolate genomic DNA from cells pellet and analyze it by PCR of CGG repeats or DNA sequencing of HyTK gene.

3.3 PCR of CGG Repeats

1. Analyze the length of $(CGG)_n$ repeats by PCR in the presence of DMSO and betaine. Use ~1:1 mixture of two polymerases: Phusion High-Fidelity DNA Polymerase and Taq polymerase to amplify longer $(CGG)_n$ repeats.
2. Set up PCR reaction in 50 μL, by adding its components in the following order: 0.5 μL Taq polymerase (5 units/μL), 0.35–0.5 μL Phusion High-Fidelity DNA Polymerase (2 U/μL), 5 μL 10× Taq buffer with $(NH_4)_2SO_4$ and 20 mM $MgCl_2$, 4 μL dNTP mixture (2.5 mM each), 25 μL 5 M betaine, 1.3 μL DMSO, 1 μL 10 pmol/μL primer mix (CGG upstream and downstream, Table 1), 1 μL genomic DNA, and 13 μL PCR grade water. Add the template and mix well (*see* **Note 7**).
3. Perform PCR cycling as follows. First cycle (initial denaturation) at 95 °C for 90 s. Subsequent 41 cycles at 95 °C for 30 s (denaturation), 65 °C 30 s (annealing), 72 °C for 2 min (extension).
4. Remove tubes from the PCR machine and add ~0.5 μL of Taq polymerase–Phusion DNA polymerase mixture per tube. Mix well.
5. Continue repeat amplification by the second round of PCR using the following cycle profile: initial denaturation at 95 °C for 90 s, 17 cycles of denaturation at 95 °C for 30 s, annealing at 65 °C for 30 s, and extension at 72 °C for 120 s. Add 5 min at 72 °C for final extension.
6. Load 20–25 μL aliquot from second round PCR reaction on the gel to visualize the amplification products by 1.5% agarose gel-electrophoresis. Run the gel at low (60 V) voltage for 2–3 h in standard 0.5 × TBE electrophoretic buffer.

3.4 Mouse Gene Inactivation by siRNAs

The transfection of small interfering RNAs (siRNA) mediated by lipid-based reagents is the method of choice for the majority of cell types. But a significant fraction of mammalian cells as well as MEL cells belong to difficult-to-transfect cell type. Accell siRNAs present lipid- and viral-independent delivery technology specially designed for the cells identified as difficult to transfect.

1. Take fresh seed stock of MEL cells with FMR1-$(CGG)_n$-HyTK cassette stored in liquid nitrogen vapor phase and grow them in T25 flask containing 15 mL of the complete media for 4–5 days without any selection.
2. Prepare a 100 μM siRNA solution in 1× siRNA buffer according to the manufacturer siRNA Resuspension Protocol (*see* **Note 8**).
3. Take fresh culture of MEL cells, spin down cells at 290 ×*g* for 2 min and aspirate the growth medium. Resuspend cells in 5–10 mL of Delivery Media in sterile 15 mL tube.
4. Count the number of cells in suspension using a cell counter.
5. Prepare at least two T25 flask with 1 mL of Delivery Media. Add nontargeting control and mouse-specific siRNAs up two final concentration 2 μM into each T25 flask.
6. Transfer ~1–2 × 10^4 cells from **step 3** to the flask containing Delivery Media with the appropriate amount of siRNA (*see* **Note 9**).
7. Grow cells at 37 °C in CO_2 incubator. After 3–4 days, add 2 mL of Delivery Media containing 2 μM siRNA (*see* **Note 10**).
8. Continue culturing cells for ~6 days. Add 6–7 mL of complete growth media with 2 μM of siRNA and expand the culture up to ~10^7 cells (*see* **Note 11**).
9. Spin down and resuspend cells from **step 6** in 40 mL of complete growth media containing 12 mM Ganciclovir. Disperse the cells into 4 × 96 well plates for both targeted and control siRNA treated cells and grow as described above in **step 5** of Subheading 3.2.
10. Count and analyze Gc^R colonies after a period of ~2–3 weeks by PCR or DNA sequencing as described above in Subheadings 3.2 and 3.3.

4 Notes

1. Avoid contact of X-tremeGENE HP DNA Transfection Reagent with the walls of the plastic tubes. It could decrease transfection efficiency.
2. The presence of serum does not affect transfection efficiency when using X-tremeGENE HP DNA Transfection Reagent.
3. We recommend picking up only one cell clump per well using EVOS™ XL Core Imaging System and bent 10 μL extra-long barrier tips. Avoid taking all cells from the single well, as it can contain a few hygromycin resistant clones.

4. Perform regular 3 cycles PCR with the same conditions for the steps 1–3: 95 °C for 1 min 30 s (initial denaturation) (1 cycle), 95 °C for 30 s (denaturation), 60 °C 30 s (annealing), 72 °C for 1 min (extension) 30 cycles and then 5 min at 72 °C for final extension.
5. Try to use fresh cell stocks as much as possible for your experiments. Prolonged culturing of cell lines prior to the selection step can result in the accumulation of duplicate GcR clones, as revealed by sequencing of their HyTk reporters.
6. You need carefully approach the bent tip to the single colony under the microscope and suck it into the tip, followed by transferring to 24-well plate.
7. Betaine increases viscosity of the PCR mixture. Thus, it is crucial to pipette up and down PCR mixture at least ten times after adding DNA samples.
8. Dharmacon Accell siRNA Resuspension Protocol includes four steps:
   (a) Resuspend siRNA using the appropriate volume of 1× siRNA Buffer or RNase-free solution.
   (b) Pipette solution up and down 3–5 times while avoiding introduction of bubbles.
   (c) Place the solution on an orbital mixer/shaker for 70–90 min at 37 °C (recommended) or at room temperature.
   (d) Briefly centrifuge to collect solution to bottom of the tube/wells.
9. Important! Do not apply hygromycin selection in these steps.
10. Increase concentration of siRNA twofold from that recommended by Dharmacon (1 μM) to improve gene silencing without affecting the cells viability.
11. Cells start growing very fast after addition of complete media, so it takes 2–3 days to reach the population size of ten million cells.

References

1. Paulson H (2018) Repeat expansion diseases. Handb Clin Neurol 147:105–123
2. Mirkin SM (2007) Expandable DNA repeats and human disease. Nature 447:932–940
3. Usdin K, NCM H, Freudenreich CH (2015) Repeat instability during DNA repair: insights from model systems. Crit Rev Biochem Mol Biol 50:142–167
4. Jin P, Warren ST (2000) Understanding the molecular basis of fragile X syndrome. Hum Mol Genet 9:901–908
5. Imbert G, Feng Y, Nelson DL et al (1998) FMR1 and mutations in fragile X syndrome: molecular biology, biochemistry and genetics. In: Wells RD, Warren ST (eds) Genetics instabilities and hereditary neurological disorders. Academic Press, San Diego, pp 27–53

6. Kunst CB, Warren ST (1994) Cryptic and polar variation of the fragile X repeat could result in predisposing normal alleles. Cell 77:853–861
7. Hagerman RJ, Hagerman PJ (2002) The fragile X premutation: into the phenotypic fold. Curr Opin Genet Dev 12(3):278–283
8. Sherman SL (2000) Premature ovarian failure among fragile X premutation carriers: parent-of-origin effect? Am J Hum Genet 67:11–13
9. Man L, Lekovich J, Rosenwaks Z et al (2017) Fragile X-associated diminished ovarian reserve and primary ovarian insufficiency from molecular mechanisms to clinical manifestations. Front Mol Neurosci 10:290
10. Kenneson A, Zhang F, Hagedorn CH et al (2001) Reduced FMRP and increased FMR1 transcription is proportionally associated with CGG repeat number in intermediate-length and premutation carriers. Hum Mol Genet 10:1449–1454
11. Raca G, Siyanova EY, Mirkin SM (2000) Janus effects of premutation size CGG repeats on gene expression. Am J Hum Genet 67:366
12. Tassone F, Hagerman RJ, Taylor AK et al (2000) Elevated levels of FMR1 mRNA in carrier males: a new mechanism of involvement in the fragile-X syndrome. Am J Hum Genet 66:6–15
13. El-Osta A (2002) FMR1 silencing and the signals to chromatin: a unified model of transcriptional regulation. Biochem Biophys Res Commun 295(3):575–581
14. Hansen RS, Canfield TK, Lamb MM et al (1993) Association of fragile X syndrome with delayed replication of the FMR1 gene. Cell 73:1403–1409
15. Kononenko AV, Ebersole T, Vasquez KM et al (2018) Mechanisms of genetic instability caused by (CGG)n repeats in an experimental mammalian system. Nat Struct Mol Biol 25:669–676
16. Lupton SD, Brunton LL, Kalberg VA et al (1991) Dominant positive and negative selection using a hygromycin phosphotransferase-thymidine kinase fusion gene. Mol Cell Biol 11:3374–3378
17. Feng YQ, Lorincz MC, Fiering S et al (2001) Position effects are influenced by the orientation of a transgene with respect to flanking chromatin. Mol Cell Biol 21:298–309
18. Ebersole T, Kim J-H, Samoshkin A et al (2011) tRNA genes protect a reporter gene from epigenetic silencing in mouse cells. Cell Cycle (Georgetown, Tex) 10:2779–2791
19. Shah KA, Mirkin SM (2015) The hidden side of unstable DNA repeats: mutagenesis at a distance. DNA Repair 32:106–112
20. Shah KA, Shishkin AA, Voineagu I et al (2012) Role of DNA polymerases in repeat-mediated genome instability. Cell Rep 2:1088–1095
21. Anand RP, Lovett ST, Haber JE (2013) Break-induced DNA replication. Cold Spring Harb Perspect Biol 5:a010397
22. Malkova A, Ira G (2013) Break-induced replication: functions and molecular mechanism. Curr Opin Genet Dev 23:271–279
23. Costantino L, Sotiriou SK, Rantala JK et al (2014) Break-induced replication repair of damaged forks induces genomic duplications in human cells. Science 343:88–91
24. Sotiriou SK, Kamileri I, Lugli N et al (2016) Mammalian RAD52 functions in break-induced replication repair of collapsed DNA replication forks. Mol Cell 64:1127–1134
25. Pasero P, Vindigni A (2017) Nucleases acting at stalled forks: how to reboot the replication program with a few shortcuts. Annu Rev Genet 51:477–499
26. Kramara J, Osia B, Malkova A (2017) Break-induced replication: an unhealthy choice for stress relief? Nat Struct Mol Biol 24:11–12

Chapter 10

Assessing Triplet Repeat Expansions in Human SVG-A Cell Culture

Gregory M. Williams and Robert S. Lahue

Abstract

Determining the molecular mechanisms that contribute to trinucleotide repeat (TNR) expansions is essential to understanding the origin of genetically inherited diseases, such as Huntington's disease, and to inform efforts in developing therapeutic treatments. As one resource to probe the mechanisms of TNR expansions, we describe an expansion assay in human tissue culture cells. The cell line SVG-A, derived from human astrocytes, has the important property of supporting expansions in culture, unlike many cell lines derived from patients. SVG-A cells are also amenable to standard genetic and biochemical techniques such as siRNA, CRISPR-Cas9 and enzymatic inhibitors. This combination of features allows for mechanistic studies of TNR expansions, using the quantitative genetic assay described here as a readout. The SVG-A assay has correctly identified key proteins that drive expansions and it has facilitated testing of enzymatic inhibitors that suppress expansions as potential therapeutics. This chapter describes how repeat expansions are detected, visualized, and quantified.

Key words Trinucleotide repeats, Expansion, Genome instability, DNA mutagenesis, Huntington's disease, Reporter construct, Polymerase chain reaction, Astrocytes, Human cells

1 Introduction

The development of suitable assays for studying TNR expansions has been a key challenge, especially in higher eukaryotic systems. While mouse studies provide the gold standard for biological relevance, PCR assays for expansions in mice typically rely on tissue samples with heterogeneous mixtures of cells. The resulting expansion pattern is thus a composite of many different genetic events. There are mathematical tools for scoring TNR instability from the PCR traces [1] although these tools have not become widely used. The issue of heterogeneity can be overcome using small pool PCR [2] but at the cost of significant time and labor. Both these approaches have sensitivity limits of ~10%. It is also cumbersome to create and test alternative repeat sequences in the same mouse

Guy-Franck Richard (ed.), *Trinucleotide Repeats: Methods and Protocols*, Methods in Molecular Biology, vol. 2056,
https://doi.org/10.1007/978-1-4939-9784-8_10,

background. The same issues have limited the use of induced pluripotent stem cells for mechanistic analysis of TNR expansions.

Our laboratory developed the use of human SVG-A tissue culture cells for studying TNR expansions [3, 4]. SVG-A cells are derived from human astrocytes and immortalized with SV40 large T antigen [5, 6]. Since expansions occur in astrocytes of HD mice and patients [7], the cells provide biological relevance. SVG-A cells have several additional important properties. First, they have been proven to support expansions of CAG/CTG repeats in culture [3, 4, 8, 9]. Using the assay described here, genetically independent expansions in SVG-A cells have been measured and validated with a sensitivity of 1–10% [8, 9]. Furthermore, the key protein factor MutSβ (Msh2-Msh3), known from knockout mouse studies to be essential for expansions, is also required for expansions in SVG-A cells [8, 9]. Thus, the mechanisms of CAG/CTG expansions in SVG-A cells appears to be similar or identical to those in mice and humans. This system makes it straightforward to test alternative sequences instead of CAG/CTG repeats; for example, a TAG repeat was evaluated and shown to be nonexpanding in SVG-A cells [3].

The second major virtue of the SVG-A system is that the cells are amenable to standard molecular biology and biochemical approaches, which include siRNA, CRISPR-Cas9 and treatments with small molecule enzyme inhibitors [4, 8, 9]. These tools allow direct investigation of protein factors that either drive or impede expansions. For example, inactivation of the *MSH3* gene using CRISPR-Cas9 generated an *MSH3*$^{-/-}$ cell line which was selectively deficient in MutSβ and also defective for expansions [9]. The *MSH3*$^{-/-}$ cell line can be supplemented with cDNAs, encoding either wild type or variant forms of Msh3, to assess their effects on expansions [9]. The ability to test genetic variants of *MSH3*, and potentially in other driver genes, is important and timely due to the recent genome wide association studies that identified human SNP variants associated with changes in age-of-onset and progression of HD and other TNR expansion diseases [10–13]. Wild-type SVG-A (*MSH3*$^{+/+}$), deficient (*MSH3*$^{-/-}$), and rescue (*MSH3*$^{-/-}$ with *MSH3* cDNA) are available from Ximbio (https://ximbio.com/). The third utility of this assay is that its quantitative features allow comparisons of expansion frequencies between different experimental conditions, for example upon knockdown of a candidate driver gene. Statistical evaluations are straightforward using standard tests. The assay also provides direct readout of expansion sizes, information that can also be valuable for addressing mechanism. We have observed expansions between +4 and +21 repeats using this system [8].

Briefly, the assay requires about 14 days (Fig. 1a) but concurrent assays can be dovetailed with suitable planning. The assay utilizes a shuttle vector, that is, a plasmid capable of replicating in *E. coli*, human cells, and yeast (Fig. 1b). Bacteria are used for standard cloning and preparation of plasmid stocks for the assay. The shuttle

A.

Day 1	Seed SVG-A cells Optional: siRNA or inhibitor treatment
Day 3	Transfect cells with shuttle vector Optional: siRNA or inhibitor treatment
Days 3 – 5	Expansions occur
Day 5	Cell lysis
Day 6	Plasmid recover and *Dpn*I digestion
Day 7	Transform yeast
Day 10	Count yeast colonies on –His plates
Day 11	Count yeast colonies on +Can plates
Day 12	Colony PCR
Day 13	Sequencing gel
Day 14	Calculate expansion frequencies

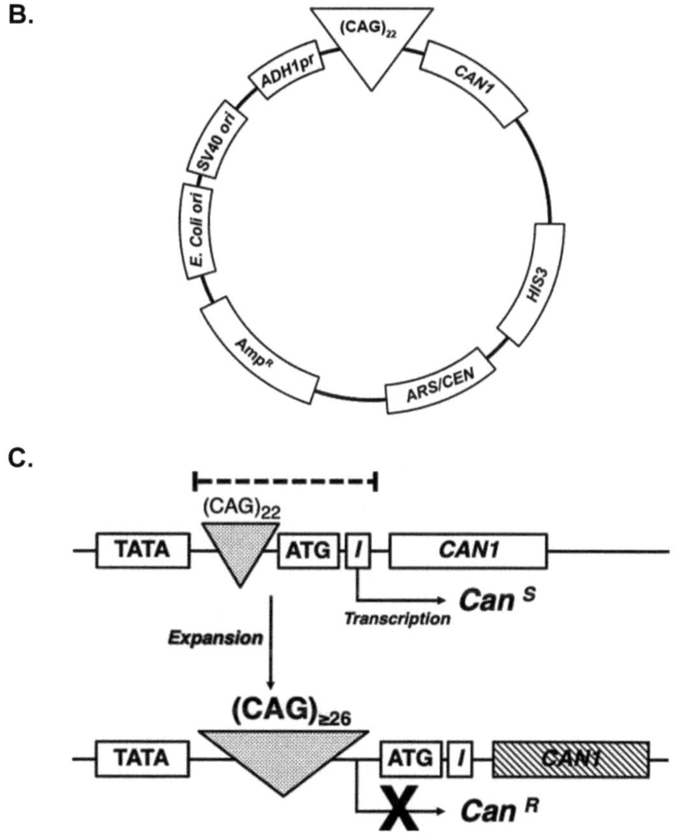

Fig. 1 Illustration of the expansion assay, the shuttle vector and the genetic selection of triplet repeat expansions. (**a**) Timeline of the shuttle vector assay. As an option, siRNA or enzyme inhibitors can be incorporated into the assay between days 1 and 3. Expansions occur between days 3 and 5. (**b**) Illustration of the genetic elements of the pBL302 shuttle vector for expansions. This ~9 kbp plasmid harbors a $(CAG)_{22}$ triplet repeat and can be replicated in bacteria (*E. coli ori*, Amp^R), yeast (*ADH1* promoter, *CAN1, HIS3, ARS/CEN*), and SV40-immortalized mammalian cells (SV40 *ori*). (**c**) The pBL302 plasmid contains a $(CAG)_{22}$ between the TATA box and the *CAN1* gene. Transcription at this locus is sensitive to the spacing between the TATA box and the preferred transcription initiation site, denoted "I". The dashed line indicates the optimal zone for initiation. With an unexpanded $(CAG)_{22}$ repeat tract, initiation at I results in functional expression of the *CAN1* gene and sensitivity to the toxic arginine analogue canavanine (Can^S). An expansion ≥4 repeats alters transcription initiation to include an out-of-frame ATG, blocking translation (indicated by "X") and resulting in canavanine resistance (Can^R; indicated by striped *CAN1*)

vector is then transfected into SVG-A cells and subsequently recovered for genetic analysis in yeast. Replication in human cells requires the presence of the SV40 large T antigen (Tag), which is expressed in SVG-A cells. Portability of the shuttle vector to alternative cell lines is made possible by shuttle vector variants that also contain the *Tag* gene [3].

The shuttle vector is transfected into SVG-A cells where the TNR, typically $(CAG)_{22}$ in our experiments, can expand (Fig. 1a). About 48 h later, the shuttle vector is purified from SVG-A cells. Digestion with the restriction enzyme *Dpn*I eliminates any shuttle vector molecules that were not metabolized in the SVG-A cells (e.g., any plasmid molecules that were not taken up during transfection and therefore are excluded from consideration) (Fig. 2a). Running an aliquot of recovered plasmid DNA digested with *Dpn*I on a standard agarose gel is a simple way to confirm that most of the purified shuttle vector underwent at least one round of DNA replication in SVG-A and is therefore resistant to cleavage (Fig. 2b). The recovered shuttle vector pool is then transformed into *S. cerevisiae* where a genetic selection (His^+ Can^R) identifies those plasmid molecules with an apparent expansion (Fig. 1c). Knowledge of the total plasmid pool (His^+) allows quantification of an observed expansion frequency.

Putative expansions are then investigated by colony PCR to visualize, validate, and size the expansions (Fig. 3). Authentic expansions are indicated in lanes indicated by asterisks in the figure. Expanded allele lengths can be estimated at ±1–2 repeats, depending on the molecular weight markers available. False positives are identified as no change to PCR product length and therefore eliminated from subsequent calculations. A more complete description of authentic and false positive events is provided in the figure legend. Background measurements allow the user to estimate any expansions that might have occurred either during workup of the shuttle vector in *E. coli* or that might arise in yeast. Background frequency is determined by direct transfection of the starting shuttle vector into yeast, followed by genetic selection and PCR analysis, as described above. Our experience is that the background level is quite low, 0.01–0.10%, such that the assay provides a suitably robust signal–noise ratio of at least tenfold and more typically100-fold or more.

The assay also allows the experimenter to use siRNA to interfere with cellular targets that may be involved in expansion mechanism (Fig. 1a). Alternatively, therapeutic approaches such as enzyme inhibitors can also be tested [4, 8]. Typically, these treatments are added prior to the transfection of the shuttle vector such that the target of the knockdown/inhibition is affected before the shuttle vector enters the cell. For protein knockdown experiments, siRNA (Dharmacon) transfections can be performed 24 h after cell seeding (*day 2*), with the second siRNA treatment along-

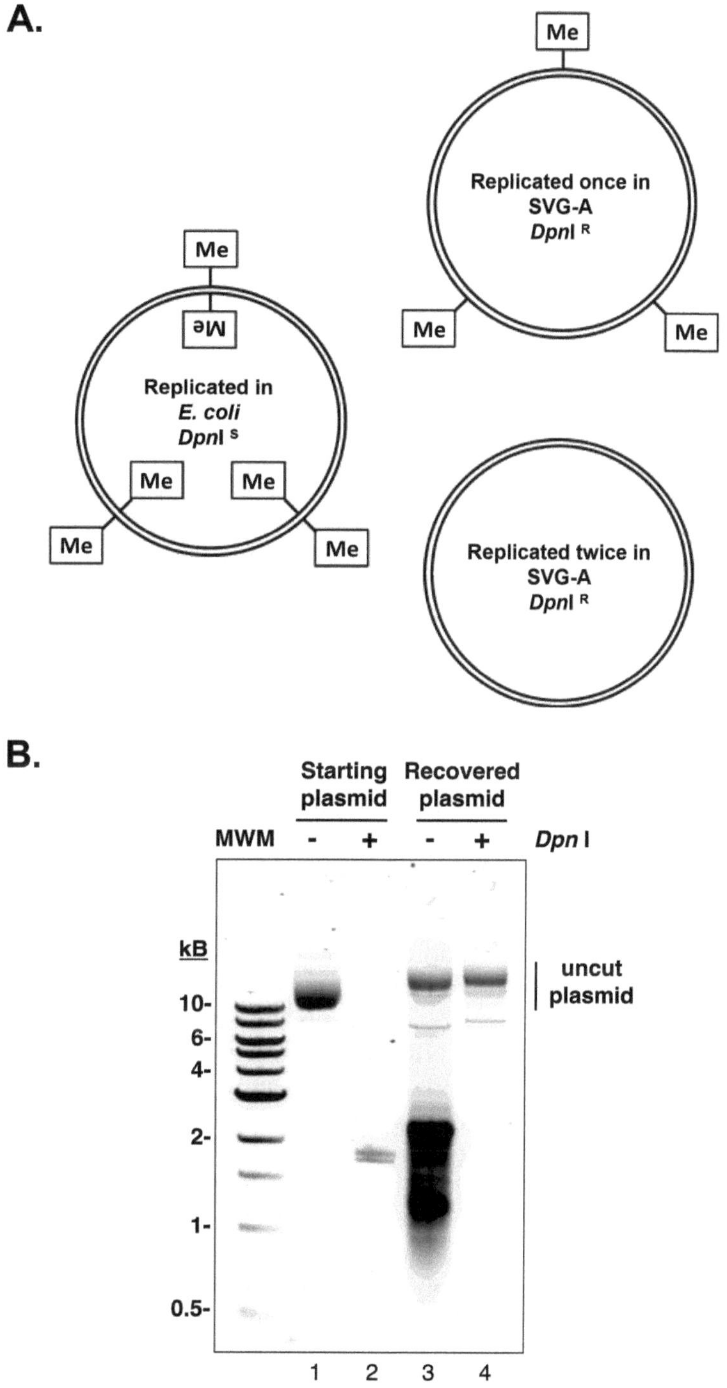

Fig. 2 *Dpn*I digestion of recovered shuttle vector. (**a**) *Dpn*I is a restriction enzyme that cuts at fully methylated GATC sites (indicated by "Me" on both strands of DNA). Prokaryotic replication results in fully methylated adenine base pairs at GATC sites throughout the DNA, so the starting plasmid is sensitive to *Dpn*I. Mammalian cells do not methylate the adenine bases at GATC sites. Thus, any reporter plasmid that replicated once or more in SVG-A cells becomes resistant to *Dpn*I digestion. (**b**) An 0.8% agarose gel showing starting (lanes 1–2) and recovered (lanes 3–4) plasmid with or without *Dpn*I digestion. Migration of uncut plasmid, either supercoiled or nicked, is indicated on the side. MWM, molecular weight markers

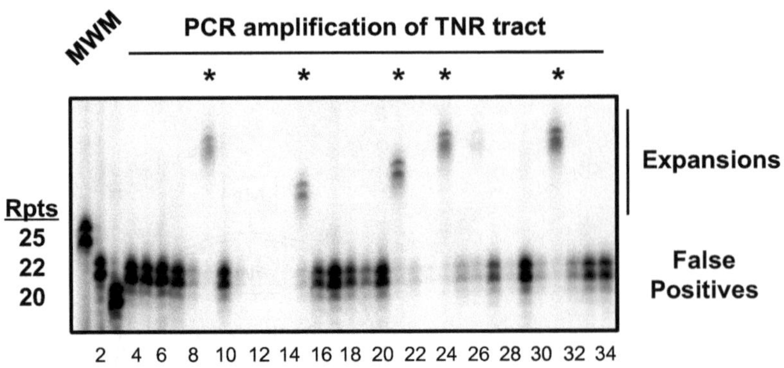

Fig. 3 Analysis of expansions. A representative sequencing gel showing PCR amplification of the reporter plasmid. Two microliters of the PCR product was loaded in each well. Molecular weight markers (MWM) in lanes 1–3 are from PCR amplification of plasmids with known CAG repeat lengths. Lanes 4–34 represent products from individual Can^R yeast colonies. Authentic expansions containing a band ≥26 repeats are denoted by asterisks at the top of the figure in lanes 9, 15, 21, 24, and 31. False-positives (Lanes 4–7, 8, 10, 11, 16–20, 22, 25–27, 29, 30, 32–24) do not show an expansion in the CAG repeat. Lane 26 was judged a false positive since >50% of the total intensity in the lane remains at the starting tract size. No product (Lanes 12–14, 23, 28) indicates that the PCR reaction was not successful. The double bands in most lanes are due to a common PCR artifact for amplification of TNR tracts

side the shuttle vector transfection (*day 3 – day 4*). Enzyme inhibitors can be added directly into the culture medium between *day 1* and the time the cells are harvested on *day 5*. A third approach is to modify the SVG-A cells via CRISPR-Cas9.

The main limitation of the SVG-A assay is that the starting TNR tract is limited to ~22 repeats. This limitation stems from the canavanine selection step. Tracts longer than 22 repeats convey resistance to the drug, so the starting tract is indistinguishable from expanded. Current indications are that expansions from 22 repeat tracts require the same factors (e.g., MutSβ) as seen for longer repeats; however, additional assays will need to be developed for utilizing longer starting TNRs. We welcome the recent publication describing an expansion assay for starting CGG tracts up to 153 repeats in murine erythroid leukemia cells [14].

2 Materials

2.1 General Reagents

1. Luria-Bertani broth (LB): 10 g Tryptone, 5 g Yeast Extract, 5 g sodium chloride. Make up to a final volume of 1 L of deionized water in a 2 L flask, autoclave at 121 °C for 20 min. For LB + Ampicillin plates, also add 20 g of agar and autoclave as stated above. Allow the flask to cool before adding Ampicillin

into the culture at a final concentration of 75 μg/mL. Stir media before pouring. Store at 4 °C until use.

2. SVG-A culture medium: Dulbecco's Modified Eagle's Medium—High Glucose supplemented with Fetal Bovine Serum (FBS) at 10% v/v, 100 mg/mL penicillin–streptomycin. Store at 4 °C until use.
3. Hank's Balanced Salt Solution with Trypsin: Hank's Balanced Salt Solution supplemented with Trypsin-EDTA solution at 10% v/v. Store at 4 °C until use.
4. 40% w/v glucose: 400 g glucose into 600 mL deionized water. Bring to a final volume of 1 L with deionized water. Autoclave at 121 °C for 20 min. Store a room temperature until use.
5. YPD medium: 20 g peptone, 10 g Yeast Extract. Make up to a final volume of 950 mL of deionized water. Autoclave at 121 °C for 20 min, store at room temperature. Before use, add 50 mL of sterile 40% glucose and mix well. For YPD plates, also add 15–20 g of agar to the solution and autoclave as stated above. Once cooled, add 50 mL of sterile 40% glucose and stir before pouring. Store at 4 °C until use.
6. Lipofectamine 2000 (Invitrogen).
7. Opti-MEM media (Invitrogen).

2.2 Isolation of Shuttle Vector

1. Hirt's lysis buffer: 10 mM Tris–Cl pH 7.5, 1 mM EDTA, 0.6% SDS. Filter-sterilize with 0.2 μm filter. Store at room temperature.
2. 5 M NaCl: Add 292.2 g sodium chloride to 600 mL of deionized water, dissolve with stirring at 55 °C. Bring up to a final volume of 1 L with deionized water, autoclave at 121 °C for 20 min. Store at room temperature.
3. 1× TE: 10 mM Tris–HCl pH 8.0, 1 mM EDTA pH 8.0. Autoclave.
4. RNaseA (10 mL): Dissolve 100 mg RNaseA in 7 mL 1× TE pH 7.5. Bring final volume up to 10 mL with 1× TE pH 7.5. Aliquot into microtubes and boil for 10 min. Store at −20 °C.
5. Proteinase K.
6. Amicon Ultra Centrifugal Filter (Ultracel 50 K Filter).
7. Ethanol.
8. *Dpn*I restriction enzyme (NEB).

2.3 Yeast Transformation

1. 10× TE: 100 mM Tris–HCl pH 7.5, 10 mM EDTA pH 7.5. Autoclave. Store at room temperature.
2. 50% Polyethylene glycol (PEG, 200 mL): Add 100 g PEG (molecular weight MW = 3350) to 100 mL of deionized water. Apply low heat to dissolve. Bring up total volume to 200 mL

with deionized water. Filter-sterilize with 0.2 μm filter. Store at room temperature (*see* **Note 1**).

3. 1 M Lithium acetate (LiAc, 200 mL): Add 20.4 g LiAc (molecular weight MW = 102.02) to 100 mL of deionized water, dissolve by stirring. Adjust pH to 7.5 with diluted acetic acid. Bring up total volume to 200 mL with deionized water. Filter-sterilize. Store at room temperature.
4. LiAc/TE Mix (10 mL): 1 mL of 1 M LiAc, 1 mL of 10× TE, 8 mL of sterile deionized water. Vortex to mix (*see* **Note 2**).
5. 40% PEG Mix (10 mL): 1 mL of 1 M LiAc, 1 mL of 10× TE, 8 mL of 50% PEG solution. Vortex to mix (*see* **Note 3**).
6. Sonicated salmon sperm DNA (10 mg/mL).
7. Histidine amino acid dropout Mix (−His): 2.5 g adenine, 1.2 g arginine, 6.0 g aspartic acid, 6.0 g glutamic acid, 3.6 g leucine, 1.8 g lysine, 1.2 g methionine, 3.0 g phenylalanine, 22.5 g serine, 12.0 g threonine, 2.4 g tryptophan, 1.8 g tyrosine, 9.0 g valine, 1.2 g uracil, 2.5 g isoleucine. Homogenize components using a coffee grinder and place in a cylindrical glass storage bottle. Add 3–5 clean marbles to the bottle and mix overnight on an end-over-end shaker to assure complete homogenization.
8. Histidine/Arginine amino acid dropout Mix (−His −Arg): Follow the same procedure as above (Subheading 2.3, **item 6**) but *do not* add in the 1.2 g of arginine. This mix is suitable to make the −His +Canavanine selective plates (*see* **Note 4**).
9. Synthetic Complete lacking Histidine (SC −His) dropout plates: Add 1.3 g of the His amino acid dropout mix to 100 mL of sterile deionized water and dissolve with low heat and stirring. Filter-sterilize the mixture using a 0.2 μm filter and save for later. Separately, add 1.7 g Yeast Nitrogen Base without amino acids or ammonium sulfate, 5 g ammonium sulfate, 20 g of glucose, and 15–20 g of agar into ~600 mL of deionized water in a 2 L flask. Mix with stirring, then bring volume up to 900 mL with deionized water. Add aluminum foil to the top of flask and autoclave at 121 °C for 25 min. Allow the media to cool to ~55 °C in a water bath. When cooled, add the 100 mL of -His amino acid dropout liquid to the flask and allow a few minutes to mix well prior to pouring into petri dishes (*see* **Note 5**).
10. Media lacking histidine and arginine but containing canavanine (SC −His +CAN): Follow the same procedure outlines as above (Subheading 2.3, **item 8**), making sure to start with −His −Arg dropout mix. Once the autoclaved media cools to ~55 °C, add the 100 mL of −His −Arg amino acid dropout liquid to the flask. Next, add in L-Canavanine at a final concentration of 100 μg/mL. Stir to thoroughly mix solution.

Pour ~25 mL per plate, allow plates to dry on the bench overnight in stacks of 3–5 to reduce condensation formation. Store at 4 °C until needed. Warm plates in 30 °C incubator before use.

2.4 Polymerase Chain Reaction (PCR)

1. Yeast colony lysis buffer (10 mL, 100 reactions): 9 mL sterile deionized water, 500 μL of 1 M DTT (50 mM final concentration), 500 μL 10% Triton-X (0.5% final concentration). Mix well. Use 100 μL per colony lysis reaction.
2. Formamide stop reaction solution (200 mL): 0.1 g bromophenol blue, 0.1 g xylene cyanol, 8 mL 0.5 M EDTA (pH 8.0), 192 mL formamide (Sigma). Mix well, aliquot into microtubes and store at −20 °C until needed (*see* **Note 6**).
3. PCR primers: forward CY5 5′-labeled primer oBL251 and reverse CY5 5′-labeled primer Can1Rev (Table 1).
4. TNR PCR Master Mix (100 reactions): 200 μL MyTaq Buffer (Bioline), 255 μL molecular biology grade water, 20 μL of forward primer oBL251 (at 50 pmol/μL), 20 μL of reverse primer Can1REV (at 50 pmol/μL), 5 μL MyTaq Enzyme (Bioline). Add 5 μL of TNR PCR Master Mix to each well of a 96-well PCR plate along with 5 μL of Yeast colony Lysis.

2.5 Urea Sequencing Gel

1. 10× TBE running buffer (2 L): 14.9 g EDTA disodium salt dihydrate, 216 g Tris base, 110 g boric acid (Sigma). Make up to a final volume of 2 L with deionized water. Dissolve components on a stir plate with low heat. Store at room temperature.
2. SequaGel Diluent (2 L): 901 g of urea. Make up to a final volume of 2 L with deionized water. Store at room temperature.
3. 10× SequaGel Buffer (1 L): 450.5 g urea. Make up to a final volume of 1 L with 10× TBE.
4. 10% w/v ammonium persulfate (APS): 1 g APS into 10 mL of deionized water. Store at 4 °C (short term storage) or aliquot into microtubes and store long term at −20 °C (*see* **Note 7**).
5. 6% sequencing gel (70 mL): 45.8 mL SequaGel diluent, 16.8 mL UreaGel (National Diagnostics), 7 mL of 10× SequaGel Buffer, 400 μL 10% APS, 40 μL TEMED (*see* **Note 8**).
6. Whatman #1 filter paper.

Table 1
Primers used in this study

oBL251	GATGTTACTTGGGGAGAGGTGCGATAAT
Can1Rev	TGCTTCTCCTCTATGTCGGCGTCT
TNR tract sequencing primer (Subheading 3.1)	GATGTTACTTGGGGAGAGGTGCGATAAT

3 Methods

3.1 Plasmid Isolation

Isolating a large amount of TNR reporter plasmid at one time ensures that the starting material is consistent throughout several experiments. The isolated plasmid can then be submitted for DNA sequencing of the TNR tract and the CAN1 reporter gene, ensuring that both are free of mutations. We routinely used a sequencing primer whose 3′ end anneals 51 bp upstream of the first CAG triplet (Table 1).

1. Isolate DNA using a standard plasmid preparation kit such as the Qiagen EndoFree Plasmid Maxi Kit. Streak out the *E. coli* harboring the plasmid of interest to single colonies on LB plates supplemented with 75 μg/mL ampicillin. Place the plate into a 37 °C incubator to grow overnight.
2. The following day, use a single colony to inoculate a 5 mL LB + ampicillin liquid media in a 13 mL snap cap tube. Grow this culture at 37 °C with 200 rpm shaking for approximately 12 h.
3. The next morning, inoculate a flask containing 600 mL of LB supplemented with 75 μg/mL ampicillin with 1 mL of the overnight culture and place in a 37 °C incubator, shaking at 200 rpm. Using a spectrophotometer, measure the OD_{600} of the culture every hour until the culture reaches an $OD_{600} = 0.3$. From this point out, measure the OD_{600} every 15–20 min until the culture reaches a final OD_{600} of 0.6 (*see* **Note 9**).
4. Cultures at a final $OD_{600} = 0.6$ can then be used for large-scale plasmid isolation using the Qiagen EndoFree Plasmid Maxi Kit or an equivalent kit.

3.2 SVG-A Cell Culture Conditions

The glial cell line SVG-A are adherent astrocytes that have been immortalized with SV40 Large T Antigen [5, 6]. All steps are routine human tissue culture procedures performed under a laminar flow hood. SVG-A cells are typically passaged every 36–48 h depending on seeding density, and are cultured in T75 flasks containing 10 mL of complete DMEM media at 37 °C in a humidified 5% CO_2 atmosphere (*see* Subheading 2.1). SVG-A cells should be cultured in the appropriate flasks/dishes that have an adherent surface (e.g., Sarstedt Standard or Cell+ vent cap flasks). SVG-A cells are not as adherent as other cell lines. Special care should be taken to minimize the disturbance of cells adherent to the bottom surface of the flask. It is best to not add any solutions directly onto the cells. Rather, add the solution to the opposite surface of where the cells are adhered. When working with 60 mm dishes containing adherent cells, tilt the dish and add the media to the sidewall, then gently level the plate so the 1× PBS slowly comes in contact with the cell surface. Carefully reverse this process to remove the PBS wash. All media used in cell culture should be warmed in a 37 °C water bath before use, and all waste materials including liquids should be disposed of properly.

Remove flasks from the 37 °C incubator and assess the confluency of the culture using a brightfield microscope under 4–10× magnification. Cultures should be grown to 60–90% confluency before splitting. Before splitting or seeding any cells, make sure to check (a) the cells are adhered to the bottom of the flask; (b) the cells are beginning to take on their star-shaped morphology, and (c) the media is not contaminated with any microorganism.

1. Bring culture into the hood and remove the DMEM culture media by pipetting.
2. Invert the flask and add 5 mL of Hanks Balanced Salt solution to the bottom of the flask. Tip the flask back down to rinse the remaining serum from the cell surface. Invert the flask once again and remove the Hanks solution with a serological pipetman (*see* **Note 10**).
3. Add 5 mL of Hanks + Trypsin (45 mL Hanks +5 mL Trypsin) to bottom of the flask. Turn the flask horizontal again, allowing the Hanks + Trypsin to come in contact with the cells, covering the entire adherent cell surface. Allow 1–2 min for the cells to be trypsinized, not exceeding 5 min. This step removes the cells from the adherent surface, releasing them into the liquid media. To avoid clumping of cells, do not agitate the flask while waiting for them to detach from the adherent surface. Cells that are difficult to detach may be placed at 37 °C to facilitate dispersal.
4. Add 10 mL of complete DMEM into the flask to stop the trypsinization reaction (*see* **Note 11**). Use the complete DMEM to wash all cells from the bottom of the flask. Take ~13 mL of the cell resuspension and add it to a 15 mL conical tube.
5. Centrifuge the cell suspension for 5 min at 320 × *g*. In the interim, add 10 mL of complete DMEM to a sterile T75 flask, making sure to completely wet the bottom of the flask with the complete DMEM.
6. Decant and dispose of the supernatant, retaining the cell pellet. Resuspend the pellet in 5–10 mL of fresh complete DMEM. Count cells using a hemocytometer or any available cell counter. In a T75 flask, seed cells at a final concentration of 4.0×10^5–1.0×10^6 cells per mL in 10 mL of DMEM (*see* **Note 12**).

7. Place the flask horizontal once again, and gently rotate in a figure-eight motion to mix cells in the media. Remove cells from the hood and place into 37 °C incubator for ~48 h. Make sure that the adherent surface of the flask is in the correct orientation (in contact with the shelf) when culturing cells.

3.3 SVG-A Cell Seeding and Shuttle Vector Transfection

It is best to work with SVG-A cells that were passaged within ~48 h of the following steps (i.e., are 70–80% confluent). For transient transfections, cells are typically seeded in 60 mm dishes that have an adherent surface.

1. *Day 1* (Fig. 1a): SVG-A cells are seeded into 60 mm dishes and allowed 36–48 h to adhere to the dish and replicate before they are transiently transfected with the TNR reporter plasmid. SVG-A cells are trypsinized, pellet, and resuspended in the appropriate volume of media as per Subheading 3.2.
2. From the cell resuspension, determine the number of cells in the culture using either a hemocytometer or any available cell counter. If possible, calculate the cell culture viability (calculated by dividing the number of live cells by the total number of cells counted), as a cell viability >85% is necessary to continue the assay and greatly increases the chances of successful transfection.
3. Prepare a cell dilution in a new 15 mL conical tube at a concentration of 3.0×10^5–4.0×10^5 viable cells per 1 mL. Add 1 mL of cell dilution to a 60 mm dish already containing 3 mL complete DMEM (*see* **Note 13**). The total volume of complete DMEM media in the 60 mm dish will be 4 mL.
4. After adding cells to the 60 mm dishes, gently rotate the dishes in a figure-eight motion to mix cells in the media. Place the plates in the 37 °C incubator for ~48 h to settle and adhere to the culture flask.

3.4 Transient Transfection of TNR Shuttle Vector

1. *Day 3*: 36–48 h after seeding, assess the health and confluency of the cells under a brightfield microscope. The cell culture should appear 30–50% confluent. Two sterile microtubes are required for each 60 mm dish that is being transfected. In the first tube, dilute 10 μL of the transfection reagent Lipofectamine 2000 in 250 μL of Opti-MEM media. Incubate at room temperature for 5 min (*see* **Note 14**).
2. In the second Eppendorf tube, dilute 1–7 μg of the TNR shuttle vector in 250 μL of Opti-MEM media.
3. Combine the two tubes (Lipofectamine + TNR shuttle vector) and incubate for 20 min at room temperature to allow complex formation.

4. During the incubation, remove the 60 mm dishes containing the seeded SVG-A cells from the incubator. Remove the complete DMEM media and rinse the cells with 1 mL of Opti-MEM media. Add 3 mL of Opti-MEM media to each 60 mm dish, making sure not to agitate the cells seeded on the adherent surface. Place the dishes back into the 37 °C incubator to warm until **step 3** above is complete.
5. Add the 510 μL Lipofectamine + TNR shuttle vector complex to cells drop-wise, making sure to evenly distribute the complex across the dish (*see* **Note 15**). Place 60 mm dishes back into the 37 °C incubator for 6 h.
6. Gently remove the Opti-MEM media from the 60 mm dish using a serological pipette. Rinse the cells with 1 mL of complete DMEM to remove any residual Opti-MEM. Add 4 mL of fresh complete DMEM to the dish (*see* **Note 16**).
7. Place dishes back into the 37 °C incubator for 48 h, allowing for replication of the TNR reporter plasmid.

3.5 Isolation and Recovery of Shuttle Vector from SVG-A Cells

1. *Day 5*: Remove the transfected 60 mm dishes from the 37 °C incubator and assess the health and confluency of the cells under a brightfield microscope. The cell culture should appear 90–100% confluent and still adherent to the 60 mm dish (*see* **Note 17**).
2. Aspirate off the DMEM media using a serological pipette. Add 1 mL of ice cold, filter-sterile 1× PBS to the 60 mm dish, then carefully remove the PBS and discard it into liquid waste.
3. Add 1 mL of ice cold, filter-sterile Hirt's lysis buffer to each 60 mm dish. Swirl the lysis buffer in the dish to thoroughly cover the entire cell surface. The lysate should become quite viscous, indicative of the genomic DNA being released. From this point onward, take extra care with the lysate to assure that the DNA is not sheared. Never pipet or vortex the lysate.
4. Using a cell scraper, gently scrape the cell lysate toward one side of the dish. Pour the lysate (do not pipet) into a 1.5 mL microtube.
5. Add 250 μL of 5 M NaCl to the lysate. Gently mix by inversion 4–5 times. Do not vortex lysates as this could once again shear the DNA. Place these tubes at 4 °C overnight (*see* **Note 18**).
6. *Day 6*: Place the tubes in the 37 °C water bath for ~5 min to help eliminate the flocculent SDS precipitate clouding the lysate. Spin the tubes in the table top microcentrifuge for 40 min at 22,000 × *g* at 4 °C. Lipids, proteins, and genomic DNA should pellet at the bottom of the tube. Carefully decant the supernatant in a new microtube making sure not to disturb the pellet.

7. To digest any residual protein, add Proteinase K to the supernatant at a final concentration of 100 μg/mL. Gently invert the microtube 4–5 times to mix and incubate at 50 °C for at least 2 h.
8. Add the digested lysate to an Amicon Ultra Centrifugal Filter (Ultracel 50 K Filter) and centrifuge at 2800 × *g* for 10 min at 4 °C (*see* **Note 19**).
9. Remove the centrifugal filter from the collection tube. Carefully invert the centrifugal filter into a new collection tube, and centrifuge at 1000 × *g* for 5 min at 4 °C to recover retentate.
10. Transfer the retentate into a fresh microtube and add 2 volumes (typically 1 mL) of 100% ethanol. Mix by inversion 4–5 times and place the samples into the −80 °C freezer for 1 h to precipitate DNA (*see* **Note 20**).
11. Centrifuge the samples at 22,000 × *g* for 30 min at 4 °C. A small pellet should appear at the bottom of the tube.
12. Decant the supernatant and wash the DNA pellet with 1 mL of 70% ethanol, and centrifuge again at top speed for 5 min at 4 °C. Decant the supernatant and repeat the wash step a second time.
13. Decant the ethanol supernatant ethanol and air dry the pellet in the fume hood. Resuspend the dry pellet in 50–100 μL of 1 × TE (pH 8.0).
14. In a microtube, digest 50 μL of recovered plasmid DNA with *Dpn*I (NEB) at 37 °C for 1–3 h. A standard digestion reaction would include: 50 μL recovered plasmid DNA, 6 μL 10× NEB Cutsmart Buffer, 1 μL RNaseA (10 mg/mL), and 3 μL *Dpn*I enzyme (20 units/μL). After 1–3 incubation, heat-inactivate the enzyme at 80 °C for 20 min.
15. Quantify a small aliquot of the digested DNA by UV absorbance or by electrophoresis on a 0.8% agarose gel.

3.6 Transformation of Shuttle Vector into Yeast by Lithium Acetate

1. *Day 6*: Grow a single yeast colony in 5 mL of YPD liquid media overnight at 30 °C with shaking.
2. *Day 7*: From the overnight culture, inoculate a fresh YPD culture and incubate in a 30 °C shaker until the culture reaches mid-logarithmic growth at an OD_{600} = 0.5–0.8 (approximately 2.0 × 10^7 cells/mL). This cell density ensures an optimal transformation efficiency (*see* **Note 21**).
3. Collect the cells by centrifugation (2700 × *g* for 5 min) and discard the supernatant. Wash the pellet in 1 mL sterile dIH_20. Transfer the resuspension to a microcentrifuge tube.
4. Collect the cells by centrifugation (2700 × *g* for 5 min) and discard the supernatant. Gently resuspend the cells with 1 mL

LiAc/TE mix. Collect the cells by centrifugation once again and resuspend the pellet in 250 μL LiAc/TE mix.

5. For each transformation, mix 50 μL of the yeast suspension, ~150 ng of plasmid and 10 μL sonicated salmon sperm DNA (10 mg/mL) [15]. Always do a negative control with no plasmid DNA added.
6. Gently mix, add 600 μL 40% PEG mix.
7. Incubate reactions in a 30 °C shaker for 30–60 min. Longer incubation times are fine.
8. Remove transformations and heat shock the reactions in a 42 °C water bath for exactly 15 min.
9. Add 3 mL of YPD at 30 °C to each transformation mix in a 13 mL snap cap tube and shake at 30 °C for 4–6 h.
10. Centrifuge cultures at 2700 × *g* for 5 min. Resuspend the pellet in 1 mL of sterile dIH2O to remove the remainder of YPD. Centrifuge the cells again for 2 min at 2700 × *g*.
11. Resuspend the washed pellet in 100–200 μL of dIH_2O and plate the appropriate dilutions onto your SC–His–Arg+Can and SC–His media plates. 50–100 μL of undiluted cells onto the +Can plates should yield ~5–50 colonies, and 20–50 μL of a 1:10 dilution of the resuspension onto SC–His plates should yield between 50 and 500 colonies. Cells can be spread with sterile glass beads or by glass rod. Incubate in 30 °C cabinet for ~3 days (*see* **Note 22**).
12. *Days 10–11*: Count the number of colonies on SC–His (total transformants) and SC–His–Arg+Can (potential expansions) plates. Calculate the apparent expansion frequency as per Subheading 3.9.

3.7 PCR Amplification of TNR Fragment

1. *Day 12*: Single-colony PCR amplification is used to validate expansions and to determine the size of the expanded triplet repeat (±1–2 repeats). This analysis is performed on yeast colonies that have grown on the selective plates (–His –Arg +Can). Typically 10–15 canavanine-resistant colonies from each transformation are examined by PCR.
2. Add 100 μL of yeast colony lysis buffer into each well of a 96-well PCR plate.
3. Pick a single yeast colony off of the selective plates using a sterile 200 μL tip or sterile wooden stick and transfer it into a single well. Make sure the colony is resuspended thoroughly in the lysis buffer.
4. Vortex the plate briefly, then incubate the plate at 37 °C for 30 min. After incubation, vortex the plate again and incubate at 95 °C for 8 min, inhibiting the cell lysis reaction. Both incubations can be performed in a thermocycler.

5. After the heating step, the plate can be vortexed one final time (*see* **Note 23**).
6. PCR can be performed in 96-well PCR plates by adding 5 μL of the TNR PCR master mix (*see* Subheading 2.4) and 5 μL of the yeast colony lysis from the previous step. Make sure to include a negative control as well as $(CAG)_{20}$, $(CAG)_{22}$, and $(CAG)_{25}$ marker controls. CY5 5′-labeled primers that flank the triplet repeat tract (Table 1) are used under the following thermocycling conditions: 1 cycle of 2 min at 95 °C, 30 cycles of 1 min at 95 °C (denaturation), 1 min at 60 °C (annealing), and 1 min at 72 °C (elongation). A final elongation step of 72 °C for 5 min. PCR reactions can be stored at −20 °C until ready to be analyzed on a 6% denaturing gel (Fig. 3).

3.8 Sequencing Gel and Analysis of TNR Tracts

1. *Day 13*: 6% denaturing polyacrylamide gels (approximately 42 cm high × 37 cm wide) are used to analyze triplet repeat size. PCR amplification of the reporter plasmid pBL302 using primers oBL251 and Can1Rev results in a ~160 bp fragment (unexpanded TNR tract). Authentic expansions result in a larger amplicon. A stop reaction step must be performed with the PCR samples before loading them onto the gel. Add 5 μL of Formamide stop reaction solution (Subheading 2.4) to each PCR reaction, and heat at 95 °C for 8 min.
2. Pour a 6% sequencing gel by adding the components (Subheading 2.5) into a squeeze bottle and gently mix by inverting. Slowly add the sequencing gel mixture between the horizontal glass plates, moving in a side-to-side motion. If bubbles occur, they can be carefully tapped out using a rubber mallet. Continue to add the sequencing gel mixture until the entire space between the pieces of glass is full. Insert the gel comb.
3. Allow 30 min for the gel to polymerize.
4. Place the gel into the running apparatus and fill the top and bottom wells with 1× TBE buffer. Prewarm the gel up by running it at 50–60 W for 1 h, making sure the voltage does not surpass 2000 V. The outside glass of the gel should be warm to the touch.
5. Load 2 μL of the stopped PCR reactions per well (*see* **Note 24**). For ample separation of sample size, run the sequencing gel for 3–4 h at 40–70 W making sure that the voltage does not surpass 2000 V. The bromophenol blue dye front (dark blue) will migrate out of the gel, while the xylene cyanol dye front (light blue) should finish approximately ¾ of the way down the gel.
6. Disconnect the power and place the gel on Styrofoam blocks. Gently pry apart the two plates with a plastic spatula and lift off

one plate. Place a piece of Whatman #1 filter paper directly onto the gel, gently press down and smooth to remove all air bubbles. Gently peel away the filter paper with adhered gel. Image the gel using a scanner that will excite the CY5 5′ labeled DNA (700 nm red light excitation).

3.9 Calculation of Expansion Frequency

It is essential to perform colony PCR on several different colonies to assure the expansion events that are being reported actually took place. It may be necessary to correct the calculated mutation rate based on the number of authentic expansion events that are identified by PCR and sequencing gels. An expansion in the reporter plasmid should alter the transcription of the *CAN1* gene, allowing yeast cells with the plasmid to be resistant to the toxic arginine analogue L-Canavanine. "False-positives" are yeast colonies that have taken up the reporter plasmid (are His^{+}) and grow in the presence of L-Canavanine (Can^{R}) but *do not* harbor expansions in the plasmid. Figure 4 and the following explain how to calculate true expansion frequency, using the results from the sequencing gel shown in Fig. 3.

1. To determine the initial background levels of false-positive colonies from your starter plasmid in yeast, transform 100–500 ng of the starting reporter plasmid pBL302 into yeast as a control alongside the transformations of the *Dpn*I digested recovered plasmid (*see* Subheading 3.6). Plate 100 μL of the undiluted transformation resuspension onto SC–His–Arg+Can plates, and 20 μL of the undiluted resuspension onto SC–His plates. Spread with glass beads and incubate at 30 °C for 3–4 days.
2. Count the number of colonies on both the SC–His and the SC–His–Arg+Can plates. The SC–His plate represents the total number of yeast cells that have taken up the plasmid (His^{+}). The SC–His–Arg+Can plates represent the number of false-positives (His^{+} Can^{R}). Divide the number of His^{+} Can^{R} by the total number of His+ colonies off of the SC–His plates. Remember to take into account the difference in plating volume. In this case, 100 μL of cells were plated onto SC–His–Arg+Can plates, and only 20 μL onto SC–His plates. Therefore, the number of colonies from the SC–His plates is multiplied by 5 (100/20 = 5). This value is the yeast background adjustment (*see* **Note 25**) (Fig. 4a).
3. From the recovered plasmid transformations, count the number of colonies from both the SC–His–Arg+Can and SC–His plates. Make sure to take into account any differences in plating volume of dilution factors. In this example, the same volume of cells were plated on both SC–His and SC–His–Arg+Can plates. To calculate observed expansion frequency, divide the number of colonies counted from the SC–His–Arg+Can plates

A. Background no SVG-A transfection

\# colonies from SC-His+Can = 5 from 100 uL undiluted sample
\# colonies from SC-His = 450 from 100 uL 5-fold diluted sample

$$\frac{\text{(\#colonies SC-His+Can) x dilution factor}}{\text{(\#colonies SC-His) x dilution factor}} = \frac{5 \times 1}{450 \times 5} = \mathbf{0.002}$$

B. Observed expansion frequency plasmid recovered from SVG-A cells

\# colonies from SC-His+Can = 31
\# colonies from SC-His = 101

$$\frac{\text{(\#colonies SC-His+Can)}}{\text{(\#colonies SC-His)}} = \frac{31}{101} = \mathbf{0.307}$$

C. Authenticated expansions from PCR/gel analysis

Total attempted PCR = 31
Total successful PCR = 26
Authentic expansions = 5

$$\frac{\text{Authentic expansions}}{\text{Successful PCR}} = \frac{5}{26} = \mathbf{0.192}$$

D. Corrected expansion frequency from B and C

Observed Expansion Freq **x** Authenticated Expansions **x** (1 – Background)

0.307 **x** 0.192 **x** 0.998 = **0.059**

Fig. 4 Sample calculation of TNR expansion frequency incorporating the results from Fig. 3. (**a**) Background calculations are performed by direct transformation of the starting shuttle vector preparation into yeast. This value takes into account any low-level frequency of expansions that occur during plasmid workup in *E. coli* or immediately upon transformation into yeast. Background frequencies are refined by taking into account PCR verification (*see* **Note 25**). (**b**) Observed expansion frequency is calculated from the colonies arising from DNA recovered from SVG-A cells. Different plating volumes or plating dilutions can be accounted for in this equation. (**c**) Authentic expansion events are calculated from the sequencing gel results (Fig. 3) and incorporate the number of real expansions and total successful PCR reactions in the experiment. (**d**) The corrected expansion frequency takes into account the observed expansion frequency, the fraction of authentic expansions and the background frequency

by the total number of colonies containing the plasmid counted from the SC–His plates. This value is the observed expansion frequency (Fig. 4b).

4. From the colonies that have grown on the SC–His–Arg+Can plates, perform PCR (*see* Subheading 3.7) and resolve the reaction on a denaturing sequencing gel (*see* Subheading 3.8).

From the sequencing gel image, count the number of true expansions (those larger than the 25 repeat marker). Count the number of PCR reactions that successfully amplified the TNR tract. Subtract the number of successful PCR reactions from the total number of attempted PCR reactions to get the 'Total Events'. Divide the number of authentic expansions by the calculated total events. This value is the authentic expansion frequency (Fig. 4c).

5. Using the values calculated above, multiply the observed expansion frequency by the authentic expansion frequency. Multiply again by (1.0 – Background). The final number is the corrected expansion frequency (Fig. 4b).

4 Notes

1. PEG solution is light sensitive. Wrap the bottle with aluminum foil to protect it from light. This solution can also become contaminated easily, so visually inspect it prior to use. If low transformation efficiencies are observed, remake the PEG solution as a first potential remedy.
2. Make this LiAc/TE mix fresh right before the transformation.
3. Make this 40% PEG mix fresh right before the transformation. Keep covered from light.
4. Canavanine is an arginine analogue that interferes with L-arginine utilization due to its structural similarity. L-arginine is dropped out of the mix and replaced with canavanine.
5. Make sure that sterile technique is used when adding the dropout mix into the flask. Flame the lips of all flasks before pouring. Pour ~25 mL per plate, allow plates to dry on the bench overnight in stacks of 3–5 to reduce condensation formation. Store at 4 °C until needed. Warm plates in 30 °C incubator before plating.
6. Formamide is carcinogenic and should only be pipetted in the fume hood.
7. 10% APS has a short lifespan at 4 °C (~3–4 weeks). If there is an issue with gel polymerization, this would be the likely culprit.
8. APS is an oxidizing agent that catalyzes the polymerization of acrylamide in the mix. TEMED helps speed up this polymerization. Thus, make sure to add the 10% APS and TEMED last to the sequencing gel mix to assure it does not polymerize before it can be poured.

9. This culture should be closely monitored to assure that it does not reach stationary phase ($OD_{600} > 0.8$), as plasmids containing repetitive sequences such as TNRs may undergo contraction events when the cells proceed to stationary phase [16].
10. The complete DMEM culture media contains a trypsin inhibitor so that the cells can adhere to the bottom of the flask. Using Hanks to wash the cells removes the remaining DMEM, allowing for the trypsinization reaction to occur.
11. The trypsin inhibitors in the DMEM inhibit any further trypsinization. Make sure to add at least twice the volume of complete DMEM as the Hanks + Trypsin.
12. This final resuspension step will vary depending on the confluency of the cells and the time interval since the prior cell passage. The pellet is usually resuspended in 10 mL of DMEM, and 0.5 mL – 2.0 mL are usually added to 10 mL of fresh DMEM in a T75 flask. Adding 1 mL of a higher dilution of the cell pellet, (i.e., 1:8–1:10) to a T75 flask containing 10 mL complete DMEM will result in few cells being added to the flask, and thus a longer incubation period to reach confluency. These dilutions may be changed depending on confluence. Ideally, count the cells before they are added to the flask.
13. Always add media to the dish/flask before you add your cells. Adding cells directly to a dry surface can inhibit cell adherence.
14. Opti-MEM is a reduced-serum media that works well with cationic lipid transfection reagents such as Lipofectamine.
15. Adding the incubated shuttle vector complex in a dropwise manner assures the cells on the bottom of the dish are not disturbed.
16. Opti-MEM media does not contain FBS and can be toxic to the cells at longer exposure times.
17. If the cells appear to be peeling off the bottom of dish, the cells are likely overly confluent and may have been initially seeded at too high a density. The number of cells seeded at Subheading 3.3 may need to be adjusted relative to culture conditions or the amount of time the SVG-A cells are incubated at 37 °C.
18. The addition of a high salt buffer helps remove any proteins that may be bound to DNA and keeps those proteins in the aqueous layer of the lysate so that they do not precipitate with DNA in alcohol precipitation step of the protocol.
19. Typically, the Proteinase K digested supernatant from a 60 mm dish is approximately 1.1 mL in volume. The maximum volume capacity of the Amicon filters is ~500 μL. Thus, two filters are required for each sample. It is not advised to load more than 500 μL per filter as the filter can get clogged and retain DNA/protein that is smaller than the 50 K cutoff.

20. Extending the −80 °C ethanol precipitation overnight may improve the plasmid recovery, but also adds an extra half day to the assay. There is also no need to add further salt to your sample, as there is NaCl present from the previous steps.
21. It is useful to set up more than one yeast dilution the morning of the transformation to assure the cells are grown to the correct OD_{600}. 10 mL of culture is required for each plasmid to be transformed. A 1:30 or 1:50 dilution using a saturated overnight culture will usually reach mid-log phase in 3 h.
22. When first performing this assay, it is useful to plate a few different dilutions to assure there are a sufficient number of cells to count. For example, plating 50 μL of undiluted cells, 20 μL of 1:10 dilution of cell, and 20 μL of 1:100 diluted cells on both selective and permissive plates. These numbers/dilutions may be different base on transformation efficiency.
23. Yeast colony lysis plates can be stored at 4 °C until required for PCR amplification.
24. The Formamide Stop Reaction Solution contains two different loading dyes to help visualize loading and migration of samples through the gel.
25. We often observe that background assays yield Can^R colonies but that PCR analysis shows no authentic expansions. A maximum background frequency (e.g., ≤ value) can be estimated by assuming that, if one more background Can^R colony had appeared, it would be authentic. The calculation should therefore be 1/((total successful PCR) + 1). For the example (*see* Fig. 4), five background colonies were tested; therefore the authenticated expansion frequency is ≤1/6 or ≤0.167. The maximum background frequency becomes 0.002 × (≤0.167) = ≤0.0003.

Acknowledgments

This work was supported by Government of Ireland Postdoctoral Fellowship GOIPD/2018/291 from the Irish Research Council (to Gregory M. Williams) and by Science Foundation Ireland grant 16/BBSRC/3395 (to Robert S. Lahue).

References

1. Lee J-M, Zhang J, Su AI et al (2010) A novel approach to investigate tissue-specific trinucleotide repeat instability. BMC Syst Biol 4:29–44
2. Gomes-Pereira M, Bidichandani SI, Monckton DG (2004) Analysis of unstable triplet repeats using small-pool polymerase chain reaction. Methods Mol Biol 277:61–76
3. Claassen DA, Lahue RS (2007) Expansions of CAG-CTG repeats in immortalized human astrocytes. Hum Mol Genet 16:3088–3096
4. Debacker K, Frizzell A, Gleeson O et al (2012) Histone deacetylase complexes promote trinucleotide repeat expansions. PLoS Biol. https://doi.org/10.1371/journal.pbio.1001257

5. Major EO, Miller AE, Mourrain P et al (1985) Establishment of a line of human fetal glial cells that supports JC virus multiplication. Proc Natl Acad Sci U S A 82:1257–1261
6. Major EO, Traub RG (1986) JC virus T protein during productive infection in human fetal brain and kidney cells. Virology 148:221–225
7. Shelbourne PF, Keller-McGandy C, Bi WL et al (2007) Triplet repeat mutation length gains correlate with cell-type specific vulnerability in Huntington disease brain. Hum Mol Genet 16:1133–1142
8. Gannon A-MM, Frizzell A, Healy E et al (2012) MutSβ and histone deacetylase complexes promote expansions of trinucleotide repeats in human cells. Nucleic Acids Res 40:10324–10333
9. Keogh N, Chan KY, Li G-M et al (2017) MutSβ abundance and Msh3 ATP hydrolysis are important drivers of CTG-CAG repeat expansions. Nucleic Acids Res 45:10068–10078
10. Genetic Modifiers of Huntington's Disease (GeM-HD) Consortium (2015) Identification of genetic factors that modify clinical onset of Huntington's disease. Cell 162:516–526
11. Bettencourt C, Hensmann-Moss D, Flower M et al (2016) DNA repair pathways underlie a common genetic mechanism modulating onset in polyglutamine diseases. Ann Neurol 79:983–990
12. Lee J-M, Chao MJ, Harold D et al (2017) A modifier of Huntington's disease onset at the MLH1 locus. Hum Mol Genet 26:3859–3867
13. Hensman-Moss D, Pardinas AF, Langbehn D et al (2017) Identification of genetic variants associated with Huntington's disease progression: a genome-wide association study. Lancet Neurol 16:701–711
14. Kononenko AV, Ebersole T, Vasquez KM et al (2018) Mechanisms of genetic instability caused by (CGG)n repeats in an experimental mammalian system. Nat Struct Mol Biol 25:669–676
15. Gietz RD, Woods RA (2002) Transformation of yeast by the lithium acetate/single-stranded carrier DNA/polyethylene glycol method. Methods Enzymol 350:87–96
16. Bowater RP, Rosche WA, Jaworski A et al (1996) Relationship between *Escherichia coli* growth and deletions of CTG-CAG triplet repeats in plasmids. J Mol Biol 264:82–96

Chapter 11

Isolation and Analysis of the CGG-Repeat Size in Male and Female Gametes from a Fragile X Mouse Model

Xiaonan Zhao, Huiyan Lu, Pradeep K. Dagur, and Karen Usdin

Abstract

Analysis of individual gametes has a number of applications in the study of the mechanism of repeat expansion in mouse models of the fragile X-related disorders, as well as in mouse models of other repeat expansion diseases. This chapter describes the techniques required to isolate oocytes and male gametes of different stages of maturity, along with the techniques required to accurately determine the repeat number in these gametes.

Key words Oocyte, Sperm, Germ cell, Fluorescence-activated cell sorting, Single cell analysis, Small pool PCR

1 Introduction

The fragile X-related disorders (FXDs) are members of the repeat expansion diseases in which the expansion-prone repeat tract, located in exon 1 of the *FMR1* gene, consists of >54 CGG-repeats [1]. Expansion occurs primarily on intergenerational transmission with some additional somatic instability apparent in some individuals. We have made use of a mouse model of these disorders to try to understand the expansion mechanism responsible [2–6]. The ability to isolate and accurately determine the repeat number present in the gametes in this mouse model has helped in our understanding of the timing of expansion and provided important clues as to the underlying mechanism [7]. In addition, the fact that we have found that expansion in male gametes is limited to the premeiotic stages of spermatogenesis [7], allows us to study the effect of various DNA repair/recombination mutations on intergenerational expansion even in animals that are sterile by isolating and analyzing the repeat size in immature gametes. Furthermore, the ability to analyze the repeats in individual gametes using single cell PCR greatly expedites the study of genetic factors important for intergenerational expansion without requiring the production of

Guy-Franck Richard (ed.), *Trinucleotide Repeats: Methods and Protocols*, Methods in Molecular Biology, vol. 2056, https://doi.org/10.1007/978-1-4939-9784-8_11,

large numbers of offspring. Single cell or small pool PCR is also useful for the analysis of somatic instability in these animals, since it gives a more realistic measurement of the extent of expansion and contraction than does the analysis of bulk DNA [8]. This chapter will provide detailed protocols for the isolation of male and female gametes from mice and for the analysis of the repeat in these gametes in either bulk DNA or the DNA from single cells.

2 Materials

2.1 Oocyte Collection

1. Female FX mice (*see* **Note 1**).
2. Needles (26-gauge), 1 mL sterile syringe.
3. Forceps, fine forceps, fine scissors.
4. 35-mm petri dish
5. Oocyte handling pipette (consisting of hand-held pipette assembly and pulled capillary).
6. Stereomicroscope.
7. Pregnant Mare Serum Gonadotropin (PMSG), store the solution in aliquots at −20 °C for up to 1 month (*see* **Note 2**).
8. Human chorionic gonadotropin (hCG), store the solution in aliquots at −20 °C for up to 1 month (*see* **Note 2**).
9. M2 medium.
10. M2 with hyaluronidase.
11. Dulbecco's Phosphate buffered saline (DPBS; without calcium or magnesium).

2.2 Male Gamete Collection

1. Male FX mice (*see* **Note 3**).
2. Forceps, fine forceps, fine scissors, needles (26-gauge).
3. 35-mm petri dish
4. 70-μm cell strainer
5. 5 mL tube with cell strainer cap
6. Fluorescence activated cell sorter (FACS).
7. Dulbecco's Phosphate buffered saline (DPBS; without calcium or magnesium).
8. DMEM Dulbecco's modified Eagle medium (DMEM; 4.5 g/L glucose).
9. Collagenase type IV dissolved in DMEM to a final concentration of 10 mg/mL. Sterilize by passing through a 0.22-μm filter. Store the solution in aliquots at −20 °C.
10. DNase I (10 U/μL).
11. Dispase (1 U/mL), store the solution in aliquots at −20 °C.

12. Fetal bovine serum (FBS; heat inactivated), store the solution in aliquots at −20 °C.
13. Penicillin-Streptomycin (Pen Strep; 10,000 U/mL).
14. Dimethyl sulfoxide (DMSO).
15. Hoechst 33342 (10 mg/mL).
16. Collagenase/DNase solution: Thaw collagenase IV stock solution and dilute with DMEM to a final concentration of 1 mg/mL. Add 10 U/μL DNase I to make a final concentration of 100 U/mL. Store at 4 °C for up to a week.
17. Dispase/DNase solution: Thaw dispase stock solution and add 10 U/μL DNase I to a final concentration of 100 U/mL. Store at 4 °C for up to a week.
18. MEF growth medium: Add FBS into DMEM to a final concentration of 10% (v/v) FBS. Add 10,000 U/mL Pen Strep to make a final concentration of 10 U/mL. Store at 4 °C for up to 2 weeks.
19. Cell freezing medium: Add FBS and DMSO into DMEM to a final concentration of 10% (v/v) FBS and 10% (v/v) DMSO. Store at 4 °C for up to 2 weeks.
20. Cell sorting buffer: Add FBS into DPBS to a final concentration of 5% (v/v) FBS. Store at 4 °C for up to 2 weeks.
21. 2× cell staining buffer: Add 10 mg/mL Hoechst 33342 into cell sorting buffer to a final concentration of 10 μg/mL Hoechst 33342. Prepare fresh.

2.3 DNA Isolation and Determination of Repeat Number

1. Proteinase K (20 mg/mL, RNA grade). Add Proteinase K into equal volume of DPBS to make a final concentration of 10 mg/mL.
2. Dithiothreitol (DTT) dissolved in sterile distilled H_2O to a final concentration of 1 M. Sterilize by passing through a 0.22-μm filter. Store the solution in aliquots at −20 °C for up to 1 year.
3. Buffer ATL (Qiagen).
4. Sodium chloride (5 M NaCl).
5. Ethanol and 70% (v/v) ethanol.
6. Cell lysis buffer: Add 20 mg/mL Proteinase K and 1 M DTT into ATL buffer to a final concentration of 0.55 mg/mL Proteinase K and 30 mM DTT. Prepare fresh.
7. Tris–HCl (1 M, pH 9.0).
8. Magnesium chloride ($MgCl_2$; 1 M).
9. Ammonium sulfate ($(NH_4)_2SO_4$) dissolved in sterile double-distilled H_2O to a final concentration of 2.2 M. Sterilize by

passage through a 0.22-μm filter. Store the solution at room temperature.

10. Triton X-100.
11. Betaine dissolved in sterile distilled H_2O to make a 5 M solution. Sterilize by passage through a 0.22-μm filter. Store the solution in aliquots at 4 °C for up to 1 year (*see* **Note 4**).
12. Dimethyl sulfoxide (DMSO).
13. dNTP set (50 mM each of dATP, dCTP, dGTP, and dTTP): Add the dNTP mix into 4 volumes of sterile double-distilled H_2O to a final concentration of 10 mM each, store the solution in aliquots at −20 °C (*see* **Note 5**).
14. dCTP (100 mM).
15. dGTP (100 mM).
16. Testicular cell lysis buffer: Add 20 mg/mL Proteinase K and 1 M DTT into ATL buffer to a final concentration of 0.55 mg/mL Proteinase K and 30 mM DTT.
17. 10× Q5 CGG PCR buffer [9]: Add 1 M Tris–HCl (pH 9.0), 1 M $MgCl_2$, 2.2 M $(NH_4)_2SO_4$, and Triton X-100 into sterile double-distilled H_2O and make final concentration of 500 mM Tris–HCl, 15 mM $MgCl_2$, 220 mM $(NH_4)_2SO_4$, 2% Triton X-100. Store at room temperature.
18. 2× Betaine–DMSO mix: Add 1 volume of DMSO into 25 volume of Betaine to make a final concentration of 4.8 M betaine, 4% DMSO.
19. dCTP/dGTP mix: Add equal volumes of dCTP and dGTP into 2 volumes of sterile double-distilled H_2O to make a final concentration of 25 mM each. Store the solution in aliquots at −20 °C (*see* **Note 5**).
20. Q5 Hot Start High-Fidelity DNA Polymerase (2000 U/mL, New England Biolabs).
21. 2× KAPA2G Fast HotStart Genotyping Mix (KAPA Biosystems).

3 Methods

Carry out all procedures in biosafety cabinets maintaining sterile working procedures. All biomedical/biohazard reagents and waste must be handled according to institutional lab safety guidelines. The methods described here are suitable only for collecting cells for genomic DNA analysis, not for other purposes like in vitro fertilization.

3.1 Oocyte Collection

This procedure is a slight modification of a previously published procedure [10].

1. Intraperitoneal injection of female mice with five international units (IU) PMSG (*see* **Note 6**).
2. Intraperitoneal injection of female mice with five IU hCG 47 h after PMSG injection (*see* **Note 6**).
3. Thirteen hours after hCG injection, euthanize the females by CO_2 inhalation. Place the animal(s) in the home cage and introduce 100% carbon dioxide by a fill rate of about 10–30% of the cage volume per minute with carbon dioxide [11].
4. Quickly dissect out the oviducts with a small section of the uterus and transfer to a clean 35-mm petri dish with pre-warmed M2 media. The ampullae of the oviducts should be much enlarged.
5. Transfer one oviduct in a new 35-mm petri dish with M2 with hyaluronidase medium. Under the stereomicroscope with 20× magnification, use fine forceps to grasp the ampullae, and use another fine forceps or 26-gauge needle to tear the ampullae to release the cumulus oocyte masses.
6. Incubate the oocytes in M2 with hyaluronidase medium for 2–5 min to allow the cumulus cells to dissociate.
7. Use an oocyte handling pipette to pick up the oocyte and transfer them to a new 35-mm petri dish containing several drops (100 μL/drop) of fresh M2 medium to rinse off the hyaluronidase solution, cumulus cells and debris.
8. Transfer individual oocytes into an 0.5 mL PCR tube containing 10 μL DPBS and freeze at −80 °C.

3.2 Testicular Cell Collection

This procedure is a slight modification of a previously published procedure [7, 12].

1. Euthanize the male mice by CO_2 inhalation as described above and quickly dissect out the testes.
2. Place the testes in a 60-mm petri dish containing DPBS.
3. Use two pairs of fine forceps to grasp and remove the tunica albuginea.
4. Cut the testes into small pieces and treat with 4 mL collagenase/DNase solution, incubate at 37 °C for 20 min in a CO_2 incubator.
5. Use a truncated 1000 μL tip to gently pipette and separate the seminiferous tubules.
6. Transfer the seminiferous tubules into 15 mL conical tube, centrifuge at 200 × *g* for 5 min at room temperature.
7. Carefully remove the supernatant, add 10 mL DPBS and gently pipette to wash the seminiferous tubules.

8. Centrifuge at 200 × *g* for 5 min at room temperature.
9. Repeat **steps** 7 and **8** three times to remove cell debris.
10. Add 4 mL Dispase/DNase solution, incubate at 37 °C for 20 min in a CO_2 incubator, with gentle pipetting of the cells every 5 min.
11. Filter the mixture through a 70-μm cell strainer.
12. Centrifuge at 500 × *g* for 5 min at room temperature.
13. Carefully remove the supernatant. If possible, the cells should be processed immediately for staining and sorting as described in Subheading 3.3. If necessary, the cells can be frozen as described in **steps 14** and **15** and recovered for later analysis.
14. Slowly resuspend cells in 6 mL prechilled (4 °C) cell freezing media, transfer to six cryovials (1 mL/vial, about 1 × 10^7/mL, *see* **Note** 7).
15. Transfer the cryovials to the prechilled (4 °C) StrataCooler Cryo preservation module. Place the module in a −80 °C freezer overnight. Transfer the vials to liquid nitrogen for long-term storage.

3.3 Staining of Testicular Cells Prior to Isolation by Fluorescence Activated Cell Sorter (FACS)

Different testicular cell types were isolated by flow cytometry using a modification of a previously published procedure [13].

1. Warm the MEF growth media at 37 °C.
2. If cells are fresh prepared, go to **step 6**.
3. Otherwise, remove the frozen vials of testicular cells from liquid nitrogen and thaw in a 37 °C water bath until completely unfrozen, usually about 3–5 min (*see* **Note 8**).
4. Transfer the cells into a 15 mL conical tube with 10 mL prewarmed MEF growth media.
5. Centrifuge the cells at 200 × *g* for 5 min at room temperature. Carefully remove the supernatant.
6. Add 10 mL DPBS and pipette to gently wash the cells.
7. Centrifuge at 200 × *g* for 5 min at room temperature.
8. Carefully remove the supernatant and add 10 mL prewarmed cell sorting buffer (*see* **Note 9**).
9. Count the cells and adjust the cell number to 2 × 10^6/mL using cell sorting buffer (*see* **Note 9**).
10. Add equal volume of 2× cell staining buffer to stain cell at a final concentration of 5 μg/mL Hoechst 33342. Incubate at 37 °C for 45 min, gently shaking the dish every 5 min.
11. Centrifuge at 200 × *g* for 5 min at room temperature.
12. Carefully remove the supernatant and resuspend cell in 3 mL testicular cell sorting buffer, cells are now ready for sorting (*see* **Note 10**).

3.4 Testicular Cell Sorting

This protocol describes the use of a FACSARIA™ (SORP) (BD) fluorescence activated cell sorter (FACS) system to isolate different murine male gametes. Note that other cell sorters may also be used, according to manufacturer recommendations.

1. Startup and QC the cytometer as per the manufacturer's instructions.
2. Create a new template. The instrument must have a 488-nm blue laser to measure the scatter properties and a 355 nm UV laser (at 60 mW or higher) to excite the Hoechst dye. Select the instrument settings to include the height, area and width parameters of forward scatter (FSC), side scatter (SSC) and two detectors from the UV laser – one with a bandpass filter of 450/20 nm (Blue shift of HOECHST emission) and the other at 640/20 nm (Red shift of HOECHST emission), The fluorescence detectors should be on linear scale, not log (*see* **Note 11**).
3. Once the right parameters have been selected for collecting data for the HOECHST and FSC/SSC parameters, make a series of dot plots including (1) a plot showing FC vs SSC, (2) a plot showing FSC width vs FSC area, (3) a one parameter plot showing the 450/20 fluorescence, and (4) a dot plot showing 450/20 fluorescence vs the 640/20 fluorescence (Fig. 1).
4. Immediately prior to running the samples on the sorter, transfer cell to a 5-mL tube with cell strainer cap to removes any residual clumps of cells.
5. Load the stained and filtered sample on sample port of sorter and start collecting data. Run the samples at a relatively slow acquisition rate (approximately 5000 cells per second to give tight coefficients of variations in the analysis of the samples). While instrument is acquiring data in real-time, adjust the voltages of the FSC and SSC detectors to place the cells on scale. Subsequently adjust the voltages to the 450/20 and 640/20 detectors to visualize 1C, 2C, and 4C populations on linear scales, after excluding doublets using width and area parameters. The populations can be viewed on either the one parameter plot of the 450/20 detector or on the dot plot of the 450/20 vs 640/20 detectors. The first peak (one parameter plot) or major cluster (on the bivariate dot plot) is the 1C population (population 1 and 2), the 2C peak (population 3) is at 1.8–2 times intensity of 1C signal and 4C (population 4) as 1.6–2 times of the 2C signal intensity. Initial gates were established signals using identically processed and stained samples obtained from FX mouse and control mouse lacking haploid population (Fig. 1E, F).

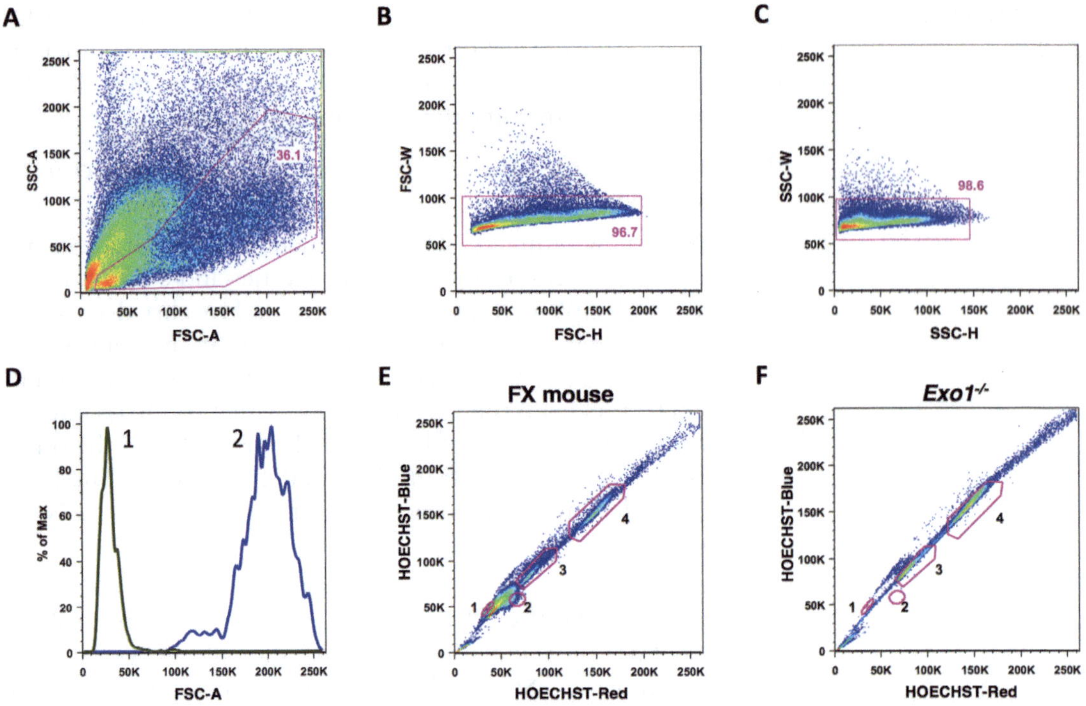

Fig. 1 Gating scheme to purify different testicular cells types. Live cells were differentiated from dead cells and debris based on scatter properties (**A**). Further doublets were removed on the basis of width parameters of the FSC detector (**D**) and then the SSC detector (**C**). The 450/20 (Blue shift) and 640/20 (Red shift) signals were then used to identify the 1C (population 1 and 2), 2C (population 3) and 4C (population 4) cell clusters (**E**, **F**). Among the 1C population (first cluster population 1 and 2) gates were made to distinguish the smaller elongating spermatids from the larger round spermatids (**D**)

6. The 1C population was further sub gated into two populations based on relative size using FSC parameter (1C Higher FSC and 1C Lower FSC) (Fig. 1D).
7. After establishing 1C higher FSC, 1C lower FSC, 2C and 4C gates, those populations are sorted at a flow rate between 5000 and 10,000 events per second and collected in DNase, RNase free sterile 1.8 mL microcentrifuge tubes containing 100 μL of cell sorting buffer.
8. Take 20 μL of sorted cells and place on a slide. Examine the purity of each subpopulation using fluorescence microscopy. The excitation and emission wavelength of Hoechst 33342 are 352 nm and 455 nm respectively. The blue fluorescence may be efficiently excited with a xenon or mercury-arc lamp or with a UV laser, and be detected using the common DAPI filter or blue GFP filters (*see* **Note 12**).
9. Centrifuge each of the cell subpopulations at 200 × *g* for 5 min at room temperature. Carefully remove the supernatant.
10. The cell pellet can be used directly for genomic DNA (gDNA) preparation or frozen at −80 °C.

3.5 Sperm Collection

1. Warm DPBS at 37 °C.
2. Euthanize the male mice by CO_2 inhalation as described in Subheading 3.2 and quickly dissect out the cauda epididymis with part of the vas deferens.
3. Place the epididymis with the vas deferens in a 35-mm petri dish with 1 mL prewarmed DPBS, remove as much fat and blood vessels as possible and rinse with prewarmed DPBS (*see* **Note 13**).
4. Place the epididymis with vas deferens in a new 35-mm petri dish with 2 mL prewarmed DPBS.
5. Use forceps to gently squeeze out the sperm from the vas deferens.
6. Use a 30-gauge needle on a syringe to make 5–10 slit on the cauda epididymis (*see* **Note 14**).
7. Incubate the dish at 37 °C for 30 min. Gentle shake the dish every 5 min. Sperm will swim out from the slit and the solution will become cloudy.
8. Gently shake the dish and collect 1 mL suspension into a 1.5 mL microcentrifuge tube (*see* **Note 15**).
9. Centrifuge at 300 × *g* for 5 min at room temperature.
10. Carefully remove the supernatant. The pellet should be white and without visible red blood cells at the bottom (*see* **Note 16**).
11. Gently tap the tube one or two times to loosen the pellet.
12. Slowly add 1 mL prewarm DPBS along the tube wall.
13. Incubate the tube at 37 °C for 20 min and allow the sperm to swim out.
14. Collect 500 μL supernatant into a new 1.5 mL microcentrifuge tube.
15. Centrifuge at 300 × *g* for 5 min at room temperature.
16. Carefully remove the supernatant. If there is visible red blood cell at the bottom, repeat the swim out **steps 11–16** until there is no visible red blood cell at the bottom.
17. The sperm pellet can be used directly for gDNA preparation or frozen at −80 °C.

3.6 DNA Isolation from Oocytes

1. Take out the tubes with individual oocytes from −80 °C and incubate at 37 °C for 10 min.
2. Place the tube on dry ice for 10 min.
3. Repeat **steps 1** and **2** three times.
4. Add 2.5 μL 10 mg/mL Proteinase K to the tube to make a final concentration of 2 mg/mL Proteinase K.

5. Incubate at 55 °C for 2 h.
6. Incubate at 95 °C for 10 min.
7. The oocyte DNA in a total volume of 12.5 μL can be used directly for PCR or frozen at −20 °C.

3.7 DNA Isolation from Testicular Cells and Sperm

1. Add 300 μL cell lysis buffer to each tube of the sorted testicular cells and the sperm sample. Either fresh prepared or frozen samples can be used.
2. Vortex for 10 s to mix the sample.
3. Incubate at 55 °C overnight.
4. Spin down the liquid that has accumulated in the lid at 300 × *g* for 1 min.
5. Add 90 μL 5 M NaCl, gently invert the tube to mix.
6. Centrifuge at 13,000 × *g* for 10 min at room temperature.
7. Transfer as much of supernatant as possible to a new 1.5 mL microcentrifuge tube, taking care not to transfer the debris.
8. Add an equal volume of ethanol and invert gently to mix.
9. Precipitate the gDNA at −20 °C for 1 h (*see* **Note 17**).
10. Centrifuge at 13,000 × *g* for 10 min at room temperature.
11. Carefully remove the supernatant and add 800 μL 70% ethanol to wash the pellet.
12. Centrifuge at 13,000 × *g* for 10 min at room temperature.
13. Carefully remove the supernatant and leave the lid open for 5 min to dry the pellet.
14. Add 5–100 μL PCR grade H_2O to dissolve the DNA pellet. Incubate at 55 °C for 15 min (*see* **Note 18**).
15. Genomic DNA samples can be used directly for PCR or frozen at −20 °C.

3.8 Analysis of the Repeat Number in Male Gametes

1. To analyze the repeats in individual gametes, determine the DNA concentration and dilute to 3 pg/μL. Use 1 μL as the template to carry out nested PCR using the small pool PCR/Nested PCR strategy described in Subheading 3.10 below.
2. To analyze the repeats from bulk gDNA from sperm or different testicular cell samples, dilute the gDNA to a concentration of 100 ng/μL. Use 1 μL to do a single round of PCR as described in **steps 3–6** of Subheading 3.10.

3.9 Analysis of the Repeat Number in Oocytes

Use the small pool PCR/nested PCR strategy described in Subheading 3.10 to amplify the repeats from individual oocyte samples using 4 μL of the oocyte DNA solution for each reaction.

Table 1
Primers used in this study

Name	Sequence
Not_mFraxC	AGTTCAGCGGCCGCGCTGGGAGCGTTTCGGTTTCACTTCCGGT
Not_FraxR4	CAAGTCGCGGCCGCCTTGTAGAAAGCGCCATTGGAGCCCCGCA
FraxM5	CGGGGGGCGTGCGGTAACGGCCCAA
FAM-FraxM4	FAM-CTTGAGGCCCAGCCGCCGTCGGCC

Dissolve the primers in PCR grade H_2O at a concentration of 100 μM. Store the solution in aliquots at −20°C

3.10 Small Pool PCR/Nested PCR Analysis of Repeat Number

1. Carry out the first round of PCR using the Not_mFraxC and Not_FraxR4 primer pair (Table 1) in a 20 μL reaction. The PCR mix contains 1× Q5 CGG PCR buffer, 1× Betaine–DMSO mix (2.4 M Betaine, 2% DMSO), 0.2 mM dNTPs plus an additional 0.1 mM dCTP/dGTP, 0.5 μM of each primer and 0.02 U/μL of the DNA Q5 polymerase. The first round PCR parameters should be 98 °C for 10 min, 33 cycles of (98 °C for 30 s, 59 °C for 30 s, and 72 °C for 2.5 min), followed by 72 °C for 10 min (Table 1).
2. Amplify 1 μL of the first round PCR reaction or in the case of bulk DNA analysis, 1 μL of a 100 ng/μL gDNA solution, using the FAM-FraxM4 and FraxM5 primer pair (Table 1) in a 21 μL reaction (*see* **Note 19**). The PCR mix contains 1× KAPA2G Fast HotStart Genotyping Mix, 1× Betaine–DMSO mix (2.4 M Betaine, 2% DMSO), 0.5 μM each of the primers FraxM4 and FraxM5. Subject the PCR mix to amplification using the following cycling parameters: 95 °C for 10 min, 35 cycle of (95 °C for 30 s, 65 °C for 30 s, and 72 °C for 70 s), followed by incubation 72 °C for 10 min. The 70 s annealing step can be extended to 1.5 min for amplification of alleles with >300 repeats.
3. Resolve the PCR products by capillary electrophoresis on an ABI Genetic Analyzer. The resultant fsa files can be analyzed using GeneMapper or equivalent software. An R script that can be used for this purpose is available on request [9]. Repeat sizes are calculated using the formula: repeat number = (size of PCR products − 49 bp)/3 (*see* **Note 20**).

4 Notes

1. All experiments involving live rodents must adhere to national and institutional regulations.
2. Store PMSG and hCG in a single use aliquot, avoid freeze-thaw cycles.

3. In addition to the FX male mice, male mice, for example *Exo1*$^{-/-}$ mice [4, 7], which do not complete meiosis and therefore lack haploid sperm can be used as a sorting control to confirm the specificity of the haploid population isolated.
4. To make 20 mL 5 M betaine weigh 13.5 g betaine and add 8 mL sterile double-distilled H_2O. Once most of the betaine has dissolved, make the volume up to 20 mL and wait until the betaine has dissolved completely.
5. Store the dNTPs and dCTP–dGTP mix in small aliquots at −20 °C and discard after three freeze–thaw cycles.
6. The dose needed of each gonadotropin is strain-dependent. Generally, doses of 2.0–5.0 IU per mouse of each gonadotropin and ages of 21–35 days (body weights of 12–14 g) will give the best yield of oocytes.
7. Normally a total number of 5–7 × 10^7 testicular cells can be collected from a 6-month old FX male mouse by this method. The *Exo1*$^{-/-}$ males have smaller testes and fewer testicular cells. The total testicular cell number is ~3–5 × 10^6.
8. Thawing procedure is time and temperature-sensitive. For better recovery of cryopreserved cells, this step should be performed at 37 °C as gently and quickly as possible.
9. Reduce the volume of cell sorting buffer if total testicular cell number is low. If the cell number is lower than 2 × 10^6/mL, use 1 mL for staining.
10. A good concentration of cells for sorting is about 1–2 × 10^7/mL. If the cell number is less than this, use at least 500 μL for sorting.
11. It is advisable to shut down the 407 nm LASER in order to avoid any partial excitation of HOECHST dye by the violet LASER line.
12. Subpopulation 1 included elongated spermatids and spermatozoa with a 1C DNA content, and subpopulation 2 included postmeiotic haploid round spermatids with a 1C DNA content. Subpopulation 3 included secondary spermatocytes, germinal stem cells and some somatic cells with a 2C content. Subpopulation 4 contains prophase spermatocytes with a 4C DNA content. The purity of subpopulations 1, 2, and 4 should be over 90%.
13. Instead of removing the blood vessels attached to the cauda epididymis, forceps can be used to gently squeeze out the blood from blood vessels. This step can remove most of the blood, but at the risk of some sperm loss.
14. Do not mince the cauda epididymis. Minimizing trauma will avoid contamination with somatic cells.

15. Gently shake the dish and tilt the dish a bit to allow the epididymis and vas deferens to slip to the bottom of the dish. Avoid the tissue debris while collecting the suspension. Up to 1.8 mL can be collected.
16. Visible red blood cells may appear at the bottom of the pellet if the blood vessels were not removed properly. Repeating the next swim out steps (**11–16**) will improve the purity of sperm sample.
17. The DNA pellet can be very small and hard to see in the tube if total cell number is less than 100,000. Addition of 1 μL of pellet paint (EMD Millipore) helps in the visualization of the DNA.
18. Adjust the volume of water base on the size of the pellet. Normally add 100 μL for sperm sample and add 5 μL water for samples with less than 100,000 cells.
19. These primers are specific for the FXD mouse generated in our laboratory [14]. Primers specific for other mouse models should aim to have a similar Tm.
20. The number 49 is the number of bases that flank the repeats in amplicons generated by the FraxM5 and FAM-FraxM4 primer pair. This number may change if other primers are used.

Acknowledgments

The authors would like to thank Dr. John Philip McCoy, Jr. (NHLBI) for his careful reading of the manuscript. This work was made possible with funding to KU from the Intramural Program of NIDDK, NIH (DK057808).

References

1. Lozano R, Rosero CA, Hagerman RJ (2014) Fragile X spectrum disorders. Intractable Rare Dis Res 3(4):134–146
2. Lokanga RA, Senejani AG, Sweasy JB et al (2015) Heterozygosity for a hypomorphic Polbeta mutation reduces the expansion frequency in a mouse model of the fragile X-related disorders. PLoS Genet 11(4):e1005181
3. Lokanga RA, Zhao XN, Usdin K (2014) The mismatch repair protein MSH2 is rate limiting for repeat expansion in a fragile X premutation mouse model. Hum Mutat 35(1):129–136
4. Zhao X-N, Zhang Y, Wilkins K et al (2018) Mlh3 promotes while Exo1 protects against repeat expansion in mouse model for the fragile X-related disorders. PLoS Genet 14(10):e1007719
5. Zhao XN, Usdin K (2018) FAN1 protects against repeat expansions in a fragile X mouse model. DNA Repair (Amst) 69:1–5
6. Zhao XN, Lokanga R, Allette K et al (2016) A MutSbeta-dependent contribution of MutSalpha to repeat expansions in fragile X premutation mice? PLoS Genet 12(7):e1006190
7. Zhao XN, Usdin K (2018) Timing of expansion of fragile X premutation alleles during intergenerational transmission in a mouse model of the fragile X-related disorders. Front Genet 9:314
8. Zhao X-N, Gazy I, Hayward BE et al Repeat Instability in the Fragile X-related disorders: lessons from a mouse model. Brain Sci 8:E52
9. Hayward BE, Zhou Y, Kumari D et al (2016) A set of assays for the comprehensive analysis of

FMR1 alleles in the fragile X-related disorders. J Mol Diagn 18(5):762–774

10. Nagy A, Gertsenstein M, Vintersten K et al (2003) Manipulating the mouse embryo: a laboratory manual. CSH Press, Woodbury
11. Danneman PJ, Stein S, Walshaw SO (1997) Humane and practical implications of using carbon dioxide mixed with oxygen for anesthesia or euthanasia of rats. Lab Anim Sci 47(4):376–385
12. Guan K, Wolf F, Becker A et al (2009) Isolation and cultivation of stem cells from adult mouse testes. Nat Protocol 4(2):143–154
13. Hayama T, Yamaguchi T, Kato-Itoh M et al (2016) Practical selection methods for rat and mouse round spermatids without DNA staining by flow cytometric cell sorting. Mol Reprod Dev 83(6):488–496
14. Entezam A, Biacsi R, Orrison B et al (2007) Regional FMRP deficits and large repeat expansions into the full mutation range in a new fragile X premutation mouse model. Gene 395(1–2):125–134

Chapter 12

In Vitro Synthesis and RNA Structure Probing of CUG Triplet Repeat RNA

Remco T. P. van Cruchten and Derick G. Wansink

Abstract

Aberrant RNA structure plays a central role in the molecular mechanisms guided by repeat RNAs in diseases like myotonic dystrophy (DM), *C9orf72*-linked amyotrophic lateral sclerosis (ALS) and fragile X tremor/ataxia syndrome (FXTAS). Much knowledge remains to be gained about how these repeat-expanded transcripts are actually folded, especially regarding the properties specific to very long and interrupted repeats. RNA structure can be interrogated by chemical as well as enzymatic probes. These probes usually bind or cleave single-stranded nucleotides, which can subsequently be detected using reverse transcriptase primer extension. In this chapter, we describe methodology for in vitro synthesis and structure probing of expanded CUG repeat RNAs associated with DM type 1 and approaches for the associated data analysis.

Key words CUG repeat, *DMPK*, In vitro transcription, Myotonic dystrophy, RNA folding, RNA structure, Hairpin, SHAPE, RNase T1, DMS

1 Introduction

Key toxic effects of repeat RNAs are thought to originate from peculiarities in their structure, which often appear as hairpin or stem loop-like folds [1]. Among these effects are prolonged nuclear residence and interactions with RNA-binding proteins, usually visualized as the so-called foci in microscopy, as well as the more recently described repeat-associated non-AUG (RAN) translation [2, 3]. RNA structure information can also be helpful in rationally targeting these toxic transcripts with antisense oligonucleotides (AONs) or small molecules [4, 5].

In vitro RNA structure is generally investigated using chemical or enzymatic probes that either bind or cleave the RNA at single-stranded or flexible nucleotides. These sites can be identified via fragment analysis or termination of reverse transcriptase (RT) primer extension (RT stop) [6]. Probes used for RNA structure probing are often nucleotide specific. This can be an advantage for

Guy-Franck Richard (ed.), *Trinucleotide Repeats: Methods and Protocols*, Methods in Molecular Biology, vol. 2056, https://doi.org/10.1007/978-1-4939-9784-8_12,

repeated sequences, since every induced RT stop event inevitably leads to a decrease in signal intensity downstream to that site. However, for in-depth analysis of short repeats, a more promiscuous probe might be the best choice. During the past decade, selective 2′ hydroxyl acylation analyzed by primer extension (SHAPE) has rapidly become popular as a technique that interrogates every nucleotide [7]. For an overview of RNA structure probes we refer to Weeks [6].

In this chapter, we focus on probing the structures of CUG repeats in vitro using the SHAPE reagent 2-methylnicotinic acid imidazolide (NAI; modifies A, C, G, and U), dimethyl sulfate (DMS; modifies A and C) and RNase T1 (cleaves 3′ of G), after which RT stops are measured using capillary electrophoresis (CE). We consider this technique as the method of choice for RNA structure probing when the cellular expression level of the repeat-containing transcript of interest is low and when analysis of specific model molecules is desired, for example a range of repeat lengths. For an overview of the entire procedure *see* Fig. 1.

Next to elucidation of basic RNA structure, this technique can be used to study the influence on RNA structure of ionic conditions (e.g., Mg^{2+} concentration) and the binding of ligands

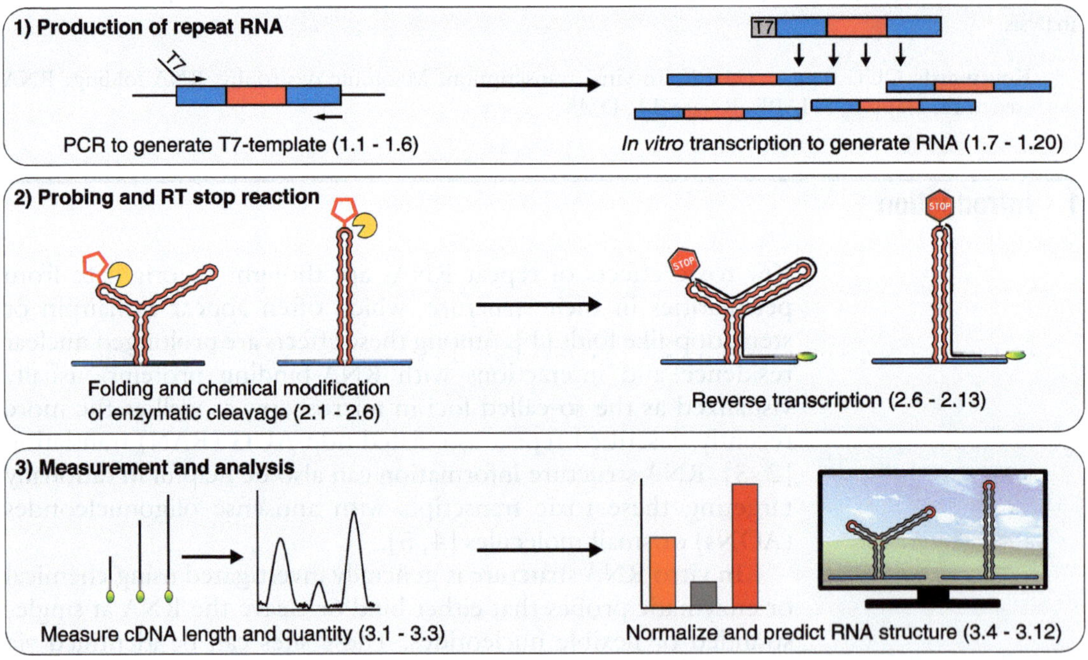

Fig. 1 Overview of the RNA structure probing method. (1) A transcription template is generated via PCR, and subsequently used to generate a large amount of RNA (repeat sequence in red, flanking sequences in blue). (2) This RNA is folded in vitro and subjected to chemical modification or enzymatic cleavage, both of which result in termination of reverse transcription that is performed with fluorescently labeled primers. (3) The length and amount of cDNA are measured via capillary electrophoresis and the obtained data is normalized to use in prediction of RNA structure

(e.g., small molecules, antisense oligonucleotides, proteins). We expect this protocol to work well for CAG repeats also (e.g., dentatorubral-pallidoluysian atrophy, Huntington's disease, and spinocerebellar ataxia types 1, 3, 6, and 7), whereas GGGGCC (*C9orf72* amyotrophic lateral sclerosis-frontotemporal dementia) or CGG (fragile X-associated tremor/ataxia syndrome) repeats might be more difficult because of their high GC content.

Deducing a RNA structure from reactivity data is not trivial, and there are often multiple nonmutually exclusive solutions to the puzzle of fitting a structure to reactivity data [8]. Here, we discuss two methods of data analysis. One should however keep in mind that each particular research aim may require a distinct method and that there are often multiple ways to analyze the data in a scientifically justified manner. Fortunately, for most repeats the basic structural features are known, which can serve as a convenient starting point [1].

2 Materials

Make sure to use only RNase-free materials and solutions. It is advised to purchase certified RNase-free chemicals and dedicate these and specific labware to RNA work only. Always wear gloves when handling RNA and keep RNA on ice or at −80 °C whenever possible, but try to prevent repeated freeze–thaw cycles.

2.1 PCR and In Vitro Transcription

1. Phusion High Fidelity DNA Polymerase (Thermo Scientific or New England Biolabs (NEB)) and dNTPs.
2. Forward primer with T7-promoter overhang and reverse primer (*see* **Note 1**).
3. Thermocycler machine.
4. Standard agarose gel necessities for TAE-buffered gels.
5. DNA/RNA (gel-)purification/concentration kit (e.g., Macherey-Nagel's Nucleospin® Gel and PCR cleanup kit).
6. 5 mM Tris–HCl pH 7.6, 0.5 mM EDTA pH 8.0 (0.5× TE).
7. UV-Vis spectrometer to measure DNA and RNA concentration (e.g., NanoDrop).
8. In vitro transcription kit such as NEB's HiScribe™ T7 High Yield RNA Synthesis Kit.
9. DNase I, RNase-free.
10. RNase-free water, ideally DEPC-treated.
11. 0.5 M EDTA.
12. 0.1 M NaOH.
13. 2× denaturing RNA loading dye (~95% formamide + dye, e.g., Thermo 2× RNA Loading Dye)

14. RNA ladder.
15. 3 M NaOAc (pH 5.2).
16. 70 and 100% EtOH.
17. Cooled microcentrifuge.
18. −20 °C freezer.

2.2 Probing and RT Stop Reaction

1. 5 mM Tris–HCl pH 7.6, 0.5 mM EDTA pH 8.0 (0.5× TE).
2. Thermocycler machine.
3. RNA folding buffer: 333 mM HEPES (pH 7.6), 20 mM $MgCl_2$, 333 mM NaCl.
4. RNA structure probe of choice. For example:
   (a) NAI (in vivo SHAPE Reagent, Merck, or can be synthesized according to Spitale et al. [9]) diluted in anhydrous DMSO.
   (b) DMS, diluted in ethanol. Caution: highly toxic (*see* **Note 2**).
   (c) RNase T1, diluted in 10 mM Tris–HCl (pH 7.5).
5. 3 M NaOAc (pH 5.2).
6. 0.1 M EDTA.
7. Glycogen.
8. 70% and 100% EtOH.
9. ß-mercaptoethanol (when using DMS).
10. Reagents for phenol–chloroform extraction and isopropanol (when using RNase T1 or ligands that require additional purification).
11. −80 °C freezer.
12. Cooled microcentrifuge.
13. RNase-free water, ideally DEPC-treated.
14. Fluorescently 5′-labeled reverse primer. Check the detector set of the CE machine for suitable fluorophores. For the ABI3730, we found 6-FAM and HEX to work well.
15. SuperScript III reverse transcriptase (Thermo/Invitrogen), 10 mM dNTPs (*see* **Note 3**).
16. ddGTP solution (not required for basic optimization experiments).
17. 4 M NaOH.
18. 4 M HCl.
19. Highly deionized formamide (e.g., Hi-Di, ABI/Thermo Scientific) (*see* **Note 4**).
20. Microcentrifuge heat block.

21. GeneScan™ 500 LIZ™ dye Size Standard (ABI/Thermo Scientific) or another suitable CE size standard.
22. High-resolution CE machine (*see* **Note 5**).

3 Methods

3.1 Production of Repeat RNA

When setting up an experiment to determine the structure of a repeat-containing RNA, the first consideration is the composition of this RNA. The longer the repeat, the more difficult various steps in the procedure will become.

Questions to be answered prior to start of the analyses are: What repeat lengths are sufficient to answer the particular research question? Will the RNA contain a pure or an interrupted repeat, such as occurs in a subset of DM1 patients [10]? Since repeat-flanking segments in a transcript might influence the structure of the repeat part [11, 12], how much of these sequences need to be integrated in the model RNA?

We generated RNAs consisting of pure CUG repeats of up to 200 triplets flanked by in total ~900 nucleotides [12], but in general studies describing interactions of repeats with flanking sequences spanning >100 nucleotides are rare. By attaching long flanking regions and determining the structure of these as well, valuable information can be obtained about possible interactions of the repeat with these other parts of the transcript.

When designing a transcription template, keep in mind that 3′ of the region of interest there should be a spacer or natural sequence of at least 15–20 nucleotides, followed by a unique sequence to locate the primer for the RT step (*see* **Note 6**).

Obtaining pure transcription templates carrying long repeats can be troublesome, because of difficulties with PCR and the instability of repeats during cloning in bacteria (usually contractions). This instability can, however, also be used to your advantage, for example to easily create an array of different repeat lengths by clonal selection of bacteria after transfection with a long-repeat plasmid. Also, PCR-based methods can be considered to synthetically produce repeat DNA [13].

1. Assemble and perform PCR reactions according to Tables 1 and 2. Optimization may be required (*see* **Note 1**).
2. Separate the PCR products on a long (>15 cm) EtBr-stained agarose gel (e.g., 1.2%) for 90–120 min (*see* **Note** 7).
3. While minimizing UV exposure, slice out the bands of the expected product and recover the DNA from the gel with the NucleoSpin® Gel and PCR Clean-up kit.
4. Elute twice with a small volume 0.5× TE (pH 8) (e.g., 15 μl), to ensure the highest possible concentration.

Table 1
Composition of PCR reaction ligating a T7 promoter

5× Phusion HF buffer	5 µl
10 mM dNTPs	0.5 µl
10 µM forward primer with T7 promoter	1 µl
10 µM reverse primer	1 µl
Template, e.g., 1 ng plasmid	… µl
Phusion polymerase 2 U/µl	0.5 µl
Water	To 25 µl

Table 2
Suggested cycling conditions for PCR ligating a T7 promoter

98 °C	30 s	–
98 °C	15 s	30 cycles
Appropriate annealing temperature for the primers used	20 s	
72 °C	3 min	
72 °C	10 min	–

5. Measure the concentration of the obtained PCR product, for example, using UV-Vis spectrometry (*see* **Note 8**).
6. Confirm sequence composition via sequence analysis.
7. Assemble an in vitro transcription reaction at room temperature according to the Table 3, which describes a double-volume reaction compared to the kit manual of 40 µl with 500 ng template DNA (*see* **Note 9**).
8. For repeat RNAs below ~100 triplets, incubate at 37 °C for 3 h. For longer repeats perform this incubation at room temperature for 4 h (*see* **Note 10**).
9. Add 10 µl 10× DNase I reaction buffer, water to 98 µl and 2 µl RNase-free DNase I, and incubate at 37 °C for 15 min.
10. Add 1 µl 500 mM EDTA and proceed to column purification for estimation of the yield to optimize gel purification.
11. Perform the clean-up according to the manufacturer's instructions for RNA purification and elute three times with 20 µl 0.5× TE (pH 8), pooling the eluates.
12. Measure the concentration.
13. Prepare an RNase-free gel tray and running tank by soaking in 0.1 M NaOH for 1 h, followed by extensive washing with mil-

Table 3
Composition of T7 in vitro transcription reaction

25 mM NTPs	16 µl
10× transcription buffer	4 µl
DNA T7 template, e.g., 50 ng/µl	10 µl
Water	6 µl
T7 RNA polymerase	4 µl

liQ and drying. Cool the amount of TAE needed as running buffer to 4 °C (*see* **Note 11**).

14. Prepare an EtBr-stained TAE buffered 1% agarose gel.
15. Mix an appropriate amount of RNA with 2× denaturing RNA loading buffer to load ~2 µg per slot.
16. Heat at 70 °C for 5 min and cool on ice for 1 min.
17. Put the gel in cooled buffer just before loading, and load the RNA along with a suitable RNA ladder and run for ~1:30 h at 100 V.
18. While minimizing UV exposure, slice out the bands and recover the RNA using the NucleoSpin® Gel and PCR Clean-up kit.
19. Elute three times with 30 µl 0.5× TE (pH 8), combine the eluates, and ethanol precipitate these together by adding 0.1 vol 3 M NaOAc (pH 5.2), and 3 vol EtOH and storage at −80 °C for at least 2 h for additional purification from salts that can be carried over from the column.
20. Pellet the RNA by centrifugation at 4 °C and wash it twice with 70% EtOH. Dry the pellet and dissolve in 0.5× TE (pH 7.6), and measure the RNA concentration precisely. To check the integrity of the RNA it can be tested on agarose gel or PAGE. *See* Fig. 2 for an example.

3.2 Probing and RT Stop Reaction

1. Dissolve 0.35 picomole RNA in 12 µl 0.5× TE (pH 7.6) (*see* **Note 12**).
2. Heat at 85 °C for 5 min.
3. Cool on ice and add 6 µl RNA folding buffer (*see* **Note 13**).
4. Incubate at 37 °C for 30 min.
5. Add the reagent of choice (*see* below) and incubate for an appropriate time at 37 °C. Take along a control reaction with only the solvent. This step should be optimized for each situation. We found the following final concentrations and incubation times to work well for CUG repeat RNA with up to 200 triplets (*see* **Note 14**).

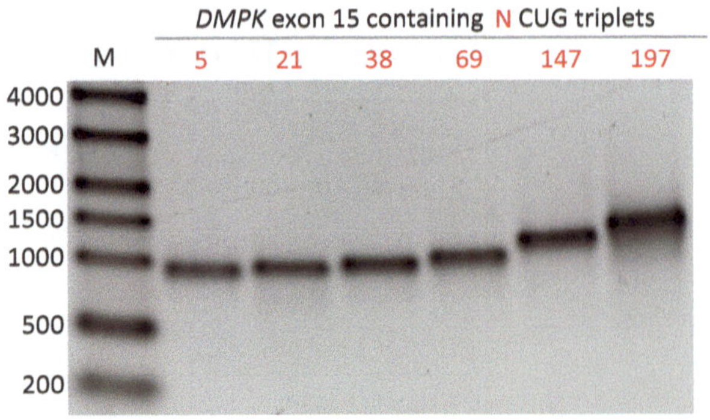

Fig. 2 A collection of repeat RNAs after purification. 150 ng RNA consisting of 5 to 197 CUG triplets flanked by ~300 (5′) and ~500 (3′) *DMPK* nucleotides (exon 15) was separated on an 1% agarose gel, post-stained with EtBr and visualized under UV

   (a) *NAI*: 20 mM for 15 min.
   (b) *DMS*: 0.25% for 6 min.
   (c) *RNase T1*: 0.01 U/μl for 10 min.

6. Quench the reaction and precipitate the RNA in a microcentrifuge tube at −80 °C overnight as described below:
   (a) *NAI*: place on ice and immediately add 0.1 vol 3 M NaOAc (pH 5.2), 0.1 vol 0.1 M EDTA, 10 μg glycogen (make mastermix) and then 3 vol 100% EtOH.
   (b) *DMS*: add 0.25 vol pure ß-mercaptoethanol and ethanol precipitate as described for quenching NAI reactions. ß-mercaptoethanol can be mixed with the precipitation reagents.
   (c) *RNase enzymes*: supplement the reaction to 100 μl with DEPC-treated water, perform a phenol–chloroform extraction and precipitate as described for quenching NAI reactions, but now with use of 1 vol isopropanol.
7. Recover the RNA by centrifugation, wash twice with 70% EtOH and dissolve in 11 μl water (*see* **Note 15**).
8. Add the RNA to 1 μl 10 μM fluorescently labeled primer and 1 μl 10 mM dNTPs in a thermocycler tube (*see* **Note 6**). To generate a ddGTP ladder, also perform this reaction using 10–20 pmol untreated RNA with 1 μl 10 mM dNTPs and 10 mM ddGTP instead of only dNTPs, using a differently labeled primer with the same sequence (*see* **Note 16**).
9. Heat at 65 °C for 5 min, then cool immediately on ice.
10. Add 4 μl 5× FSB, 1 μl 0.1 M DTT, 1 μl water, and 1 μl Superscript III (make mastermix) (*see* **Note 3**).
11. Incubate for 45 min at 55 °C, cool to 4 °C.

12. Add 1 µl 4 M NaOH, incubate at 95 °C for 5 min.
13. Cool on ice and add 1 µl 4 M HCl, 10 µg glycogen, 0.1 vol 3 M NaOAc (pH 5.2), and (make mastermix) and add (to) 2.5 vol cold EtOH in a microcentrifuge tube. Store at −80 °C for at least 2 h.

3.3 Measurement and Data Analysis: Deriving RNA Structure from CE Traces

1. Recover the cDNA by centrifugation. Wash the pellet twice with 70% EtOH and dissolve in 10 µl formamide by incubation at 65 °C for 15 min. For the ddGTP ladder, use 2 µl formamide per reaction to be measured (*see* **Note 4**).
2. Mix 7.5 µl of the cDNA sample with 2 µl ddGTP ladder and 0.5 µl GeneScan™ Size Standard.
3. Measure cDNA lengths via fragment analysis by CE (*see* **Note 5**).

Data analysis for RNA structure probing can be difficult. This is partly due to naturally occurring RT stops, induced by the structure or sequence intrinsic to the tested RNA. This requires precise alignment of the +reagent and –reagent CE traces to prevent false positives or negatives. Initial or rough data analysis can manually be performed using ABI's Peak Scanner™ 2.0 software. This is relatively straightforward and can be used to evaluate qualitative as well as quantitative differences directly based on the CE traces (*see* **Note 17**). An example is shown in Fig. 3, where the area under the curves indicates that the RNase T1-treatment used here leads to an approximate seven-fold increase of RNA cleavage or RT stop events compared to the control situation in the middle of the repeat. A high degree of RT stops in the middle of the repeat sequence arises

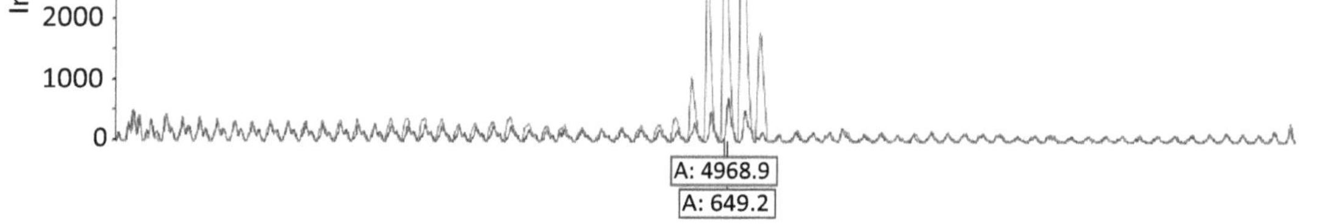

Fig. 3 Example of two CE traces in Peak Scanner™ 2.0 from *DMPK* exon 15 RNA with 69 CUG repeats probed with RNase T1 (red) and a control reaction (blue) focused on the repeat region. The area under the curve function, specified in the boxes under the X-axis, is used as estimation of intensity for two corresponding peaks. The reactivity in the middle of the repeat is typical for a single hairpin structure; lower intensity peaks in other regions may indicate the existence of structures alternative to a single hairpin

from the single-stranded loop of a single hairpin, whereas RT stops at other sites suggest the presence of branched or multiple hairpins. RT stops at the ultimate ends of the repeat are also common and are due to the slippery nature of repeat hairpins [14]. Note that naturally occurring RT stops in repeat regions are usually repetitive and low in frequency.

Although manual analysis of the electrophoresis signals can be quick and simple, it becomes labor intensive to in-depth analyze a whole transcript. Moreover, the outcome can be biased by many factors (e.g., differences in the overall signal intensity level between samples). Also, in this way the +reagent and –reagent traces are only roughly aligned and can thus be shifted, leading to imperfect background correction. A more thorough method to analyze the CE data is to use academically developed programs such as CAFA [15], RiboCat [16], HiTRACE [17], SHAPEfinder [18], or QuSHAPE [19], the latter of which will be used here. The general principle is similar for all these programs: compare the +reagent and –reagent traces and perform background subtraction, normalization and alignment steps. QuSHAPE was developed to analyze specifically SHAPE data, but we found it suitable also for other probing methods. *See* http://weeks.chem.unc.edu/qushape/ for the software and a highly informative tutorial of this user-friendly program.

4. Create a text file containing the sequence of the RNA of interest with the correct repeat length.
5. Open QuSHAPE in the Python software package (*see* www.python.org) and follow the program instructions to create a new project with the CE traces.
6. The software will show four traces, from top to bottom: +reagent, –reagent, ddNTP ladder of +reagent and ladder of –reagent capillary, and then asks to select a region of interest. For analysis of the repeat region, look for a regularly repeating pattern in the two bottom traces and select exactly the same region in both traces. Including a region 3′ to the repeat can facilitate downstream analysis (*see* **Note 17**).
7. For the next steps, *smoothening*, *mobility shift*, *baseline correction* and *signal decay correction* usually the standard settings suffice, but do critically evaluate what is happening with the traces in each step, since this influences the outcome. Consult QuSHAPE's documentation for the effect of these transformations (*see* **Note 18**).
8. The next signal alignment step is crucial, and is often troublesome for repeated sequences. After applying this step, ensure that the bottom (ddNTP) traces are exactly aligned and otherwise correct this manually via *Modify Matched Peaks*. If this is

not possible, consider that the chosen regions are not identical and correct this.

9. In the sequence alignment step again critically evaluate the outcome of the automated alignment, which is often imperfect for repeated sequences. Correct until (nearly) perfect, make especially sure there is no shift that can skew the alignment.
10. Refer to the QuSHAPE manual what type of scaling and normalization suits the project. We found *scale by windowing* and *normalization* with the suggested factor to work well.
11. Critically evaluate the reported data by visually comparing the matched peaks. When using a nucleotide-specific probe, verify whether (essentially) only the targeted nucleotides have a high *normDiff* reactivity value. An example outcome is shown in Fig. 4 (*see* **Note 19**).
12. Visual interpretation of a graph plotting the *normDiff* reactivities can be informative, but these values can also be used as constraints in RNA folding prediction software such as *Fold* the in RNAstructure [20] package or *RNAprobing* in ViennaRNA [21]. Please refer to the documentation of these programs for details (*see* **Note 20**).

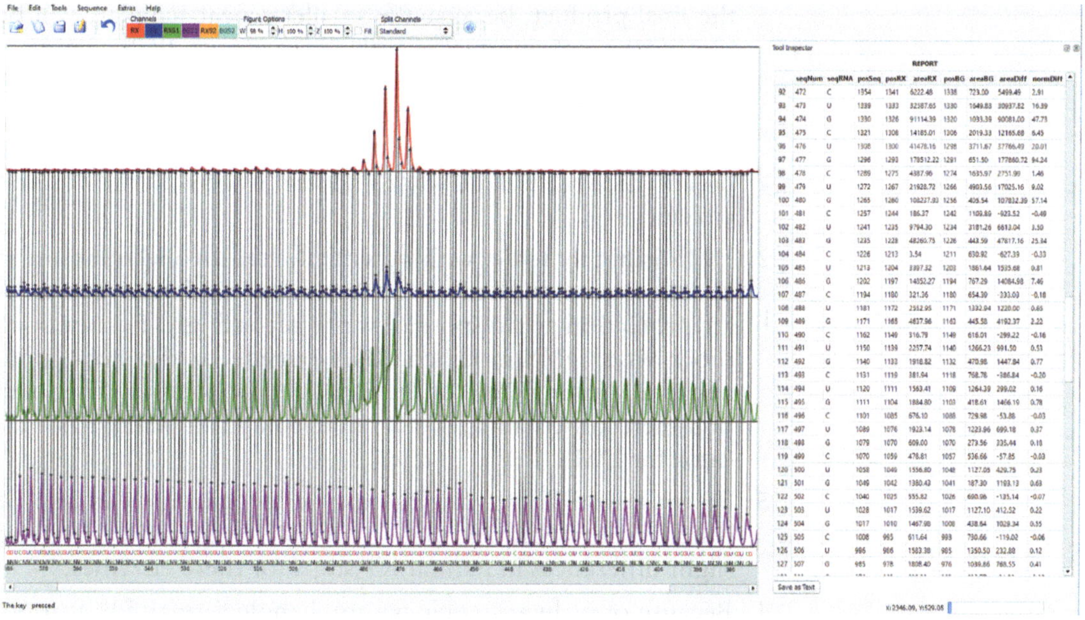

Fig. 4 Outcome of QuSHAPE analysis from a similar experiment as in Fig. 3, showing the full repeat. In red the +RNase T1 reaction and in blue the control, with their corresponding ddGTP traces in green and pink. In the right panel the normalization and quantification data

4 Notes

1. It may be necessary to perform multiple reactions in parallel to obtain sufficient PCR product, especially for repeats of >100 triplets. For repeats of <50 triplets most standard PCR protocols suffice. We obtained good results with NEB's Q5 high fidelity polymerase. To attach a 5′ T7 RNA polymerase promoter to the PCR product, introduce a 5′ overhang of TAATACGACTCACTATAGGG on the forward primer. Transcription will start at the underlined G. A SP6 promoter will also work when using an in vitro transcription system based on SP6 polymerase. PCR across repeats can be made more efficient when primers are used that are located closer to the repeat. If a pure plasmid preparation carrying the transcription template with a T7 promoter is available, a properly linearized plasmid can also be used for in vitro transcription and one can start at Subheading 3.1, **step 2** for digestion reactions or Subheading 3.1, **step 7** for pure transcription template at a concentration ≥ 25 ng/μl. PCR additives such as betaine (up to 3.5 M) or DMSO (up to 10%), and variation of the denaturation or elongation time can improve yield and must be optimized for each condition, especially for long and GC-rich repeats. A minor contamination with a short-repeat template will have a significant impact on the composition of the final product, because the smaller repeat template will be amplified much more efficiently. To generate PCR templates with long repeats, heat-pulse extension PCR [22] and optimization PCR [23] also worked for us, but the enzyme used (DyNAzyme EXT) has been discontinued by the supplier. We however found heat-pulse PCR to also work with the Phusion enzyme.
2. DMS is highly toxic, with potentially lethal concentrations in air below the odor limit. Work in a fume hood, wear appropriate protection and dispose of waste accordingly. Do not open tubes with DMS-modified RNA outside of the hood until after the washing steps of the ethanol precipitation. The smell of β-mercaptoethanol used for quenching can be used as indicator for DMS.
3. To preserve RT enzyme, the use of less enzyme can also be tested. Both SSIII and SSIV work well, although we found slight differences in natural RT stops for these enzymes.
4. Because of its hygroscopic nature, handle formamide at room temperature, make aliquots and store these under N_2 at −20 °C. Use a fresh tube for each experiment; we found the quality of CE traces to decrease strongly already after one freeze–thaw cycle.

When using an adequate amount of input RNA, one may dissolve the cDNA in a larger volume (e.g., 15 μl), as to keep the possibility for repeated measurements.

5. Most sequencing facilities offer CE measurements for a low price as GeneScan method, for example, for microsatellite repeat diagnostics. An ABI 3730 DNA Analyzer is highly suitable to this end.
6. Design the RT primers at least 20 nucleotides away from the region of interest. Optimal resolution is obtained up to 300 nucleotides from the primer, but reads over 500 nucleotides are possible. For analysis using QuSHAPE, primers with the same fluorophore are used for +reagent and −reagent reactions but other methods can require another setup. We found HEX-labeled primers to give more intense signals than 6-FAM, so use 6-FAM for ddNTP reactions to prevent bleed-through in the sample channel and to maximize the sample signal.
7. It is common that byproducts, mainly the intended product but with a short repeat, arise when performing PCR across long repeats. Usually the desired product can be isolated by using a long agarose gel and running time.
8. Since in the following steps the exact concentration is not important, duplicate measurements can be skipped to limit wasting of DNA. If the concentration is <25 ng/μl, consider performing more PCR reactions or concentrating the DNA using a commercial kit or ethanol precipitation.
9. We obtained good results with the NEB HiScribe™ kit and integrated its use in this protocol. An alternative that worked also well is Thermo Scientific's MEGAscript™ kit. Note that for templates with a long repeat the efficiency of transcription will decrease. Compensate for this by using a high amount of template (e.g., 500 ng) and/or scaling up the reaction volume.
10. The optimal temperature may depend on the composition of the template; the yield will decrease with lower temperature. If aberrant transcription products are observed while incubating at 37 °C, a lower temperature is advised.
11. For separation of small RNAs (<~600 nucleotides) polyacrylamide gel electrophoresis is advised. When the transcribed RNA is later found to be perfectly homogeneous, Subheading 3.1, **steps 13–18** can be skipped in the future to prevent loss of RNA. In that case, ethanol-precipitate the RNA as in Subheading 3.1, **step 19** and continue with Subheading 3.1, **step 20**.
12. The optimal amount of input RNA may depend on various factors. An initial optimization should be performed that suits the detection limit. This step can be scaled up when planning to measure the RNA under identical conditions from different

primer sites. In that case divide the modified RNA over multiple RT reactions in Subheading 3.2, **step 8**.

Once basic probing experiments are up and running, one may consider to include an AON in this step, to examine its effect on RNA structure [11, 12]. AONs can be designed to disrupt a predicted interaction, which should be apparent in probe reactivity of interacting nucleotides. To achieve a high spatial resolution of AON binding, consider designing AONs with LNA substitutions to obtain short AONs (e.g., 10 nucleotides) that bind with high affinity. Perform an optimization experiment to obtain a suitable dose; we found an RNA:AON ratio of 1:10 to work well. Keep in mind that a long repeat can bind many AONs, and that a covered repeat is not reactive to probes for single stranded nucleotides (*see* **Note 15**).

13. The salt concentration, especially Mg^{2+}-ions, can influence the secondary and tertiary structure of an RNA [24]. The buffer composition used in our protocol was suggested by Wilkinson et al. [25]. We found that the Mg^{2+} concentration did not overtly influence the structure of CUG repeats [12], but it could be relevant to investigate the influence of these ions on other RNAs.

    The binding site and influence on RNA structure of recombinant proteins or small molecules can also be investigated with the procedures described here. These compounds can be added in this step. Keep in mind that bound ligands can alter the structure as well as shield the RNA from the probe, effects that can be difficult to separate during data analysis (*see* **Note 1**).

14. This is a critical optimization step. A low degree of modification or cleavage leads to low sensitivity, whereas a too high degree of modification leads to signal decay and can induce folding artifacts. To be sure, test if similar results can be obtained by a higher concentration of probe and decreased incubation time and vice versa.

    Thaw and dilute the probe or enzyme right before use (e.g., during folding of the RNA).

15. When bound AONs or other ligands interfere with the RT reaction and are not removed by purification after the probing reaction, these should be removed after this step. AONs and ligands binding with moderate affinity can be removed by a denaturation step (e.g., 5 min at 85 °C) followed by immediate purification using a commercial kit such as QIAgen's RNeasy® MinElute® Cleanup kit. For AON purification, addition of a 10- to 100-fold excess of a complementary AON before this denaturation step can facilitate the purification. Proteins can be removed by phenol–chloroform extraction.

16. Since the ratio dNTP–ddNTP generates a trade-off between signal strength and read length, it must be optimized for a

specific application. With a 1:1 ratio of dGTP–ddNTPs (RT enzymes have a lower affinity for ddNTPs compared to dNTPs) we obtained good ladders with CUG repeats of up to 200 triplets. The most convenient is to prepare a solution for these reactions containing 10 mM of each dNTP and 10 mM ddGTP. The amount of RNA used in one probing experiment should suffice for two to three ladder reactions. For more precise alignment and sequencing of the RNA, parallel reactions should be performed with different ddNTPs.

17. Reagent-independent (natural) RT stops can be induced by sequence and structural features. However, a high degree of reagent-independent RT stops may also be a sign of RNA degradation. When RNA degradation is suspected, check the integrity of the RNA on gel and ensure the reagents that are used are absolutely free of RNase and divalent heavy metal ions.

    As an additional check for the sequence of the RNA, check the ddNTP trace for impurities.

    By confirming that there is a reasonable amount of full-length cDNA in the +reagent trace, one can verify that over-modification or -cleavage has not taken place for short repeats. Long repeats induce slippage of the RT which results in aberrant, mostly longer, products [26], that prohibit analysis of regions just 5′ of the repeat.
18. QuSHAPE offers the option to carry over user input and alignment data from one finished analysis to a new one, which is convenient when performing similar experiments. However, it is advisable to check every step in the process and correct imperfections.
19. When the signal–noise ratio is low, there is a high risk for false positives. For suspicious or highly important data points, we advise to refer back to the raw data.
20. Adding to the complexity of data interpretation is that folding algorithms usually generate multiple nonmutually exclusive structures, often with a similar likelihood. An RNA can very well coexist in multiple structure populations, but it can be worthwhile to identify the most prominent one(s). This requires experiments with different probes, binding by AONs or introducing mutations (*see* **Note 12**).

Acknowledgments

We wish to thank Prof. Bé Wieringa for his contribution to supervision of this study as part of R.T.P. van Cruchten's Ph.D. project and for critical reading of the manuscript.

References

1. Sobczak K, de Mezer M, Michlewski G, Krol J, Krzyzosiak WJ (2003) RNA structure of trinucleotide repeats associated with human neurological diseases. Nucleic Acids Res 31:5469–5482
2. Ciesiolka A, Jazurek M, Drazkowska K, Krzyzosiak WJ (2017) Structural characteristics of simple RNA repeats associated with disease and their deleterious protein interactions. Front Cell Neurosci 11:97
3. Zu T, Gibbens B, Doty NS, Gomes-pereira M, Huguet A, Stone MD (2010) Non-ATG – initiated translation directed by microsatellite expansions. Proc Natl Acad Sci U S A 108:260–265
4. Aartsma-Rus A, van Vliet L, Hirschi M, Janson AAM, Heemskerk H, de Winter CL et al (2009) Guidelines for antisense oligonucleotide design and insight into splice-modulating mechanisms. Mol Ther 17:548–553
5. Bernat V, Disney MD (2015) RNA structures as mediators of neurological diseases and as drug targets. Neuron 87:28–46
6. Weeks KM (2010) Advances in RNA structure analysis by chemical probing. Curr Opin Struct Biol 20:295–304
7. Merino EJ, Wilkinson KA, Coughlan JL, Weeks KM (2005) RNA structure analysis at single nucleotide resolution by selective 2′-hydroxyl acylation and primer extension (SHAPE). J Am Chem Soc 127:4223–4231
8. Lorenz R, Wolfinger MT, Tanzer A, Hofacker IL (2016) Predicting RNA secondary structures from sequence and probing data. Methods 103:86–98
9. Spitale RC, Crisalli P, Flynn RA, Torre EA, Kool ET, Chang HY (2013) RNA SHAPE analysis in living cells. Nat Chem Biol 9:18–20
10. Leeflang EP, Arnheim N (1995) A novel repeat structure at the myotonic dystrophy locus in a 37 repeat allele with unexpectedly high stability. Hum Mol Genet 4:135–136
11. Busan S, Weeks KM (2013) Role of context in RNA structure: flanking sequences reconfigure CAG motif folding in huntingtin exon 1 transcripts. Biochemistry 52:8219–8225
12. van Cruchten RTP, Wieringa B, Wansink DG (2019) Expanded CUG repeats in DMPK transcripts adopt diverse hairpin conformations without influencing the structure of the flanking sequences. RNA 25:481–495
13. Figura G, Koscianska E, Krzyzosiak WJ (2015) In vitro expansion of CAG, CAA, and mixed CAG/CAA repeats. Int J Mol Sci 16:18741–18751
14. Napierała M, Krzyzosiak WJ (1997) CUG repeats present in myotonin kinase RNA form metastable "slippery" hairpins. J Biol Chem 272:31079–31085
15. Mitra S, Shcherbakova IV, Altman RB, Brenowitz M, Laederach A (2008) High-throughput single-nucleotide structural mapping by capillary automated footprinting analysis. Nucleic Acids Res 36:1–10
16. Cantara WA, Hatterschide J, Wu W, Musier-Forsyth K (2017) RiboCAT: a new capillary electrophoresis data analysis tool for nucleic acid probing. RNA 23:240–249
17. Kim H, Cordero P, Das R, Yoon S (2013) HiTRACE-web: an online tool for robust analysis of high-throughput capillary electrophoresis. Nucleic Acids Res 41:492–498
18. Vasa SM, Guex N, Wilkinson KA, Weeks KM, Giddings MC (2008) ShapeFinder: a software system for high-throughput quantitative analysis of nucleic acid reactivity information resolved by capillary electrophoresis. RNA 14:1979–1990
19. Karabiber F, McGinnis JL, Favorov OV, Weeks KM (2013) QuShape: rapid, accurate, and best-practices quantification of nucleic acid probing information, resolved by capillary electrophoresis. RNA 19:63–73
20. Reuter JS, Mathews DH (2010) RNAstructure: software for RNA secondary structure prediction and analysis. BMC Bioinformatics 11:129
21. Lorenz R, Bernhart SH, Höner zu Siederdissen C, Tafer H, Flamm C, Stadler PF et al (2011) ViennaRNA package 2.0. Algorithms Mol Biol 6:26
22. Orpana AK, Ho TH, Alagrund K, Ridanpää M, Aittomäki K, Stenman J (2013) Novel heat pulse extension-PCR-based method for detection of large CTG-repeat expansions in myotonic dystrophy type 1. J Mol Diagn 15:110–115
23. Meng YX, Shen HR, Zhao Z, Bing Q, Li N, Hu J (2015) Optimization PCR for detection CTG/CCTG-repeat expansions in the diagnosis of myotonic dystrophies. Ann Clin Lab Sci 45:502–507
24. Draper DE (2004) A guide to ions and RNA structure. RNA 10:335–343
25. Wilkinson KA, Merino EJ, Weeks KM (2006) Selective 2′-hydroxyl acylation analyzed by primer extension (SHAPE): quantitative RNA structure analysis at single nucleotide resolution. Nat Protoc 1:1610–1616
26. Carrell ST, Tang Z, Mohr S, Lambowitz AM, Thornton CA (2018) Detection of expanded RNA repeats using thermostable group II intron reverse transcriptase. Nucleic Acids Res 46:e1

Chapter 13

FISH Protocol for Myotonic Dystrophy Type 1 Cells

Arnaud F. Klein, Ludovic Arandel, Joelle Marie, and Denis Furling

Abstract

Mutant *DMPK* transcripts containing expanded CUG repeats (CUGexp) are retained within the nucleus of myotonic dystrophy type 1 (DM1) cells as discrete foci. Nuclear CUGexp-RNA foci that sequester MBNL1 splicing factor represent a hallmark of this RNA dominant disease caused by the expression of expanded microsatellite repeats. Here we described fluorescent in situ hybridization (FISH) techniques to detect either RNA containing CUG expansion or *DMPK* transcripts in human DM1 or WT cells. In addition, we propose a combined FISH/immunofluorescence protocol to visualize the colocalization of MBNL1 with CUGexp-RNA foci in DM1 cells.

Key words Myotonic dystrophy, Nuclear RNA foci, CUG expansion, *DMPK* transcripts, MBNL1, Fluorescent in situ hybridization, Immunofluorescence

1 Introduction

Myotonic dystrophy type 1 (DM1 or Steinert's disease) is a multisystemic disorder characterized by myotonia, progressive muscle weakness and atrophy, cardiac conduction defects, and cognitive impairment together with other endocrine dysfunctions [1, 2]. The disease is caused by an abnormal expansion of a CTG repeated sequence within the 3′untranslated region (UTR) of the Dystrophia Myotonica Protein Kinase (*DMPK*) gene [3–5]. The size of the CTG tract is lower than 37 repeats in healthy individuals and can reach several thousands in DM1 patients. Moreover, CTG expansions in patients are instable at both the somatic and intergenerational levels [6]. Since the identification of this expanded microsatellite repeats, DM1 has been described as the archetype of RNA gain-of-function diseases. The mutant *DMPK* allele is transcribed however messenger RNAs containing expanded CUG repeats (*CUGexp-DMPK*) are retained into the nucleus and form discrete aggregates or foci [7, 8]. These ribonuclear foci sequester factors of the Muscleblind-like (MBNL) RNA binding protein

Guy-Franck Richard (ed.), *Trinucleotide Repeats: Methods and Protocols*, Methods in Molecular Biology, vol. 2056,
https://doi.org/10.1007/978-1-4939-9784-8_13,

family [9–11], resulting in their functional loss and thereby the disruption of RNA processing events including the misregulation of the alternative splicing of many effector genes [12–15]. More than 40 misregulated splicing events have been described in the skeletal muscle of DM1 patients and some of them were associated with symptoms [12, 16–20].

The finding of ribonuclear aggregates or RNA foci in DM1 cells was a major breakthrough in the understanding of the molecular disease process [7] and their presence in affected tissues of DM1 patients is currently a hallmark of the disease [11, 21, 22]. Nuclear CUGexp-RNA foci are also detected in both cell and animal models of the disease, and their presence, number and/or intensity are often used as a readout to assess efficacy of therapeutic approaches [23]. RNA foci are composed of mutant *CUGexp-DMPK* transcripts that are normally spliced, capped and polyadenylated [8]. However, the abnormal binding of MBNL proteins to expanded CUG repeats contributes to the nuclear retention and/or impaired cytoplasmic export of these pathologic RNA [24–26].

In this chapter, we describe in details how to perform a fluorescent in situ hybridization (FISH) staining on human DM1 or WT cells to visualize CUGexp-RNA and *DMPK* transcripts. We have adapted protocol from previous works using fluorescent probes for either FISH or single molecule inexpensive FISH (smiFISH). We also describe the preparation and the fixation of the cells prior to hybridization, and an immunofluorescence protocol to detect MBNL1 in colocalization analysis purpose. The culture conditions for myoblasts and fibroblasts are adapted from Arandel et al. [27], the FISH protocol is adapted and optimized from Taneja et al. [7, 28], the smiFISH protocol from Tsanov et al. [29]; and MBNL1 immunofluorescence protocol from Arandel et al. and Byron et al. [27, 30].

2 Materials

2.1 Preparation of Cells for Hybridization and Immunofluorescence

1. Petri dish or multiwell plates for cell culture.
2. Sterile glass coverslips (12, 14, 18, or 30 mm diameter).
3. Microscope forceps.
4. Autoclaved solution of 0.5% gelatin (in water).
5. Sterile PBS for cell culture.
6. Growth medium (GM): For primary human myoblasts: mix of 199:DMEM (1:4 ratio) supplemented with 20% FBS and 50 μg/ml gentamycin. For immortalized human myoblasts: mix of 199:DMEM (1:4 ratio) supplemented with 20% FBS,

50 μg/ml gentamycin, 25 μg/ml fetuin, 0.5 ng/ml bFGF, 5 ng/ml EGF, and 0.2 μg/ml dexamethasone. For fibroblast and immortalized fibroblasts: DMEM supplemented with 15% FBS and 50 μg/ml gentamycin.

7. Differentiation medium (DM): For primary and immortalized myoblasts: DMEM supplemented with 5 μg/ml insulin. For trans-differentiated MYOD1 fibroblasts: DMEM supplemented with 5 μg/ml insulin and 4 μg/ml of doxycycline.
8. Solution of paraformaldehyde (PFA) 4% in PBS (*see* **Note 1**).
9. Alternative fixation/permeabilization solution: −20 °C pre-chilled acetone–methanol mix (volume ration 1:1) (*see* **Note 1**).
10. 70% ethanol solution.

2.2 FISH

1. Glass slides.
2. Microscope forceps.
3. Dark chamber with flat bottom, moisten (e.g., a 150 mm petri dish with paper moisten with 40% formamide and 2× SSC) (*see* **Note 1**).
4. Prehybridization buffer: 40% formamide, 2× SSC, 0.2% BSA (store at 4 °C).
5. CAG_7 probe: 2′OMe or PNA chemistry conjugated in 5′ with a fluorochrome as Cy3, Cy5 or fluorescein (stock concentration at 100 μM in TE buffer, store at −20 °C).
6. Hybridization buffer: 40% formamide, 2× SSC, 0.2% BSA, 100 nM CAG_7 fluorescent probe.
7. PBS-T: RNase-free PBS + 0.1% Tween.
8. PBS-$MgCl_2$: RNase-free PBS + 5 mM $MgCl_2$.
9. Hoechst solution: 2 μg/ml Hoechst in PBS-T.
10. Antifading mounting medium for immunofluorescence.

2.3 smiFISH

1. Glass slides.
2. Microscope forceps.
3. Dark chamber with flat bottom, moisten (e.g., a 150 mm petri dish with paper moisten with 30% formamide and 1× SSC) (*see* **Note 1**).
4. Antifading mounting medium for immunofluorescence.
5. Probe set targeting *DMPK* transcript (*see* Table 1 for sequences and Subheading 3.3, **step 1** for preparation).
6. Fluorescent FLAP probe: DNA oligonucleotide (*see* Table 1 for sequence) conjugated to Cy3 fluorochrome at both extremities.

Table 1
Sequence and modification of the probes used in FISH and smiFISH protocols

Protocol	Name	Sequence 5′ → 3′
FISH	CAG sequence	Cy3-CAGCAGCAGCAGCAGCAGCAG
smiFISH	DMPK-probe 1	TCCGGGGGACACAGCAACCGCTGAATTTACACTCGGACCTCGTCGACATGCATT
	DMPK-probe 2	ACAGGTAGTTCTCATCCTGGAAGGCGAAGTTTACACTCGGACCTCGTCGACATGCATT
	DMPK-probe 3	CAGTCGGACCTCCTTAAGCCTCACCATTACACTCGGACCTCGTCGACATGCATT
	DMPK-probe 4	CAACTGCCGGACGTGTGCCTCTAGGTTTACACTCGGACCTCGTCGACATGCATT
	DMPK-probe 5	TTCTGGTTGTCCGTGCGGATGGCCTCTTACACTCGGACCTCGTCGACATGCATT
	DMPK-probe 6	CGCTGGAACTGCCACTTCAGCTGTTTTTACACTCGGACCTCGTCGACATGCATT
	DMPK-probe 7	CTGTCCCTGAGGGCCATGCAGGAGTATTACACTCGGACCTCGTCGACATGCATT
	DMPK-probe 8	GTGAGCCCGTCCTCCACCAAGTCGAATTACACTCGGACCTCGTCGACATGCATT
	DMPK-probe 9	TGCATGTGTCGGTGGCACCTTCGAAATCTTACACTCGGACCTCGTCGACATGCATT
	DMPK-probe 10	GCTCCTTGTAGTGGACGATCTTGCCATTTACACTCGGACCTCGTCGACATGCATT
	DMPK-probe 11	GCGTCTGCCCATAGAACATTTCATAGGCTTACACTCGGACCTCGTCGACATGCATT
	DMPK-probe 12	CATCTGCCCGCAGCTTGAGGCAAGAGTTACACTCGGACCTCGTCGACATGCATT
	DMPK-probe 13	GCCACAGCGGTCCAGCAGGATGTTGTTTACACTCGGACCTCGTCGACATGCATT
	DMPK-probe 14	GGTTTGATGTCCCTGTGCACGTAGCCATTACACTCGGACCTCGTCGACATGCATT
	DMPK-probe 15	CCGCCCACGTAATACTCCATGACCAGTTACACTCGGACCTCGTCGACATGCATT
	DMPK-probe 16	CGTCTGCTTCATCTTCACTACCGCTATTACACTCGGACCTCGTCGACATGCATT
	DMPK-probe 17	GCCCACTGCAAGAAGTCGGCCACGTATTACACTCGGACCTCGTCGACATGCATT
	DMPK-probe 18	CGCACCTTCCCGAATGTCCGACAGTGTTACACTCGGACCTCGTCGACATGCATT

Protocol	Name	Sequence 5′ → 3′
	DMPK-probe 19	GTCTCCGCCGTGGAATCCGCGTAGAATTACACTCGGACCTCGTCGACATGCATT
	DMPK-probe 20	CTCCCCAAACTTGCTCAGCAGTGTCATTACACTCGGACCTCGTCGACATGCATT
	DMPK-probe 21	CCCTCTTCAGCATGTCCCACTTGTTCTTACACTCGGACCTCGTCGACATGCATT
	DMPK-probe 22	CCCGCGTCCGATCACCTTCAGAATCTTTACACTCGGACCTCGTCGACATGCATT
	DMPK-probe 23	ACCATCCCAGTCGAGGCCAAAGAAGAAGGTTACACTCGGACCTCGTCGACATGCATT
	DMPK-probe 24	AGTAGCCCACAAAAGGCAGGTGGACCCTTACACTCGGACCTCGTCGACATGCATT
smiFISH	FLAP sequence	Cy3-AATGCATGTCGACGAGGTCCGAGTGTAA-Cy3

7. smiFISH probe: solution of *DMPK* probe-set hybridized to fluorescent FLAP probe (*see* Subheading 3.3, **step 2** for preparation),
8. FLAP hybridization reaction mix: 4 μM Probe-set, 5 μM FLAP, 1× NEB3, H_2O.
9. Prehybridization buffer: 15% formamide, 1× SSC.
10. Hybridization reaction mixes: *Mix 1*: 2× SSC, 0.68 μg/μl *E. coli* tRNA, 30% formamide, 1:25 smiFISH probe (vol:vol), H_2O. *Mix 2*: 0.4 mg/ml RNase free BSA, 4 mM VRC (Vanadylribonucleoside complex), 20% dextran sulfate, H_2O.
11. RNAse-free PBS.
12. Hoechst solution: 2 μg/ml Hoechst in PBS-T.

2.4 Immuno-fluorescence

1. Glass slides.
2. Microscope forceps.
3. Dark wet chamber.
4. Monoclonal mouse primary antibody directed against MBNL1: MB1a (DSHB) [31].
5. Secondary antibody directed against mouse IgG (H + L) conjugated to a fluorochrome.
6. Antifading mounting medium for immunofluorescence (e.g., ProLong Gold).
7. BSA (powder).
8. PBS-T: PBS + 0.1% Tween.
9. CSK buffer: 100 mM NaCl, 300 mM Sucrose, 10 mM PIPES, pH 6.8, 3 mM $MgCl_2$.
10. Blocking buffer: PBS, Tween 0.1%, 3% BSA.
11. Hoechst solution: 2 μg/ml Hoechst in PBS-T.

3 Methods

3.1 Preparation of Cells for Hybridization and Immuno fluorescence

DM1 cells (myoblasts or fibroblasts) are grown on glass coverslips coated with gelatin, prepared as follows:

1. Place a glass coverslip in the bottom of a multiwell plate or a petri dish using forceps.
2. Add gelatin solution to cover the coverslip (e.g., 1 ml/35 mm petri) and incubate for 1 h at room temperature.
3. Rinse twice with PBS.
4. Plate the cells at the required density (*see* **Note 2**).
5. Let cells grow at 37 °C and 5% CO_2 to the desired confluence (80% for proliferation or 100% for differentiation) (*see* **Note 3**).

6. Remove medium (*see* **Note 4**).
7. Carefully rinse the cells once with PBS.
8. Fix the cells with a solution of 4% PFA under chemical hood for 10 min (*see* **Note 1**).
9. Carefully rinse the cells twice with PBS.
10. Rinse the cells with EtOH 70%.
11. Incubate the cells overnight in EtOH 70% at 4 °C (For convenience, cells/coverslips can be transferred to another multiwell plate using forceps).

3.2 Fluorescent In Situ Hybridization

Before starting, turn on a hybridization oven at 37 °C and another at 45 °C, warm 50 ml of PBS-T at 45 °C and prepare the wet chamber for incubation/hybridization (*see* **Note 5** for the standard incubation temperature). Do not forget to work with *RNAse-free* solutions.

1. Carefully wash the cells twice with PBS-$MgCl_2$ for 10 min.
2. Under the chemical hood: Prepare the hybridization buffer (e.g., consider 20 μl per 12 mm coverslip, 50 μl for 30 mm) (*see* **Note 1**).
3. Place a piece of Parafilm on the bottom of the chamber.
4. Dispose a drop of hybridization buffer on the Parafilm.
5. Place the coverslip over the drop with the cells down.
6. Seal the incubation chamber with Parafilm to avoid formamide fumes.
7. Incubate the cells in the chamber at 37 °C for 90 min in a hybridization oven, in the dark (*see* **Note 6**).
8. Under the chemical hood, replace the cells/coverslip in a multiwell plate using forceps.
9. Wash the cells once with PBS-T for 5 min at RT.
10. Wash the cells once with warmed PBS-T in a hybridization oven at 45 °C for 30 min.
11. Incubate the cells once with Hoechst solution to counterstain the nucleus for 10 min.
12. Wash the cells twice with PBS-T for 10 min.
13. Mount the cells with an antifading mounting media on slide and stock the cells at least one night before visualizing the cells at the microscope (Fig. 1).

3.3 smiFISH

Single Molecule inexpensive FISH or smiFISH is a technique allowing the visualization and quantification of single mRNA molecules using gene-specific unlabelled probe set hybridized in vitro to an fluorochrome-labelled secondary detector oligonucleotide (FLAP)

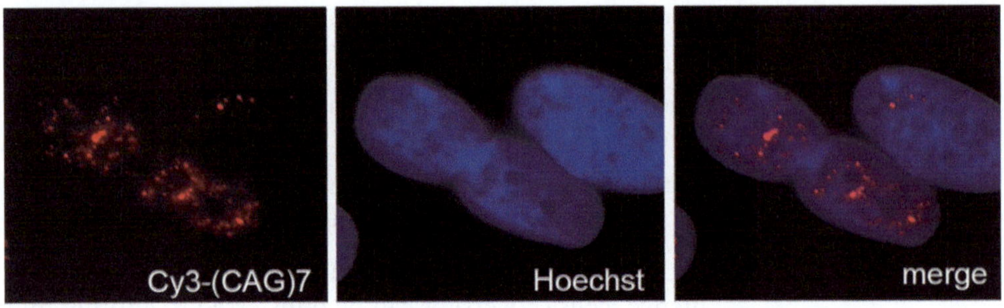

Fig. 1 RNA aggregates (or foci) of *CUGexp-DMPK* transcripts were detected by FISH using a Cy3-(CAG)7 (red) in the nucleus (Hoechst, blue) of DM1 muscle cells

(Fig. 2a). The probes used to target *DMPK* transcripts using smiFISH protocol were designed using Oligostan script included in Fish_Quant package available at https://bitbucket.org/muellerflorian/fish_quant [29]. The probes consist of 26–30 nucleotide gene-specific sequences coupled to a TTACACTCGGACCTCGTC GACATGCATT sequence, complementary to the FLAP secondary oligonucleotide (Table 1). The 24 probes target the coding region of *DMPK* transcripts (Fig. 2b). The 24 oligonucleotide probes are resuspended in TE buffer at a stock concentration of 100 μM and an equimolar mixture of the 24 oligonucleotide probes is prepared (concentration of each individual probe 4.16 μM). The probe mixture is diluted five times in TE buffer to get a 20 μM probe solution (final concentration of each individual probe 0.83 μM) and kep at −20 °C for long-term storage.

1. Prepare the FLAP hybridization reaction mix (e.g., consider 20 μl per 12 mm coverslip, 50 μl for 30 mm) in the dark (*see* **Note 6**).
2. Incubate the reaction mix in a heating block at 85 °C for 3 min.
3. Turn off the heating block and allow the tubes to cool down within the block until 35 °C.
4. Put the samples on ice.
5. The hybridized duplexes (smiFISH probes) must be kept at −20 °C in aliquots for long-term storage.
6. Prepare the cells (culture, fixation PFA 4% and permeabilization EtOH 70%) as previously described in Subheading 3.1.
7. Wash the cells twice in PBS for 10 min.
8. Under chemical hood: Incubate the cells at RT for 15 min in prehybridization buffer.
9. During the incubation prepare hybridization buffer by mixing equal volume of Mix 1 and Mix 2.

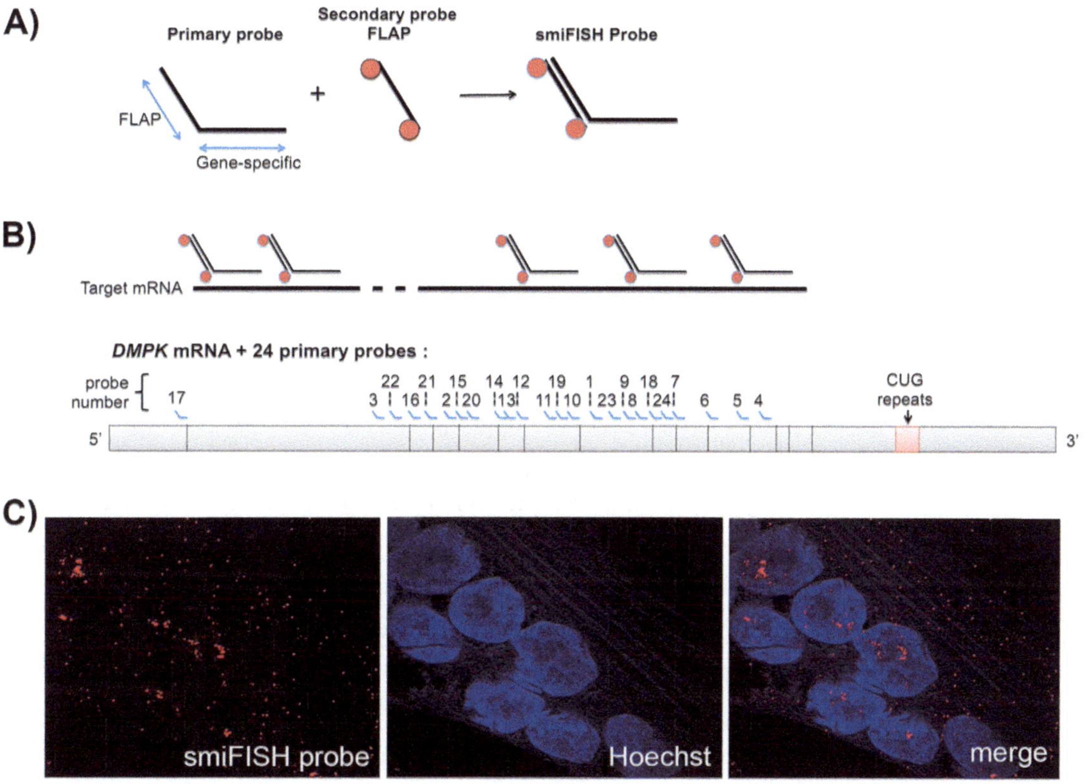

Fig. 2 Single molecule inexpensive FISH. (**A**) Schematic representation of the smiFISH principle. A set of 24 gene specific probe are hybridized in vitro to a fluorescent secondary probe via the FLAP sequence. The resulting smiFISH probes are subsequently hybridized to the targeted transcripts in cells (adapted from Tsanov et al. [29]). (**B**) Schematic representation of the 24 oligonucleotides probes on the *DMPK* transcripts. (**C**) Representative image of *DMPK* transcripts (red) observed using smiFISH technique in differentiated human WT muscle cells (nucleus in blue)

10. Place a piece of Parafilm on the bottom of the wet chamber.
11. Dispose a drop of hybridization buffer on the Parafilm.
12. Place the coverslip over the drop with the cells down.
13. Seal the incubation chamber with Parafilm to avoid formamide fumes.
14. Incubate the cells in the chamber at 37 °C overnight in a hybridization oven in the dark (*see* **Note 6**).
15. Under the chemical hood, replace the cells/coverslip in a multiwell plate using forceps.
16. Wash the cells twice with freshly prepared prehybridization buffer for 30 min.
17. Incubate the cells once with Hoechst solution for 10 min.
18. Wash the cells twice with PBS-T for 10 min.
19. Mount the cells with an antifading mounting media on slide and stock the cells at least one night before visualizing the cells at the microscope (Fig. 2c).

3.4 MBNL1 Immunofluorescence

Cells are prepared and fixed as previously described in Subheading 3.1 with a 4% PFA solution.

In alternative method, cells are fixed (and permeabilized) with an −20 °C prechilled acetone–methanol mix for 10 min at RT and washed twice with PBS-T for 10 min (as described in Holt et al. [31]). Several permeabilization methods can be used to visualize MBNL1 in human myoblasts and fibroblast depending on the state of differentiation of cells:

For undifferentiated/mononucleated cells:

1. Proceed with PFA fixation as previously described.
2. Rinse the cells with 70% ethanol solution.
3. Incubate the cells overnight in 70% ethanol solution at 4 °C.

For differentiated cells/myotubes, two alternative methods may be used. With the first method, CSK buffer is used before fixation:

1. Carefully discard the differentiation medium.
2. Rinse the cells with 4 °C chilled PBS on ice.
3. Incubate the cells with CSK buffer for 3 min at 4 °C.
4. Rinse the cells once with PBS.
5. Proceed with PFA fixation as previously described.

With the alternative method, 1% Triton is used after fixation:

1. Proceed with PFA fixation as previously described.
2. Incubate the cells with a solution of PBS containing 1% Triton for 30 min.

Subsequently proceed with blocking:

1. Rinse the cells twice with PBS-T.
2. Incubate with blocking buffer for 1 h.
3. Prepare a wet chamber with a piece of Parafilm in the bottom of the chamber.
4. Dilute the primary anti-MBNL1 antibody in blocking buffer (1/200e [31]).
5. Dispose a drop of diluted antibody on the Parafilm (as example, 10–20 μl of antibody solution per 12 mm diameter coverslip, 50 μl for a 30 mm).
6. Place the coverslip over the drop with the cells down.
7. Incubate with primary antibody in a wet chamber for 1 h.
8. Replace the cells/coverslip in the multiwell plate.
9. Wash the cells three times with PBS-T for 10 min.

10. Dilute the fluorochrome-conjugated secondary antibody in blocking buffer (1/400–1/500 with standard commercially available secondary antibodies).
11. Dispose a drop of diluted antibody on the Parafilm (as example, 10–20 μl of antibody solution per 12 mm diameter coverslip, 50 μl for a 30 mm).
12. Place the coverslip over the drop by putting the cells down.
13. Incubate the cells with secondary antibody in the dark for 1 h (*see* **Note 6**).
14. Replace the cells/coverslip in the multiwell plate.
15. Incubate the cells 10 min with a Hoechst solution.
16. Wash the cells twice with PBS-T for 10 min.
17. Mount the cells with an antifading mounting media on slide and stock the cells at least one night before visualizing the cells at the microscope (Fig. 3a).

3.5 Combined FISH and Immunofluorescence Experiments

For combined FISH/smiFISH-IF experiments (Fig. 3b), the immunofluorescence protocol starts just before the incubation with the Hoechst solution (in both the FISH and the smiFISH protocols) and is done as described in Subheading 3.4, **step 3** and subsequent (*see* **Note 7**).

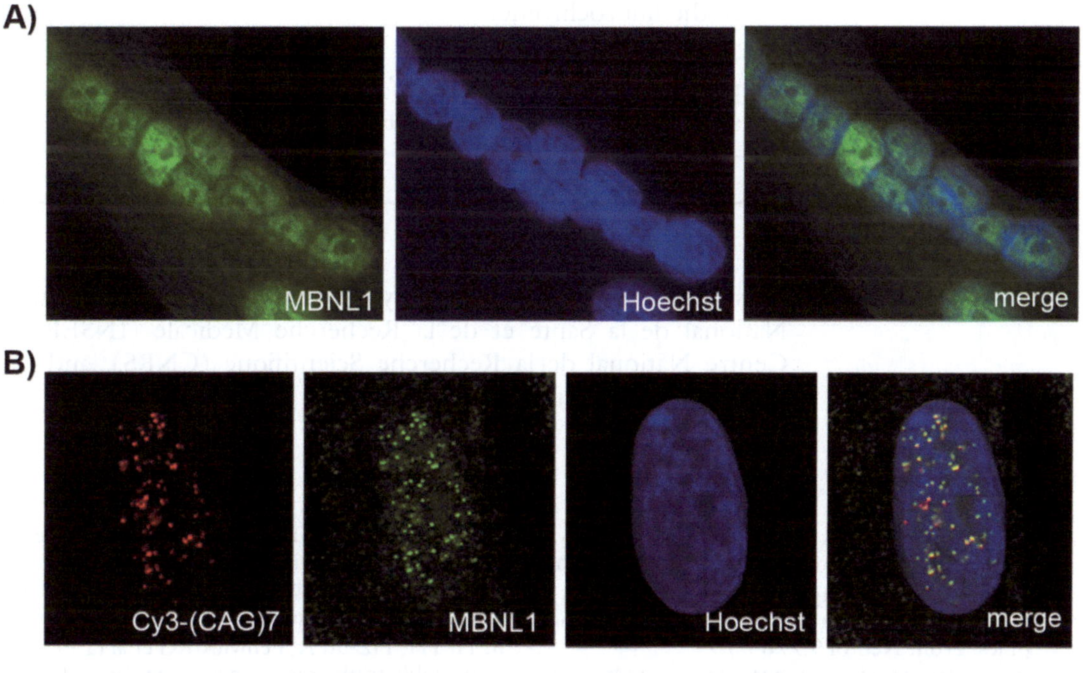

Fig. 3 Localization of MBNL1 in WT and DM1 myoblasts. (**A**) Visualization of MBNL1 (in green) using immunofluorescence technique in differentiated human WT muscle cells (nucleus in blue). (**B**) Visualization of both mutated *DMPK* transcripts using FISH technique (CAG7 probe, red) and MBNL1 using immunofluorescence technique (MB1a antibody, green) in the nucleus of DM1 myoblast (Hoechst, blue)

4 Notes

1. Every manipulation involving formaldehyde-, formamide-, or methanol-containing buffer should be performed under a chemical hood. This includes fixation of cells, preparation of hybridization buffers and hybridization steps.
2. For a homogenous repartition of the cells upon the surface of the petri, plate at high density (e.g., for immortalized myoblasts: 30,000 cells/cm^2) and let them grow for 24–48 h before fixation or switch for differentiation.
3. To induce differentiation: When the cells reached 100% confluence, remove the GM, rinse the cells once with DMEM and replace with DM. When myotubes are formed (usually between 3 and 5 days postdifferentiation) fix the cells.
4. The cells do not attach well on glass, so washing or medium changes must be done carefully to prevent cell detachment, especially for myotubes. Other coating substrates like collagen-I or Matrigel may be used instead of gelatin.
5. All incubations or washing steps should be performed at room temperature (RT), unless otherwise indicated.
6. Incubation involving fluorochrome (oligonucleotide probes or antibodies) should be performed in the dark to prevent fading of the fluorochrome.
7. The permeabilization should be adapted in accordance to the protocol used. In the case of Triton 1% permeabilization, this step could be done after the FISH/smiFISH staining.

Acknowledgments

This research was supported by Sorbonne Université, Institut National de la Santé et de la Recherche Médicale (INSERM), Centre National de la Recherche Scientifique (CNRS), and the Association Institut de Myologie (AIM).

References

1. Harper PS (2001) Myotonic dystrophy. W.B. Saunders—Harcourt Publishers, London
2. Wenninger S, Montagnese F, Schoser B (2018) Core clinical phenotypes in Myotonic dystrophies. Front Neurol 9:776–779
3. Brook JD, McCurrach ME, Harley HG et al (1992) Molecular basis of myotonic dystrophy: expansion of a trinucleotide (CTG) repeat at the 3′ end of a transcript encoding a protein kinase family member. Cell 68:799–808
4. Mahadevan M, Tsilfidis C, Sabourin L et al (1992) Myotonic dystrophy mutation: an unstable CTG repeat in the 3′ untranslated region of the gene. Science 255:1253–1255
5. Fu YH, Pizzuti A, Fenwick RG et al (1992) An unstable triplet repeat in a gene related to myotonic muscular dystrophy. Science 255:1256–1258
6. Ashizawa T, Harper PS (2006) Myotonic dystrophies: an overview. In: Genetic instabilities and neurological diseases. Elsevier, Amsterdam, pp 21–36

7. Taneja KL, McCurrach M, Schalling M et al (1995) Foci of trinucleotide repeat transcripts in nuclei of myotonic dystrophy cells and tissues. J Cell Biol 128:995–1002
8. Davis BM, McCurrach ME, Taneja KL et al (1997) Expansion of a CUG trinucleotide repeat in the 3′ untranslated region of myotonic dystrophy protein kinase transcripts results in nuclear retention of transcripts. Proc Natl Acad Sci 94:7388–7393
9. Miller JW, Urbinati CR, Teng-Umnuay P et al (2000) Recruitment of human muscleblind proteins to (CUG)(n) expansions associated with myotonic dystrophy. EMBO J 19:4439–4448
10. Fardaei M, Larkin K, Brook JD et al (2001) In vivo co-localisation of MBNL protein with DMPK expanded-repeat transcripts. Nucleic Acids Res 29:2766–2771
11. Mankodi A, Urbinati CR, Yuan QP et al (2001) Muscleblind localizes to nuclear foci of aberrant RNA in myotonic dystrophy types 1 and 2. Hum Mol Genet 10:2165–2170
12. Charlet BN, Savkur RS, Singh G et al (2002) Loss of the muscle-specific chloride channel in type 1 myotonic dystrophy due to misregulated alternative splicing. Mol Cell 10:45–53
13. Lin X, Miller JW, Mankodi A et al (2006) Failure of MBNL1-dependent post-natal splicing transitions in myotonic dystrophy. Hum Mol Genet 15:2087–2097
14. Ho TH, Charlet BN, Poulos MG et al (2004) Muscleblind proteins regulate alternative splicing. EMBO J 23:3103–3112
15. Konieczny P, Stepniak-Konieczna E, Sobczak K (2014) MBNL proteins and their target RNAs, interaction and splicing regulation. Nucleic Acids Res 42:10873–10887
16. Nakamori M, Sobczak K, Puwanant A et al (2013) Splicing biomarkers of disease severity in myotonic dystrophy. Ann Neurol 74:862–872
17. Fugier C, Klein AF, Hammer C et al (2011) Misregulated alternative splicing of BIN1 is associated with T tubule alterations and muscle weakness in myotonic dystrophy. Nat Med 17:720–725
18. Savkur RS, Philips AV, Cooper TA (2001) Aberrant regulation of insulin receptor alternative splicing is associated with insulin resistance in myotonic dystrophy. Nat Genet 29:40–47
19. Rau F, Lainé J, Ramanoudjame L et al (2015) Abnormal splicing switch of DMD's penultimate exon compromises muscle fibre maintenance in myotonic dystrophy. Nat Commun 6:385–310
20. Freyermuth F, Rau F, Kokunai Y et al (2016) Splicing misregulation of SCN5A contributes to cardiac-conduction delay and heart arrhythmia in myotonic dystrophy. Nat Commun 7:11067
21. Jiang H, Mankodi A, Swanson MS et al (2004) Myotonic dystrophy type 1 is associated with nuclear foci of mutant RNA, sequestration of muscleblind proteins and deregulated alternative splicing in neurons. Hum Mol Genet 13:3079–3088
22. Michel L, Huguet-Lachon A, Gourdon G (2015) Sense and antisense DMPK RNA foci accumulate in DM1 tissues during development. PLoS One 10:e0137620
23. Francois V, Klein AF, Beley C et al (2011) Selective silencing of mutated mRNAs in DM1 by using modified hU7-snRNAs. Nat Struct Mol Biol 18:85–87
24. Smith KP, Byron M, Johnson C et al (2007) Defining early steps in mRNA transport: mutant mRNA in myotonic dystrophy type I is blocked at entry into SC-35 domains. J Cell Biol 178:951–964
25. Querido E, Gallardo F, Beaudoin M et al (2011) Stochastic and reversible aggregation of mRNA with expanded CUG-triplet repeats. J Cell Sci 124:1703–1714
26. Dansithong W, Paul S, Comai L et al (2005) MBNL1 is the primary determinant of focus formation and aberrant insulin receptor splicing in DM1. J Biol Chem 280:5773–5780
27. Arandel L, Polay Espinoza M, Matloka M et al (2017) Immortalized human myotonic dystrophy muscle cell lines to assess therapeutic compounds. Dis Model Mech 10:487–497
28. Taneja KL (1998) Localization of trinucleotide repeat sequences in myotonic dystrophy cells using a single fluorochrome-labeled PNA probe. BioTechniques 24:472–476
29. Tsanov N, Samacoits A, Chouaib R et al (2016) smiFISH and FISH-quant—a flexible single RNA detection approach with super-resolution capability. Nucleic Acids Res 44:e165–e165
30. Byron M, Hall LL, Lawrence JB (2013) A multifaceted FISH approach to study endogenous RNAs and DNAs in native nuclear and cell structures, current protocols in human genetics. Chapter 4. Unitas 4:15–4.15.21
31. Holt I, Jacquemin V, Fardaei M et al (2009) Muscleblind-like proteins. Am J Pathol 174:216–227

Chapter 14

Real Time Videomicroscopy and Semiautomated Analysis of Brain Cell Culture Models of Trinucleotide Repeat Expansion Diseases

Sandra O. Braz, Diana M. Dinca, Geneviève Gourdon, and Mário Gomes-Pereira

Abstract

Proper brain function requires the coordinated and intricate interaction between neuronal and glial cells. Like many other neurological conditions, trinucleotide repeat expansion disorders are likely initiated by the synergistic combination of abnormalities hitting different brain cell types, which ultimately disrupt brain function and lead to the onset of neurological symptoms. Understanding how trinucleotide repeat expansions affect the phenotypes and physiology of neurons and glia is fundamental to improve our understanding of disease mechanisms in the brain and shape the design of future therapeutic interventions.

Here we describe a protocol for semiautomated videomicroscopy analysis of cultured brain cells, maintained under suitable and controlled conditions. Through real-time monitoring of basic cell phenotypes (such as proliferation, cell morphology, differentiation, and migration) this method provides an accurate primary assessment of the impact of the repeat expansion on the physiology of neurons and glia. The versatility of the system, the automated image acquisition and the semiautomated processing of the data collected allow rapid phenotypic analysis of individual cell types, as well as the investigation of cell–cell interactions. The stability of the acquisition system provides reproducible and robust results. The raw data can be easily exported to other software to perform more sophisticated imaging analysis and statistical tests. In summary, the methods described offer versatile, reproducible, and time-effective means to dissect the impact of the repeat expansion on different brain cell types and on intercellular interactions.

Key words Real-time videomicroscopy, Primary cell cultures, Neuron, Astrocyte, Oligodendrocyte, Trinucleotide repeat expansion, Cell phenotypes, Semiautomated analysis

1 Introduction

Trinucleotide repeat expansion diseases comprise neuromuscular, neurodevelopmental and neurodegenerative disorders [1, 2], which are usually associated with cognitive deficits and behavioral changes. Today we know that repeat expansions mediate disease

Sandra O. Braz and Diana M. Dinca contributed equally to this work.

Guy-Franck Richard (ed.), *Trinucleotide Repeats: Methods and Protocols*, Methods in Molecular Biology, vol. 2056,
https://doi.org/10.1007/978-1-4939-9784-8_14, © Springer Science+Business Media, LLC, part of Springer Nature 2020

etiology through a variety of mechanisms, including loss of function (e.g., fragile X syndrome, FXS; and Friedreich ataxia, FRDA) [3, 4], toxic gain of function of polyglutamine tracts (e.g., Huntington disease, HD) [5], and RNA toxicity (e.g., myotonic dystrophy type 1, DM1) [6]. On top of these mechanisms, the accumulation of toxic homopolypeptides by repeat-associated non-AUG (RAN) translation may also play a determinant pathogenic role [7].

Mouse models have been crucial to decipher the molecular pathogenesis of trinucleotide repeat expansion diseases, notably in the brain, where they recreate the intricate and multidirectional interactions between different cell types [8]. However, the broad view revealed by the analysis of tissue samples, does not grant sufficient resolution to focus on pathological events occurring in specific cell populations. This is particularly relevant in conditions in which it is conceivable that disease susceptibility and the cascade of pathogenic events vary between different cell types and/or subpopulations. Cell type selective pathogenesis in trinucleotide repeat expansion disorders is illustrated by the preferential degeneration of medium spiny neurons in the striatum of HD patients [9] and by the pervasive loss of Purkinje cells in many spinocerebellar ataxias (SCAs) [10], while other neuronal types remain relatively spared. Rat primary cultures corroborated the increased vulnerability of striatal neurons to expanded huntingtin, relative to cortical neurons [11]. More recently, the generation of human iPSC-derived Purkinje cells confirmed the burden of SCAs to this neuronal cell type [12].

In spite of the neuronal damage that precedes the neurological manifestations of trinucleotide repeat expansion diseases, a less "neurocentric" view of brain pathology is emerging, pointing to the key role of glial cells. It has been reported that astrocyte dysfunction prevents normal neuronal development and proper synaptogenesis in FXS [13, 14] and FRDA [15, 16]. Astrocyte deficits may also cause Purkinje cell hyperexcitability in SCA7 [17] and DM1 [18]. Signs of astrocyte pathology were also reported in HD [19], fragile X-associated tremor/ataxia syndrome (FXTAS) [20] and SCA1 [21]. In addition to astrocytes, oligodendrocytes are also affected by trinucleotide repeat expansions. The dysfunction of this glial cell type was documented in mouse models of HD and FXS, and it was characterized by delayed and reduced myelination in association with defective maturation of oligodendrocytes [22, 23]. The involvement of microglia in trinucleotide repeat expansion diseases has been less explored. Nonetheless, microglia activation was reported in HD patients, as well as in mouse models of HD [24, 25] and SCA1 [21]. In HD models, microglia activation is accompanied by abnormal cell morphology and defective migration response to chemotaxis [26].

Together these findings demonstrate the diverse response of different brain cells to disease, and the critical insight that can be gained from the analysis of individual cell types. Understanding the disease mechanisms that operate in different cell populations and underlie the complex neurological symptoms is crucial for future therapeutic developments. Cell culture techniques provide a powerful setting to address this question. While homogenous cell cultures can reveal the impact of the disease on the phenotype and physiology of different cell types, mixed cultures (established through the combination of different cells) can help untangle the mechanisms of intercellular miscommunication in the brain and their contribution to disease. These studies were traditionally performed on cultured cells fixed at different time points. Although informative, this strategy presents two main limitations: (a) the readouts represent isolated snapshots of physiological processes that are continuously ongoing and they may therefore miss relevant events; (b) the methodology is time-consuming, involving cell manipulation, cell labeling, signal detection, data collection and laborious data analysis.

The alternative is to perform prolonged recordings of live cell phenotypes, by real-time semiautomated videomicroscopy. The success of this methodology depends on the maintenance of well-defined and suitable culture conditions, which must guarantee cell function and stability over long periods of time. This requirement is particularly important for brain cells, given their high sensitivity to environmental changes: subtle uncontrolled fluctuations may have deleterious consequences to cell homeostasis and affect the quality and reproducibility of the results. The advanced Incucyte® live-cell analysis system (Essen Bioscience) reduces these technical challenges and maximizes the quality and reproducibility of the data collected. The video system is incorporated in a regular CO_2 incubator, allowing the cells to be kept in their optimal temperature and humidity throughout the experiment. Image acquisition is automatic: once the experimenter has defined the acquisition settings he/she can walk away, leaving the cells unperturbed. The semiautomatic analysis of the Incucyte® system is another major strength: the system offers predefined analysis settings that can be adapted by the scientist to better fit the type of cells and the biological process being studied. Once defined, the same settings and analysis can be immediately applied to the images as they are acquired by the video system—the computerized workflow translates into real-time results and traceability of eventual problems, therefore saving precious time.

The methods described here provide a videomicroscopy semiautomated approach to assess the primary impact of the disease on different cell lineages of the brain (neurons, astrocytes and oligodendrocytes), using proliferation, differentiation, cell adhesion, morphological complexity and migration (among others) as basic readouts of cell dysfunction. The results generated offer meaningful clues to design future experiments and extend the analysis of the disease mechanisms operating in individual cell populations, through more refined approaches. In spite of our focus on brain cells, the protocols can be easily adapted and applied to a myriad of other cell types.

2 Materials

2.1 Specific Equipment and Reagents

1. IncuCyte Zoom videomicroscope equipped with IncuCyte® Scratch Wound Cell Migration Software Module (9600-0012, Essen Bioscience) and IncuCyte® NeuroTrack Software Module (9600-0010, Essen Bioscience).
2. Computer equipped with Incucyte Zoom software, FIJI-ImageJ software [27] and DiPer program [28].
3. IncuCyte® Cell Migration Kit (4493, Essen Bioscience).
4. IncuCyte® ImageLock Plates (4379, Essen Bioscience).
5. IncuCyte® NeuroLight Red Lentivirus—Synapsin Promoter (4584, Essen Bioscience).
6. GentleMACS Dissociator (130-093-235 or superior, Miltenyi).
7. Neural tissue dissociation kit (130-092-628, Miltenyi) and magnetic anti-CD140a microbeads (130-092-628, Miltenyi).
8. Equipment maintenance: 0.5% Alconox, 1% Virkon, double distilled H_2O and 70% Ethanol.

2.2 Mouse Experiments

For experiments involving animal models you must follow the institutional, national and/or international guidelines for ethical conduct in the care and use of animals.

2.3 Cell Culture Media and Coating Reagents

1. Dissection medium for neurons and astrocytes: Leibovitz's L-15 Medium, 30 μM glucose.
2. Dissection medium for OPC: Hank's balanced salt solution (HBSS) without Ca^{2+} and Mg^{2+}.
3. Neuronal medium: Neurobasal-A, 1× B27 supplement, 0.5 mM L-Glutamine, 0.25 μg/mL Amphotericin B, 100 U/mL penicillin and 100 μg/mL streptomycin.
4. Astrocytes medium: DMEM low glucose, 10% fetal bovine serum (FBS) and 0.05 mg/mL Gentamycin.
5. OPC medium: DMEM F-12, 1% N2 supplement, 2% B27 supplement, 50 U/mL penicillin and 50 μg/mL streptomycin, 0.01% bovine serum albumin, 40 ng/mL FGF2 and 20 ng/mL PDGF-AA.

6. Oligodendrocytes medium: DMEM F-12, 1% N2 supplement, 2% B27 supplement, 50 U/mL penicillin and 50 μg/mL streptomycin, 50 μg/mL insulin, 40 ng/mL triiodothyronine, and 1 ng/mL CNTF.
7. Coating: 0.1 mg/mL of poly-D-lysine (PDL) and 10 μg/mL laminin (*see* **Note 1**).

3 Methods

3.1 Primary Mouse Cell Cultures

Different protocols are available in the literature and can be used to establish primary cultures of mouse neurons, astrocytes and oligodendrocytes. We briefly describe below the protocols used in our laboratory to ensure healthy and reproducible cell cultures prior to cell seeding (*see* **Note 2**).

3.1.1 For Primary Neuron Cultures

1. Prepare primary dissociated cell cultures of cortical neurons from embryonic day (E) 16.5 mouse embryos (*see* **Note 3**). Dissect the brain and place it on a dish with dissociation medium for neurons, under a stereoscope.
2. Separate the cortices from the rest of the brain and carefully remove the meninges with the help of micro tweezers.
3. Maintain the cortices in dissection medium on ice until end of the dissection.
4. Wash the cortices twice with neuronal medium, previously warmed at 37 °C.
5. Incubate the cortices in neuronal medium containing 0.05% of trypsin and 10 U/mL of DNaseI 15 min at 37 °C, shaking gently the tube every 5 min.
6. Wash the cell suspension twice with neuronal medium supplemented with 5% FBS to inhibit further tissue digestion by trypsin.
7. Dissociate the cells passing them through a 21 G needle, wash twice in neuronal medium, collecting the cells at 200 × *g* for 5 min at room temperature (RT) in between washes.
8. Count cells (*see* **Note 4**) before plating at appropriated cell density in PDL and laminin-coated 96-well plates (*see* **Note 5**) in prewarmed neuronal medium containing 5% FBS.
9. Replace the medium 4 h after plating with neuronal medium supplemented with 100 μM AraC and withdraw the FBS to avoid astrocytes proliferation (*see* **Note 6**).
10. Change half of the medium every 3–4 days (*see* **Note 7**).

3.1.2 For Primary Astrocyte Cultures

1. Prepare primary dissociated cell cultures of cortical astrocytes from postnatal day (P) 1 pups (*see* **Note 3**). Dissect the cortices as described above.
2. Wash the tissue twice with 1 mL of astrocytes medium and mechanically dissociate, passing through 21 G needle twice and then three times through a 26 G needle, waiting 2–3 min for the sedimentation of the fragments in between each dissociation.
3. Centrifuge the cell suspension at 200 × *g* for 5 min at RT, remove the supernatant and resuspend the cells in 10 mL of prewarmed astrocytes medium.
4. Plate the cells in a T75 dish at 300,000 cells/mL.
5. On the following day, change the medium (*see* **Note 7**) to remove dead cells.
6. Primary astrocytes adhere, grow and proliferate on both coated and uncoated dishes (*see* **Notes 1** and **6**).
7. Incubate the cells for 2 weeks in astrocytes medium, changing the medium every 3 days (*see* **Note 8**).

3.1.3 For Primary Oligodendrocyte Progenitor Cell (OPC) Cultures

1. Prepare dissociated cell cultures of cortical OPC from P0 to P2 mice (*see* **Note 3**). Perform the dissection as described above using dissection medium for OPC.
2. Dissociate the tissue using the neural tissue dissociation kit and following the manufacturer's protocol. Dissociate the tissue by cycles of mechanic and enzymatic dissociation to produce a single cell suspension, then filter the suspension through a 70-μm strainer and wash with HBSS with Ca^{2+} and Mg^{2+}.
3. Centrifuge the cell suspension at 300 × *g* for 10 min at RT, remove the supernatant and resuspend the cells in a 1× PBS with Ca^{2+} and Mg^{2+}, supplemented with 5% BSA (BSA buffer).
4. Isolate the OPC using magnetic anti-CD140a (PDGFRα) labelled microbeads (protocol adapted from Dincman et al. [29]).
5. After blocking, incubate the cells with the magnetic microbeads to allow the binding of the PDGFRα$^+$ cells, then wash the cells in BSA buffer and collect at 300 × *g* for 10 min at RT, to eliminate cell-free microbeads.
6. To separate the OPC, pass the cell suspension trough a column attached to a magnetic field, where the PDGFRα$^+$ cells are retained.
7. Remove the column from the magnetic field and flush the cells in OPC medium.

8. Count OPC and plate them at a density of 9,000–15,000 cells/cm^2 in PDL and laminin-coated 96-well plates (*see* **Note 5**) and keep in OPC medium to proliferate (*see* **Note 9**).
9. Two days later, replace the medium with oligodendrocytes medium, in order to induce the differentiation of OPC into oligodendrocytes (*see* **Note 6**).

3.2 Cell Proliferation (Astrocytes and OPC)

In this protocol, cell proliferation is estimated by the percentage of well surface area occupied by cells (i.e., confluence) over time.

1. Seed the astrocytes and OPC at 20,000 or 50,00 cells/well, respectively (*see* **Note 10**), on 96-well plates (*see* **Note 5**) and keep the cells in their corresponding culture media.
2. Set the system to acquire a phase-contrast picture (*see* **Note 11**) every 45 min over 50 h for astrocytes, or every 2 h during 7–8 days for oligodendrocytes, selecting the "Standard" type of scan and using the 20× objective (*see* **Note 12**). Change the cell medium every 2–3 days (*see* **Notes 6** and **13**).
3. Set the image analysis by first creating a collection of images (*see* **Note 14**) representative of the phenotypes to be monitored throughout the experiment. Select the first picture and click on "Create or Add to Image Collection" (Fig. 1, option A), select the "Basic Analyzer" job type mode and add the image to the new image collection. Select another 4–6 new images (*see* **Note 15**) and add them to the same image collection.
4. Using this collection of images, define the settings to be applied to the analyses. Under the option "New Processing Definition" (Fig. 1, option B) run the "Preview Current" command to automatically generate the "Confluence Mask" that will contour and cover the surface of what the software considers to be cells in the first picture selected.
5. Since the automatic mask is unlikely to fit all the cell shapes/densities through time and/or all cell conditions (Fig. 2a), adjust this mask in order to fully outline the shape of the cells. To do so, use the filters named "Cell/Background," "Size," and "Eccentricity," which are available on the "Segmentation Adjustment" panel (*see* **Note 16**).
6. Apply the defined settings to all the image collection by selecting the option "Preview All," and check if the mask fits perfectly the majority of the cells in the different images of the image collection previously chosen (Fig. 2b).
7. Initiate the analysis by selecting "Launch New Analysis Job" (Fig. 1, option C). The software will apply the defined settings to all the pictures acquired from the plate over time (*see* **Note 17**).

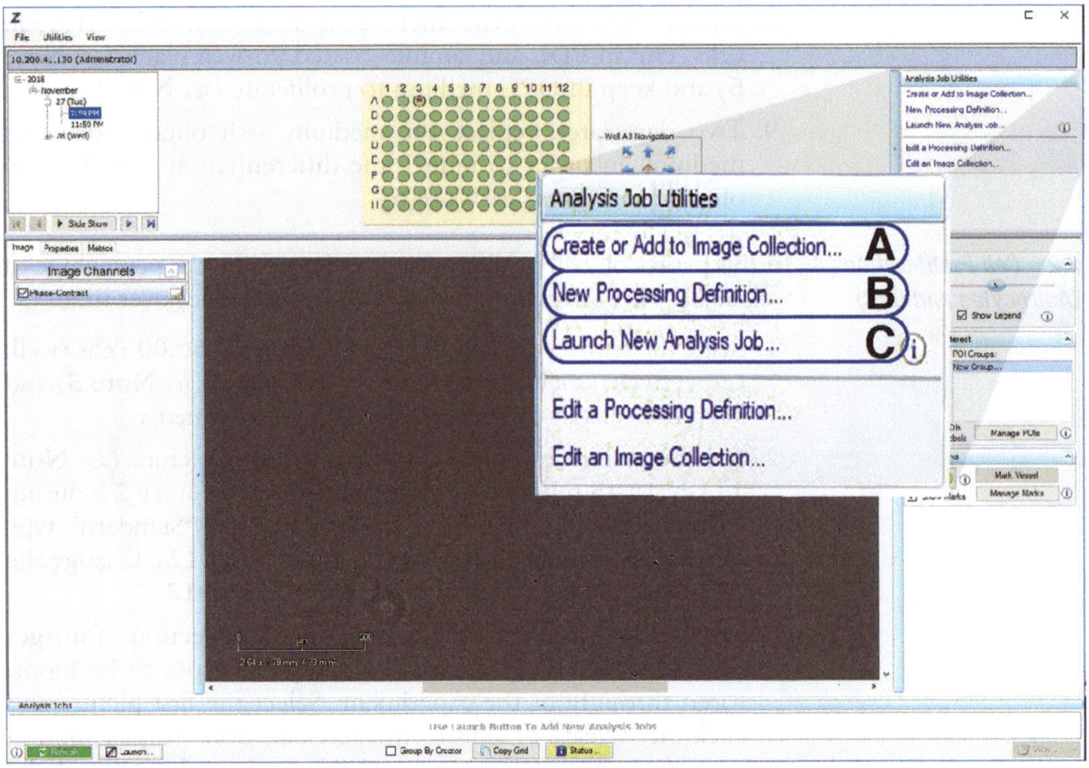

Fig. 1 Incucyte® Zoom software interface. Software interface screenshot showing the panel for the definition of the semiautomated analysis. The process starts with the creation of an image collection (option A), followed by the definition of the analysis settings that will be applied to all the images subsequently acquired (option B). Finally the analysis in launched (option C)

8. The results will estimate cell proliferation, measured as the percentage of cell confluence (*see* **Notes 18** and **19**) or as a phase-contrast object (cell) count (*see* **Notes 11** and **20**) during the time-course of the experiment. The results are plotted as the percentage of confluence over time for each well, or as the average of technical/biological replicates (Fig. 2c) (*see* **Note 21**).

3.3 Wound Healing Migration (Astrocytes and OPC)

This analysis evaluates the capacity on the cells to migrate toward and fill an empty space created by a wound on a cell monolayer. It estimates the percentage of the wound surface occupied by migrating cells over time.

1. Seed 20,000 astrocytes or 10,000 OPC per well (*see* **Note 10**), on a 96-well plate Incucyte® Image Lock (*see* **Notes 1**, **22**, and **23**) and keep the cells in their medium. Incubate the cells for 1–2 days to obtain a confluent monolayer of astrocytes, or a 70–90% confluent layer of OPC.
2. Place the open plate on the base of the Incucyte® Wound Maker (*see* **Note 24**) and carefully introduce the wound maker

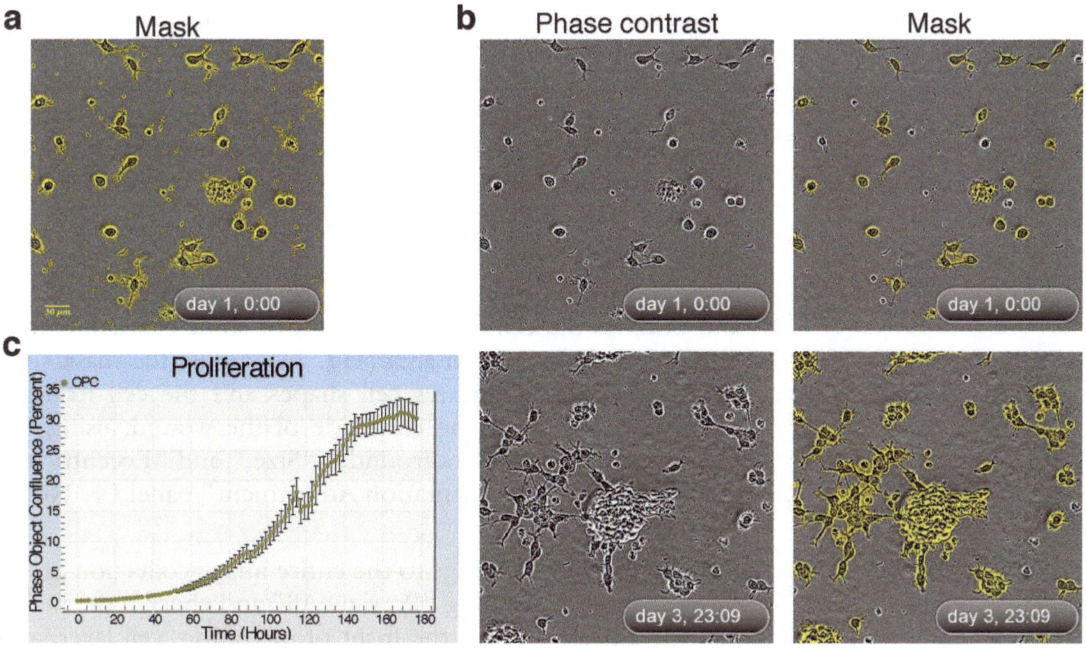

Fig. 2 Live-cell monitoring of OPC proliferation. (**a**) Phase contrast image showing a poor fit of a merged "Confluence Mask" (yellow) on OPC imaged 1 day after plating. The confluence mask is inadequately counting small cell debris and plate/coating imperfections as objects (cells), also including some space between adjacent cells. (**b**) Phase contrast images of OPC on day 1 and 3 after plating. Adequate confluence masks (yellow) faithfully delineate the shape of living cells, excluding cell debris, imperfections, and space between cells. (**c**) The quantitative analysis of cell proliferation is plotted as the percentage of confluence (surface of the well occupied by cells) over 180 h

pin block into the wells. Perform the wound on the bottom of the wells by pushing and holding the lever (*see* **Note 25**). Wash the cells gently with prewarm astrocyte or OPC medium twice, to remove any cell debris remaining in the wound (while avoiding to disturb the cells) and refill the wells with 100 μL of medium (*see* **Note 7**) using a multichannel micropipette.

3. Set the system to acquire a phase-contrast picture (*see* **Note 11**) every 45–60 min over 3 days (*see* **Note 22**), selecting the "Scratch Wound" on the "Scan Type" dropdown and using the 10× objective.
4. Set the image analysis by creating a representative set of images taking into account the phenotype to be analyzed over time (*see* **Note 14**). To this end, select the first picture and click on "Create or Add to Image Collection" (Fig. 1, option A), select the "Scratch Wound" option on the job type mode and add the image to the new image collection. Select another 4–6 new images (*see* **Note 15**), including the first scan (time 0) after wounding, which will be used to define the initial mask for the surface of the wounded (cell-free) area. Add the images to the previous image collection.

5. Using this collection of images, define the settings to be applied to the analyses. Under the option "Process Definition" (Fig. 1, option B) run the "Preview Current" command on the first picture to automatically generate the "Confluence Mask" (which will cover and contour the surface of what the software supposes to be a cell layer (Fig. 3a-1)) and the "Scratch Wound Mask" (which will cover the cell-free space created by the scratch (Fig. 3a-3)).
6. Since the automatic mask may not be able to perfectly detect and outlines the cell layer limits and/or some cell debris may remain on the wounded area (Fig. 3a), adjust the mask so it fully covers and delineates cell shapes and the cell front of migration (Fig. 3a-2) on each side of the wound, using the filters named "Cell/Background," "Size," and "Eccentricity" available on the "Segmentation Adjustment" panel (*see* **Notes 16** and **26**).
7. Apply the defined settings to the entire image collection previously created by running "Preview All" and check if the masks provide a perfect fit for the front of migration, cell layer, and wounded space for the majority of the different images previously selected (Fig. 3b).
8. Initiate the analysis by clicking on the "Launch New Analysis Job" (Fig. 1, option C). The software will apply the settings previously defined to all the pictures acquired on the plate (*see* **Note 17**).
9. The results will estimate the rate of occupancy of the space left empty following the scratch. They can be represented by one of three measurements: (a) wound width over time (distance between the front of migration of each side of the cell-free space); (b) wound confluence over time (the percentage of the wound initial surface occupied by the cells) or (c) relative wound density (RWD, the percentage of the cell density in the wound relative to the percentage of cell density in the regions surrounding the wound) (*see* **Notes 21** and **27**) (Fig. 3c).

3.4 Single Cell Tracking (Astrocytes)

This analysis allows the drawing of the migration path, the measurement of speed, directionality and displacement of individual astrocytes by manually tracking the position of the nucleus in each image, using Fiji and the open-source DiPer computer software [28].

1. Following the wound healing assay, export migration videos from the IncuCyte® in uncompressed AVI format and open them using Fiji (*see* **Note 28**). Make sure to export at least one video (or one image) with the embedded scale, to be able to use it for setting the scale in Fiji (*see* **Note 29**). The image visualization the videos can be modified to facilitate tracking (*see* **Notes 30** and **31**).

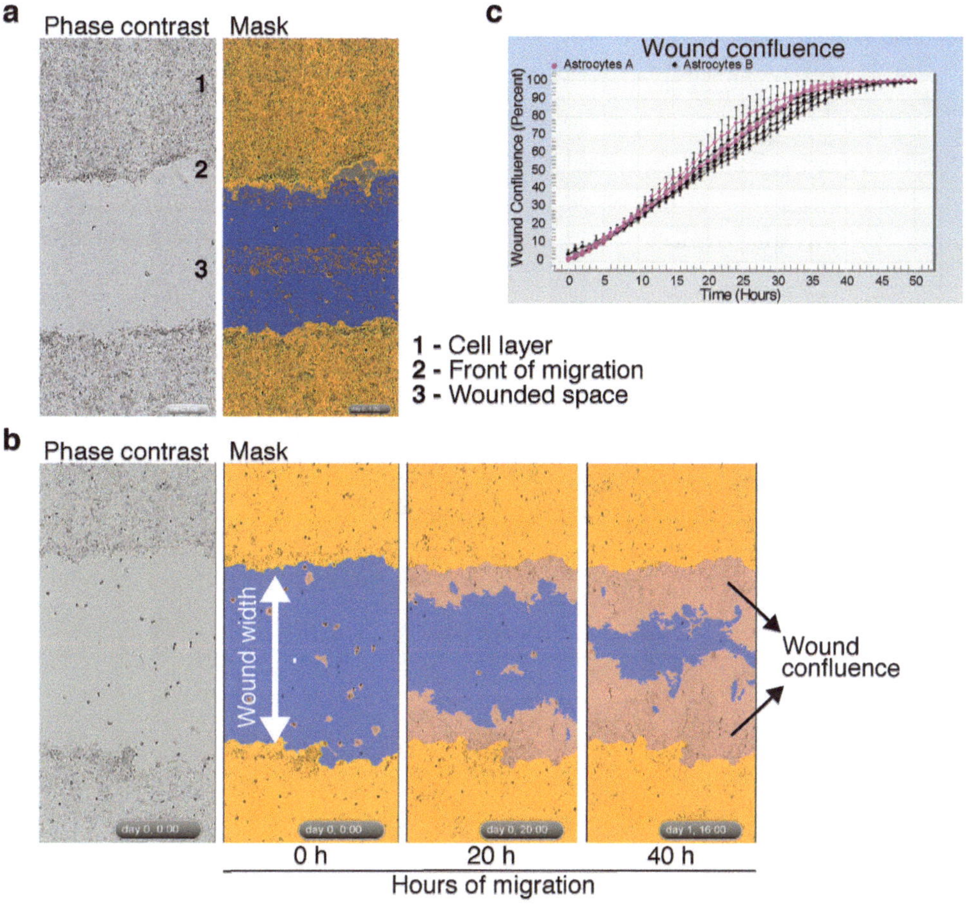

Fig. 3 Astrocyte migration capacity tested by an automated wound healing assay. (**a**) Phase contrast image of a cell monolayer after scratching, using the Incucyte® Wound Maker. The picture shows the cell layer (1), front of migration (2) and wounded space (3) on the left. The image on the right shows a merged bad fitting "Confluence mask" (yellow), covering only part of the front of migration and inadequately including empty wounded space without cells. (**b**) Phase contrast image of a scratched astrocyte monolayer and the fitting "Confluence Masks" (yellow) over time. The merged images show the "Confluence Mask" overlaying the cell layer and outlining some isolated cells left in the wounded space, while excluding cell debris. The "Scratch Wound Mask" (blue) is confined to the wounded space, free of cells. The wound width (white double arrowhead) decreases as the wound confluence increase over 40 h following the initial scratch. (**c**) The speed of collective migration of the astrocytes is estimated by the increase in wound confluence over time. Several biological replicates of astrocytes of individual mice (pink and black) are plotted

2. After setting the scale (*see* **Note 28**) use the "Manual Tracking Fiji" plugin to track the nucleus of at least 40 astrocytes per video. Insert the time interval in the corresponding panel of the Tracking window, and the x/y calibration (corresponding to the pixel width, which can be found when setting the scale in Fiji). Start tracking by clicking "Add track" (Fig. 4a) and following the advancement of one selected cell. This will measure the position of the astrocytes on the X and Y coordinates, the distance and the velocity of the astrocytes (Fig. 4b).

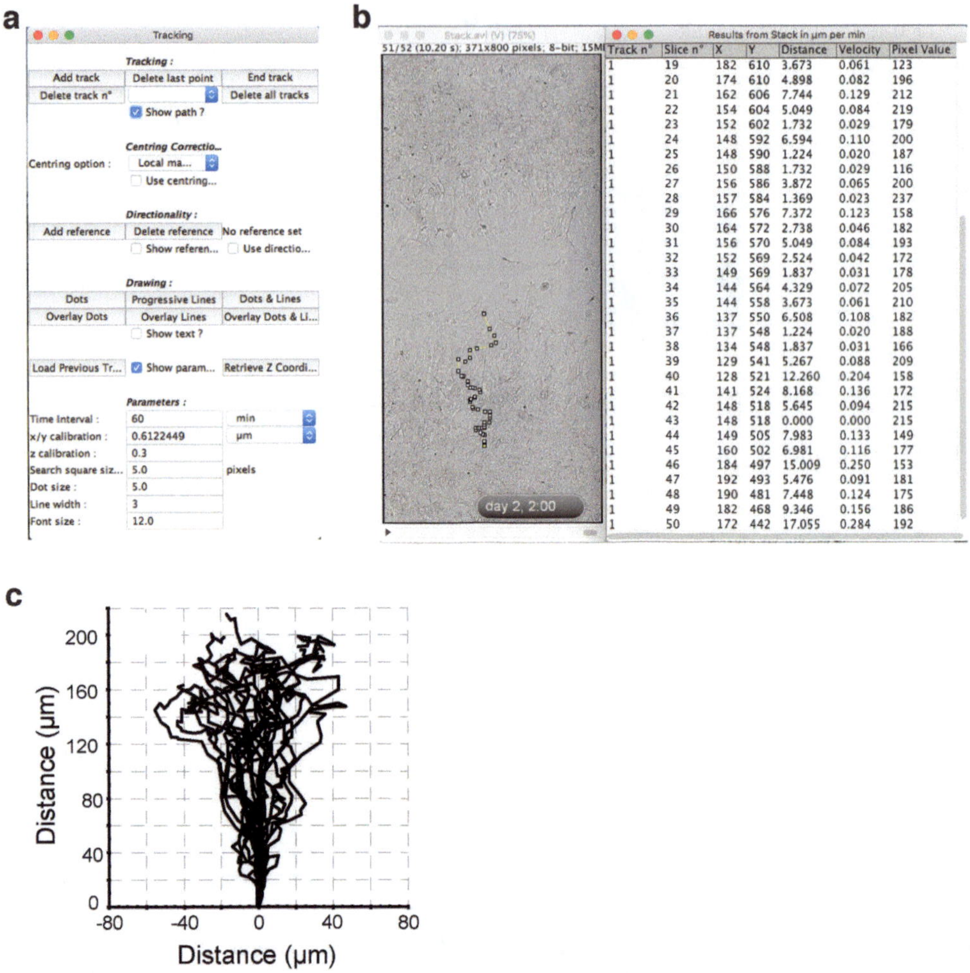

Fig. 4 Individual cell tracking procedure to study the speed, directionality and displacement of individual astrocytes. (**a**) Screen shot of the "Manual Tracking" plugin window showing the tracking options and parameters to set up prior to the analysis. (**b**) Example of one astrocyte path tracked throughout 50 h of migration and the raw data retrieved by the plugin. (**c**) Example of the projection of the migration trajectory of 20 astrocytes on the X/Y coordinates (in µm) obtained using the DiPer macros in Microsoft Excel

3. The distance and velocity results can be directly analyzed using the appropriate statistical program, or they can be used to calculate more complex parameters using the DiPer open-source macros for Microsoft Excel [28]. These macros allow the calculation of cells directionality (defined as the straight line between the start and the end point of the migration trajectory divided by the total length of the trajectory), or the mean square displacement (which will assess the area explored by the migrating cells over time), as well as plotting each cell trajectory, individually or collectively, on X/Y axes, emanating from the original starting point of displacement (Fig. 4c).

3.5 Morphological Complexity (Neurons and Oligodendrocytes)

In the following protocols the analyses measure the changes in length and branching of neurites and oligodendrocyte processes over time.

3.5.1 Neurite Development

1. Seed primary neurons at 30,000 cell per well on a coated 96-well plate and keep the cells in neuronal medium (*see* **Notes 1**, **5**, and **10**). Incubate the plates at 37 °C overnight before placing them in the Incucyte® 16 h later (in the next morning).
2. Set the system to acquire one phase-contrast picture (*see* **Note 11**) every 3 h over 7 days, using the "Standard" type of scan and the 20× objective, (*see* **Notes 12** and **32**).
3. Set the image analysis, starting by creating a representative set of images taking into account the cell morphology to be analyzed during the course of the experiment (*see* **Note 14**). To this end, select the first picture and click on "Create or Add to Image Collection" (Fig. 1 option **A**), select the mode "Neurotrack" as job type and add the image to the new image collection. Select another 4–6 new images (*see* **Note 15**) and add them to the previous collection.
4. Using this collection of images, define the settings to be applied to the analyses. Under the option "Process Definition" (Fig. 1, option B) run the "Preview Current" on the first picture to automatically generate the "Phase Cell-Body Cluster Mask" and a the "Phase Neurite Mask" (*see* **Note 33**). The first will cover and contour only the cell-body surface, while the second will trace what the software assumes to be neurites (cell processes).
5. Due to the complexity of the neuronal cultures, the automatic mask may not be able to perfectly trace all neurites. In that case, select "Phase Neurites (Analyze)" and adjust the masks in order to fully cover and delineate the cell shape. To this end, use the filters "Cell/Background," "Size," and "Eccentricity" to adjust the "Phase Cell-Body Cluster Mask" (*see* **Note 16**), and the neurite sensitivity parameters (*see* **Note 34**) for the "Neurite Mask" refinement. These option and filters are available on the "Cell-body Cluster" and "Neurite" parameter panels.
6. Apply the defined settings to all the image collection by running "Preview All" and check if the masks faithfully reproduce the complexity of the neuronal cell shape (Fig. 5a).
7. Initiate the analysis selecting the "Launch New Analysis Job" (Fig. 1, option C) and select the "NeuroTrack" job type. The software will apply the settings previously defined to all the pictures acquired on the plate throughout the experiments (*see* **Note 17**).

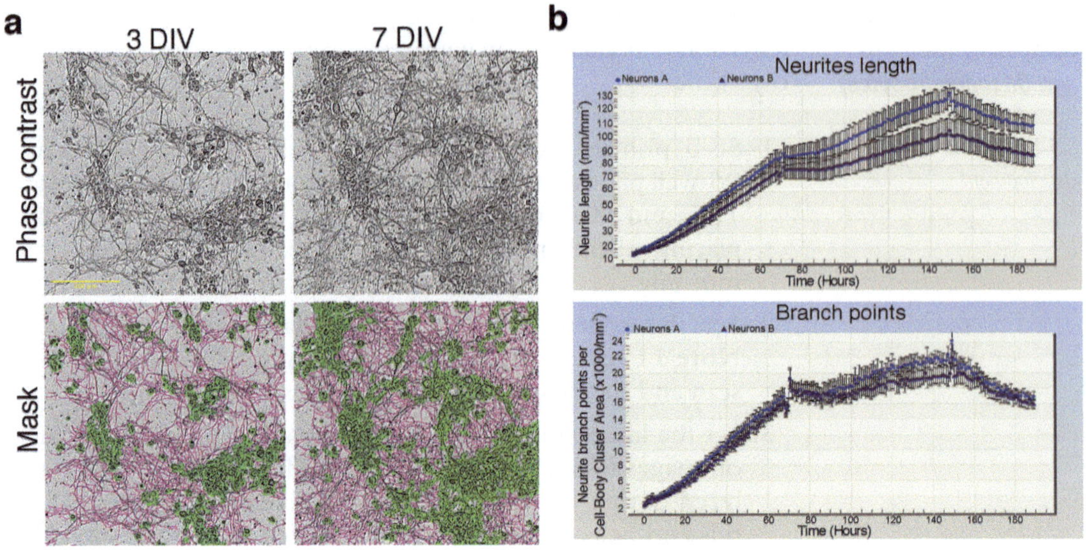

Fig. 5 Semiautomated and label-free measurement of neuritogenesis. (**a**) Phase contrast (top) and respective blended mask (bottom) images of neurons at 3 and 7 days of in vitro (DIV) development. The mask images show the perfect fitting of the "Phase Cell-Body Cluster Mask" (green) on neuronal cell bodies. The appropriate "Phase Neurite Mask" (pink) traces neurite development and growth over time. (**b**) The length of neurites (mm per mm^2 of plate surface) is automatically measured and plotted over time, during the entire course of the experiment. The number of branch points over time is counted and normalized relative to the area occupied by the cell bodies. Neurons derived from two different mice are plotted. Inflection points illustrate the moments when the medium of the cells was changed

8. The results will measure the changes in neurite length and number of branching points per well surface over time (Fig. 5b) (*see* **Notes 21** and **35**).

3.5.2 Process Extension

1. Seed OPC at 5,000 cell/well on coated 96-well plates and keep the cells in OPC medium for two days to stabilize the culture (*see* **Notes 1**, **5**, and **10**).
2. Set the system to acquire one phase-contrast picture every 2 h over 8–10 days, selecting the "Standard" type of scan and using the 20× objective (*see* **Notes 12** and **32**).
3. After 2 days, replace the medium with oligodendrocytes medium to induce OPC differentiation into mature, fully ramified oligodendrocytes. Change the medium every 2–3 days (*see* **Notes 7** and **13**).
4. To set the analysis, start by creating a representative set of images taking into account the changes in cell morphology that occur over time and that will be monitored over the course of the experiment (*see* **Note 14**). Proceed as described in Subheading 3.5.1, **steps 4** and **5**. Please note that the "Neurotrack" algorithm was developed to analyze neurons, so the automatic mask may not be able to perfectly detect the thin

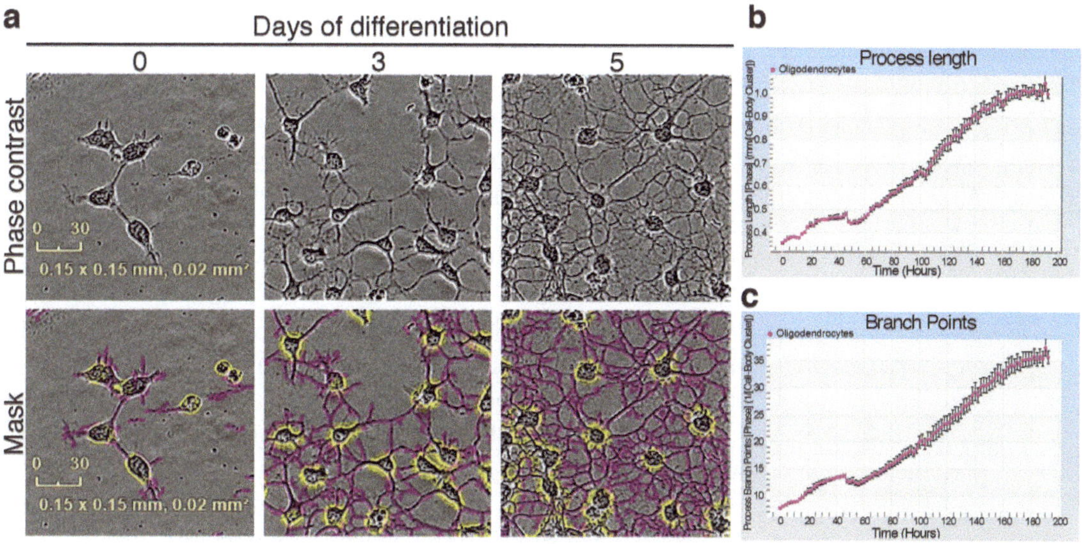

Fig. 6 Analysis of oligodendrocyte differentiation by semiautomated measurements of process extension and branching. (**a**) Phase contrast (top) and respective blended mask (bottom) images of oligodendrocytes at different stages of in vitro differentiation. The mask images show the perfect contour of the cell bodies by the "Phase Cell-Body Cluster Mask" (yellow) and the tracing of the oligodendrocyte processes and secondary branches by "Phase Neurite Mask" (pink). (**b**) The imaging system measures and plots the length of cell processes per cell body cluster over 7 days of differentiation. (**c**) The number of branch points relatively to cell body clusters is plotted over the course of the experiment

oligodendrocytes processes and secondary branching (*see* **Note 34**). To adjust the "Neurite Mask" to better fit oligodendrocyte processes and branching, set the "Neurite" parameters to maximum sensitivity (*see* **Note 36**) (Fig. 6a).

5. Launch the analyses as described in Subheading 3.5.1, **step 7**.
6. The results will show the length of the processes and the number of secondary branches per cell-body cluster, thus reflecting the cell differentiation over time (*see* **Notes 21** and **35**) (Fig. 6b, c).

3.5.3 Coculture Analyses

This type of analysis allows the investigation of neuron–glia interaction. In particular, this protocol describes how to assess the effect of astrocytes on neurite development by measuring the neurite length and branching of red fluorescent neurons over time, in the presence of astrocytes.

1. Seed primary neurons at 30,000 cell/well on a coated 96-well plate and keep the cells in neuronal medium supplemented with 5% of FBS (*see* **Notes 1**, **5**, and **10**). Incubate cells at 37 °C for 4 h.
2. Remove the culture medium. Infect neurons with IncuCyte® NeuroLight Red Lentivirus with the diluted lentivirus at a

multiplicity of infection (MOI) of 3 TU/cell (*see* **Note 37**) in 200 μL of neuronal medium. Incubate cells with the lentivirus overnight at 37 °C.

3. The next morning (after 8–10 h of lentiviral infection), remove 190 μL of lentivirus-containing medium, wash once with neuronal medium, and plate 50,000 previously cultured primary astrocytes in 200 μL of neuronal medium per well, on top of neurons. Perform half-medium changes every 3 days (*see* **Notes 7** and **13**).
4. Place the plate on the Incucyte® imaging system and set the scan to acquire one image every 3 h with the 20× objective for 10 days, selecting both phase contrast and red fluorescence channels and using the "Standard" type of scan (*see* **Notes 10** and **12**).
5. Two days after the beginning of the acquisition (when the Neurolight red signal in the neurites is sufficiently bright) optimize the "z" focus of the Incucyte ® objective manually, by moving its scale ring (usually 1.2 it is a good starting point). Test the "z" focus by clicking on "Scan on Demand" and scan some wells of the plate each time you move the ring, until you get a good image resolution of the red neurites across the entire plate.
6. Set the image analysis. Start by creating a representative set of red fluorescent images taking into account the cell morphology and cell structures to be monitored over time (*see* **Note 14**). To this end, select the first picture and click on "Create an Image Collection" (Fig. 1, option A), select the mode "Neurotrack" as job type and add the image to the new image collection. Select another 4–6 new images (*see* **Note 15**) and add them to the previous collection.
7. Using this collection of images, define the settings to be applied to the analyses. Under the option "Process Definition" (Fig. 1, option B) run the "Preview Current" on the first picture to automatically generate the "Cell-Body Cluster Mask" and the "Color Neurites Mask." The first will cover and contour only the cell-body surface, while the second will trace what the software presumes to be neurites.
8. If the automatic mask is not able to perfectly trace all neurites, adjust it in the "Color Neurites (Analyze)" panel in order to fully cover and delineate the cell shape using the filters "Cell-Body Cluster Parameters," "Cleanup," "Cell-Body Cluster Filters," and "Neurite Parameters" for the "Color Neurites Mask" (*see* **Note 34**) (Fig. 7a, b).
9. Launch the analysis as described in Subheading 3.5.1, **steps 6** and **7**.

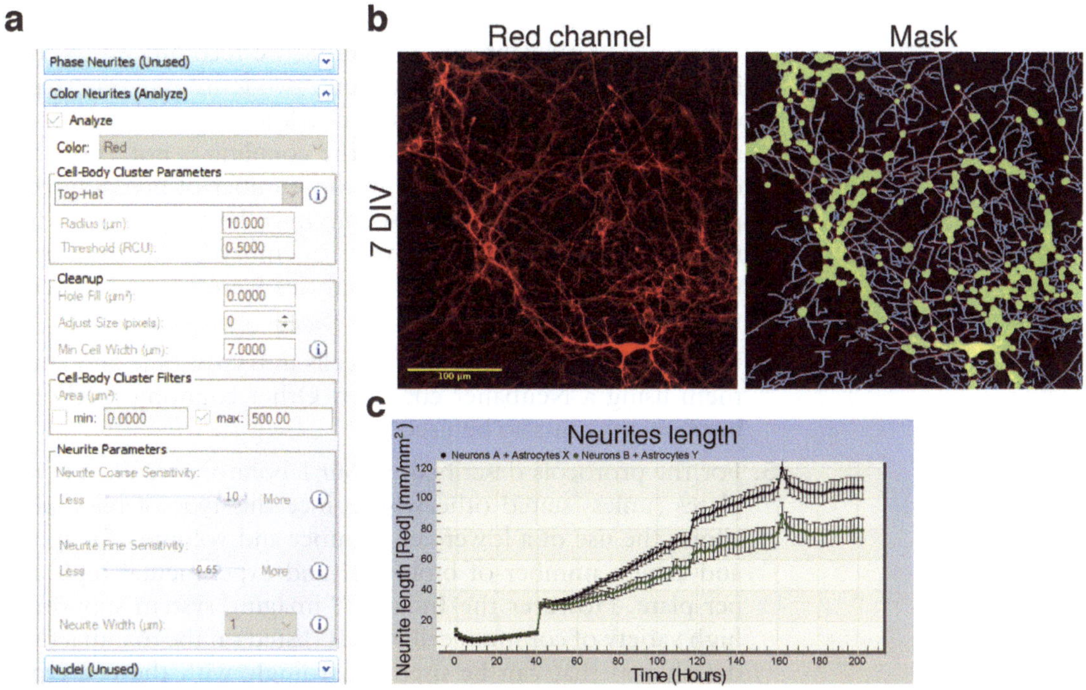

Fig. 7 Monitoring of neuronal neuritogenesis on a monolayer of astrocytes. (**a**) Screen shot of the "Color Neurites (Analyze)" panel of filters used to define and fit the settings to identify and measure correctly red-labeled neurites. The settings will be applied to the entire analysis. (**b**) Neurons imaged at 7 days in vitro (DIV) transduced with IncuCyte® NeuroLight Red Lentivirus (left) and the blended mask (right). The "Cell-Body Cluster Mask" (green) contours the cell bodies, while the "Color Neurites Mask" (blue) delineates red fluorescent neurites. (**c**) Neurite length is measured during the course of the experiment and plotted in mm per mm^2 of plate surface over time. Two different combinations of neuron and astrocyte cocultures are plotted. Inflection points illustrate the moments when the culture medium was changed

10. The results will measure the changes in the neurite length and number of branching points per well surface of the red fluorescent neurons over time (*see* **Note 35**) in the presence of unmarked cocultured astrocytes (*see* **Note 38**) (Fig. 7c).

4 Notes

1. Different extracellular matrix coating protocols and reagents can be used according with the experiment (e.g., to study cell-to-matrix interactions) and cell type used. First, coat plates with PDL for at least 20 min at room temperature and wash three times with double distilled sterile H_2O. Second, coat plates with laminin at least 3 h at 37 °C and wash the plates twice with 1× PBS.
2. The described cell culture protocols can be used to culture cells from either one single embryo/pup or pooled animals.

3. To obtain mouse embryos at E16.5 plan the mice breeding in advance. For efficient mouse mating, we recommend to cross in the same cage one male with one/two females in proestrus/estrus phase in the evening, and check for vaginal plugs in the morning of the next day. Since the coupling is not 100% efficient you may want to scale up the number of breeding couples. Also some strains/transgenic mice have lower breeding rates, which decrease the number of embryos. For the P0–P2 mice pups, one male and two females were maintained continuously in the same cage.
4. For the cell counting dilute the cells in trypan blue and count them using a Neubauer chamber. Other counting methods/instruments can also be used.
5. For the protocols described, in our laboratory we use 96-well plates (unless stated otherwise), since this type of microplate allows the use of a lower cell number and volume of reagents and a high number of biological and experimental replicates per plate. However the Incucyte® imaging system supports a high variety of common cell vessels (listed on the manufacturer datasheets) that can be used accordingly with the cell type/experiment need. In addition the system can accommodate and read six microplates simultaneously, allowing high throughput processing of samples and easy reproducibility of the results.
6. The purity of the primary cultures can be verified by immunostaining detection of cell type-specific markers, such as NeuN for neurons, GFAP for astrocytes and Olig2 for oligodendrocytes.
7. Medium should be changed with fresh prewarmed medium at 37 °C. Cell culture medium should be replaced carefully avoiding to touch or disturb the cell layer at the bottom of the plate.
8. In most experiments described we used astrocytes cultured on uncoated plates during 2 weeks in vitro, unless stated otherwise.
9. The cell density is a critical issue for the OPC culture: suboptimal densities can lead to cell death (if cell density is too low) or undesired cell differentiation (if cell density is too high). The OPC and oligodendrocytes are loosely attached to the surface of the dishes, for this reason medium changes should be performed with extra care, using prewarmed medium and gentle handling of the plates.
10. The cell densities indicated are suitable for the cell types mentioned in the protocol. However for other cell types, optimal seeding densities should be established prior to the experiment. After seeding, incubate the plates 15 min at room temperature to allow the cells to distribute evenly across the

bottom of the plate, before placing the cells in the Incucyte® incubator. Wait 15 min before starting the scan, to allow the dissipation of eventual condensation accumulated on the plate lid.

11. In addition to the acquisition of images in a stain-free manner, the system is also able to detect fluorescence, which diversifies the array of possible experiments. Notably, the fluorescent labeling of nuclear DNA is an alternative method to precisely count the number of cells and monitor cell proliferation, or the fluorescent labeling of neurites for the length and branching measurements (as described in Subheading 3.4).
12. To avoid variability resulting from scanned images collected from nonrepresentative areas of the well (in case of uneven cell distribution), it is recommended to select multiple pictures per well by editing the "Scan Pattern".
13. To change the cell medium while the experiment is ongoing, remove the plate from the machine in between two scans, change the medium and reintroduce the plate in the machine before the next scan begins.
14. The aim of creating an image collection is to have a set of representative images to train and test the settings that will be subsequently used for the analysis.
15. Although the number of pictures in the image collection is not limited, adding too many pictures slows down the process of setting definition. The selected images should represent all the possible cell variations in shape, density or other relevant parameters over time and/or across all the conditions tested. Pictures with bizarre cell density or poor image quality should not be included in the image collection and they should be disregarded in subsequent data analyses. For example, pictures taken close to the border of the well may show nonhomogeneous cell density, due to uneven seeding.
16. The "cells/background" sliding cursor is useful to distinguish more or less cells from the background. If the culture is clean from cell debris and/or the cells are flat/low contrasted, the cursors should be shifted toward the cell side to filter in the entire cell. In contrast, if the culture contains cell debris and the cell has a good phase-contrast, the cursor should be placed toward the background. Additionally, as the cell debris is normally round and of smaller size than cells, it can be filtered out by the "size" and "shape" filters—increasing the minimum "size" and "eccentricity" of the object to be considered as cells.
17. For the same group of acquisitions ("Vessel Scans") we can generate as many image collections and process definitions as we feel necessary to better adapt the analysis to the biological

process being studied. Those can be applied to all the scans at any time of the experiment while they are acquired by the imaging system, using the option "Open Ended". Adequate fitting of the mask can be checked for each individual image once the analysis is launched and finished.

18. Using the "Cell Confluence Mask" as a measurement on cells with high cytoplasm spreading and low contrast can be difficult, because different biological processes, such as cell adhesion/spreading and proliferation, cannot be easily distinguished. To overcome this potential problem cell adhesion/spreading can be discriminated from proliferation by focusing the analysis on the initial 45 min after cell seeding. Additionally it is possible to export single images from the Incucyte® software and manually analyze the cell surface with another software (e.g., freehand selection tool available in ImageJ or FIJI).

19. This is a limitation common to other methods to measure cell growth, such as the impedance-based monitoring system xCELLigence® RTCA MP system (ACEA Biosciences Inc). Although the xCELLigence® is able to detect in real-time very fast changes in cell index (based on the measurement of electrical impedance caused by the cell growth and attachment of the cells to the plate), the results are more difficult to interpret due to the lack of visual readout.

20. The software also counts the number of "objects" (cells) over time, as a measurement of cell proliferation. However, using phase-contrast pictures for this measurement can be misleading. As a result of proliferation, the cells become, naturally more confluent, and the individual cells previously identified as isolated "objects" become adjacent and make physical contact. They are no longer distinguished, as two distinct objects, but as a single one. Consequently the "cell count" provided by the software is underestimated, and it may even decrease over time, while the real cell number on the plate goes up. A proposed solution to overcome this problem is the use of fluorescent live-cell nuclear markers.

21. The results can also be illustrated by an overview of the global population dynamics in the entire plate, and individual plots can be drawn for each well of the microplate. They can also be exported as a numerical data file for subsequent statistical treatment and graphical representation by specialized software.

22. For astrocytes, uncoated plates work well and the wound takes about 50 h to close. However, the coating accelerates cell adhesion and migration, and it can help studying interactions between the cells and the extracellular matrix. For OPC the coating is necessary for cell adhesion. Although single coating with PDL can be used, allowing the wound to close over 72 h,

PDL+laminin coating increases the speed of wound healing, which is completed after 48 h. Hence, the duration of the experiment will depend on the type of coating used.

23. The use of "Incucyte® Image lock" special plate is crucial to assure that all the scans will be performed at exactly the same position throughout the experiment, since each well is marked with a cross that the IncuCyte® will use as a reference point for the positioning of the picture within the well. This will avoid variability in the scan position and therefore in the analysis.
24. Remember to clean the Incucyte® wound maker before using it with successive 5 min washes with 45 mL of double distilled H_2O and 45 mL of 70% Ethanol, using the reservoirs from the kit. While wounding the plates, all wells of the plate should contain 100 μL of medium or 1× PBS. After finishing wounding your plates, clean again the wound maker with successive 5 min washes of 45 mL of 0.5% Alconox, 1% Virkon, double distilled H_2O, and 70% ethanol. To maintain the good working conditions of the instrument it's extremely important to never turn the pin block of Incucyte® wound maker upside down, or the solutions/media will crystalize inside the pins and impair the scratching.
25. After the wound is made, lift the pin block straight up to avoid damaging the front of migration. This step will create a precise and reproducible wound throughout the 96-well plate. Using the wound maker instead of the classical pipette tip presents a great advantage since it maximizes the homogeneity of the wound between wells, it guarantees the regularity of the fronts of migration and it reduces cell lifting. Overall the process is time saving: the 96 wells of a plate can be scratched in parallel in one single passage of the wound maker.
26. Changes the filter parameters in the "Segmentation Adjustment" panel will change both "Confluence Mask" and "Scratch Wound Mask". It is not possible to apply different parameters to the different masks.
27. Although this system, like the classical wound healing assays [30], does not avoid the damage-induced cell proliferation, the analysis with RWD algorithm automatically normalizes the confluence in the wound space to the confluence in the cell layer, excluding the contribution of factors other than migration (e.g., proliferation or cell death) toward the filling of the wound.
28. To export the videos from the IncuCyte® go to "Utilities>Export Movie or Image set" and then select the right time range (from the beginning of the experiment until the moment when the wound is closed for all conditions) and the right wells. At least one video should have the scale ("Legend") and Timestamp

should be included in all videos, as a reminder for further analysis. Use "Windows AVI video (uncompressed)" format to ensure compatibility with Fiji.

29. Set the scale in Fiji by using the line tool to measure the scale on one Incucyte® image and then select "Set Scale" in the Fiji "Analyze" menu. Remember to check the "Global" box in order to apply the scale to all further images.
30. To better visualize the nucleus of the cells the stack can be flipped on the Z scale (time scale) to start the analysis from the end of the video, when the cell cytoplasm is widely spread. Once delineated, the tracking position data can be flipped back using Microsoft Excel.
31. The color of the migration images can also be processed to facilitate the visual detection of the nucleus. We recommend converting the images to 8-bit and applying the "HiLo LUT" palette.
32. Depending on the experiment the acquisition can be done over different time periods.
33. If you label neurites fluorescently, use the "Color Cell-Body Cluster Mask" and the "Color Neurite Mask" to define the settings for analysis.
34. Use the "Filtering" parameter to filter out small imperfections (e.g., due to irregular coating) or cell debris that can be mislabeled as neurites. This parameter can also be used to filter in thinner neurites/cell processes, through the selection of the "Better" or "Best" options in addition to the "Neurite Sensitivity" slider. Define the pixel size at which the cell bodies transit into neurites/cell processes using the "Neurite Width" dropdown.
35. The neurite length and branching results can be quantified relative to the area of the well, to the cell-body cluster number or area. For neurons, the quantification of the neurite length per area is normally used, when the physiological neurite dynamics is being tested, since the number of neurons and cell body area will not change over time. However, when compounds are tested, the normalizations to cell body should be considered to exclude confounding effects, such as cell death. For oligodendrocytes, it is more accurate to normalize the measurements of cell processes relative to the cell body clusters, in an attempt to minimize the influence of possible alterations in cell number. The cell-body dynamics is estimated by measuring the percentage of confluence.
36. We adapt the "Neurotrack" algorithm to measure the process extension and branching of oligodendrocytes. However neurites and axons are bigger and thicker than the oligodendro-

cytes processes. As a result the settings must be adjusted to the highest sensitivity to maximize the detection of truly thin oligodendrocytes processes and branching, while distinguishing them from cell bodies.

37. A MOI of 3 TU/cell was optimized in our laboratory to infect primary cortical neurons. For other neuronal types the optimal MOI must be determined.
38. The described protocol is useful to test, for instance, the beneficial/deleterious effect of an astrocyte monolayer of a given phenotype on neuronal differentiation, and the response to environmental stress, such as the addition of a neurotoxic compound (e.g., excess of glutamate).

Acknowledgments

We are grateful to the personnel of CERFE (Centre d'Exploration et de Recherche Fonctionelle Expérimentale, Genopole, Evry, France) and LEAT (Laboratoire d'Experimentation Animale, Imagine Institute, Paris, France) for attentively caring for the mice. We would like to thank the AFM-Téléthon (France), ANR (France) and Paris Descartes—Sorbonne Paris Cité University (France), *Imagine* Foundation (France), Fondation Bettencourt Shueller (France), and Ministère Français de la Recherche et Technologie (France) for financial support. Our research has received a state subsidy managed by the National Research Agency, under the "Investments of the Future" program, bearing the reference ANR-10-IAHU-01 and under the program ANR-10BLAN-1121-01.

References

1. La Spada AR, Taylor JP (2010) Repeat expansion disease: progress and puzzles in disease pathogenesis. Nat Rev Genet 11:247–258
2. Budworth H, McMurray CT (2013) A brief history of triplet repeat diseases. Methods Mol Biol 1010:3–17
3. Wang T, Bray SM, Warren ST (2012) New perspectives on the biology of fragile X syndrome. Curr Opin Genet Dev 22:256–263
4. Martelli A, Napierala M, Puccio H (2012) Understanding the genetic and molecular pathogenesis of Friedreich's ataxia through animal and cellular models. Dis Model Mech 5:165–176
5. Ross CA, Tabrizi SJ (2011) Huntington's disease: from molecular pathogenesis to clinical treatment. Lancet Neurol 10:83–98
6. Sicot G, Gourdon G, Gomes-Pereira M (2011) Myotonic dystrophy, when simple repeats reveal complex pathogenic entities: new findings and future challenges. Hum Mol Genet 20:R116–R123
7. Cleary JD, Ranum LP (2013) Repeat-associated non-ATG (RAN) translation in neurological disease. Hum Mol Genet 22:R45–R51
8. Braz SO, Acquaire J, Gourdon G, Gomes-Pereira M (2018) Of Mice and Men: Advances in the Understanding of Neuromuscular Aspects of Myotonic Dystrophy. Front Neurol 9:519
9. Rikani AA, Choudhry Z, Choudhry AM, Rizvi N, Ikram H, Mobassarah NJ, Tulli S (2014) The mechanism of degeneration of striatal neu-

ronal subtypes in Huntington disease. Ann Neurosci 21:112–114

10. Huang M, Verbeek DS (2019) Why do so many genetic insults lead to Purkinje Cell degeneration and spinocerebellar ataxia? Neurosci Lett 688:49–57
11. Zala D, Benchoua A, Brouillet E, Perrin V, Gaillard MC, Zurn AD, Aebischer P, Deglon N (2005) Progressive and selective striatal degeneration in primary neuronal cultures using lentiviral vector coding for a mutant huntingtin fragment. Neurobiol Dis 20:785–798
12. Wong MMK, Watson LM, Becker EBE (2017) Recent advances in modelling of cerebellar ataxia using induced pluripotent stem cells. J Neurol Neuromedicine 2:11–15
13. Jacobs S, Doering LC (2010) Astrocytes prevent abnormal neuronal development in the fragile x mouse. J Neurosci 30:4508–4514
14. Jacobs S, Cheng C, Doering LC (2016) Hippocampal neuronal subtypes develop abnormal dendritic arbors in the presence of Fragile X astrocytes. Neuroscience 324:202–217
15. Franco C, Genis L, Navarro JA, Perez-Domper P, Fernandez AM, Schneuwly S, Torres Aleman I (2017) A role for astrocytes in cerebellar deficits in frataxin deficiency: Protection by insulin-like growth factor I. Mol Cell Neurosci 80:100–110
16. Loria F, Diaz-Nido J (2015) Frataxin knockdown in human astrocytes triggers cell death and the release of factors that cause neuronal toxicity. Neurobiol Dis 76:1–12
17. Custer SK, Garden GA, Gill N, Rueb U, Libby RT, Schultz C, Guyenet SJ, Deller T, Westrum LE, Sopher BL, La Spada AR (2006) Bergmann glia expression of polyglutamine-expanded ataxin-7 produces neurodegeneration by impairing glutamate transport. Nat Neurosci 9:1302–1311
18. Sicot G, Servais L, Dinca DM, Leroy A, Prigogine C, Medja F, Braz SO, Huguet-Lachon A, Chhuon C, Nicole A, Gueriba N, Oliveira R, Dan B, Furling D, Swanson MS, Guerrera IC, Cheron G, Gourdon G, Gomes-Pereira M (2017) Downregulation of the Glial GLT1 Glutamate Transporter and Purkinje Cell Dysfunction in a Mouse Model of Myotonic Dystrophy. Cell Rep 19:2718–2729
19. Khakh BS, Sofroniew MV (2014) Astrocytes and Huntington's disease. ACS Chem Nerosci 5:494–496
20. Wenzel HJ, Hunsaker MR, Greco CM, Willemsen R, Berman RF (2010) Ubiquitin-positive intranuclear inclusions in neuronal and glial cells in a mouse model of the fragile X premutation. Brain Res 1318:155–166
21. Cvetanovic M, Ingram M, Orr H, Opal P (2015) Early activation of microglia and astrocytes in mouse models of spinocerebellar ataxia type 1. Neuroscience 289:289–299
22. Jin J, Peng Q, Hou Z, Jiang M, Wang X, Langseth AJ, Tao M, Barker PB, Mori S, Bergles DE, Ross CA, Detloff PJ, Zhang J, Duan W (2015) Early white matter abnormalities, progressive brain pathology and motor deficits in a novel knock-in mouse model of Huntington's disease. Hum Mol Genet 24:2508–2527
23. Pacey LK, Xuan IC, Guan S, Sussman D, Henkelman RM, Chen Y, Thomsen C, Hampson DR (2013) Delayed myelination in a mouse model of fragile X syndrome. Hum Mol Genet 22:3920–3930
24. Tai YF, Pavese N, Gerhard A, Tabrizi SJ, Barker RA, Brooks DJ, Piccini P (2007) Imaging microglial activation in Huntington's disease. Brain Res Bull 72:148–151
25. Franciosi S, Ryu JK, Shim Y, Hill A, Connolly C, Hayden MR, McLarnon JG, Leavitt BR (2012) Age-dependent neurovascular abnormalities and altered microglial morphology in the YAC128 mouse model of Huntington disease. Neurobiol Dis 45:438–449
26. Kwan W, Trager U, Davalos D, Chou A, Bouchard J, Andre R, Miller A, Weiss A, Giorgini F, Cheah C, Moller T, Stella N, Akassoglou K, Tabrizi SJ, Muchowski PJ (2012) Mutant huntingtin impairs immune cell migration in Huntington disease. J Clin Invest 122:4737–4747
27. Schindelin J, Arganda-Carreras I, Frise E, Kaynig V, Longair M, Pietzsch T, Preibisch S, Rueden C, Saalfeld S, Schmid B, Tinevez JY, White DJ, Hartenstein V, Eliceiri K, Tomancak P, Cardona A (2012) Fiji: an open-source platform for biological-image analysis. Nat Methods 9:676–682
28. Gorelik R, Gautreau A (2014) Quantitative and unbiased analysis of directional persistence in cell migration. Nat Protoc 9:1931–1943
29. Dincman TA, Beare JE, Ohri SS, Whittemore SR (2012) Isolation of cortical mouse oligodendrocyte precursor cells. J Neurosci Methods 209:219–226
30. Molinie N, Gautreau A (2018) Directional Collective Migration in Wound Healing Assays. Methods Mol Biol 1749:11–19

Chapter 15

Primary Cultures of Pure Embryonic Dorsal Root Ganglia Sensory Neurons as a New Cellular Model for Friedreich's Ataxia

Olivier Griso and Hélène Puccio

Abstract

Peripheral neuropathies can have various origins, from genetic to acquired causes, and affect altogether a large group of people in the world. Current available therapies aim at helping the disease symptoms but not to correct or stop the development of the disease. Primary neuronal cultures represent an essential tool in the study of events related to peripheral neuropathies as they allow to isolate the affected cell types, often originating in complex tissues in which they account for only a few percentage of cells. They provide a powerful system to identifying or testing compounds with potential therapeutic effect in the treatment of those diseases. Friedreich's ataxia is an autosomal recessive neurodegenerative disorder, which is characterized by a progressive spinocerebellar and sensory ataxia. Proprioceptive neurons of the dorsal root ganglia (DRG) are the primary affected cells. The disease is triggered by a mutation in the gene FXN which leads to a reduction of the frataxin protein. In order to study the neurophysiopathology of the disease at the cellular and molecular levels, we have established a model of primary cultures of DRG sensory neurons in which we induce the loss of the frataxin protein. With such a model we can alleviate the issues related to the complexity of DRG tissues and low amount of sensory neuron material in adult mouse. Hereby, we provide a protocol of detailed and optimized methods to obtain high yield of healthy mouse DRG sensory neuron in culture.

Key words Dorsal root ganglia, Primary cultures, Sensory neurons, Friedreich's ataxia, AAV vectors

1 Introduction

Dorsal root ganglia (DRG) sensory neuron cell cultures are an important tool for studies aiming at unveiling pathophysiological mechanisms underlying peripheral nervous system (PNS) diseases also known as peripheral neuropathies [1]. They also represent a reliable system to identify and validate new compounds with potential therapeutic effect to design treatment strategies for these diseases. The PNS includes the sensory, motor and autonomic nerves located outside the brain and spinal cord [2]. Although every component of

Guy-Franck Richard (ed.), *Trinucleotide Repeats: Methods and Protocols*, Methods in Molecular Biology, vol. 2056, https://doi.org/10.1007/978-1-4939-9784-8_15,

the PNS can be affected in peripheral neuropathies, the sensory neurons are often the primary and more severely affected sites, and the causes of peripheral neuropathies can be genetic or acquired [1]. They include diabetes associated neuropathy [3], viral infections such as human immunodeficiency virus (HIV) (such as distal symmetric polyneuropathy or DSP, antiretroviral toxic neuropathy or ATN) [4], autoimmune conditions (such as chronic inflammatory demyelinating polyneuropathy or CIDP) [5], hereditary demyelinating neuropathies (such as Charcot Marie Tooth disease type 1A or CMT1A) [6], or toxic chemotherapeutic agents (following antineoplastic therapy for example) [7]. They also include genetically acquired neurodegenerative disorder such as Friedreich's ataxia.

Friedreich's ataxia (FA) is an autosomal recessive neurodegenerative disorder, characterized by a progressive spinocerebellar and sensory ataxia associating hypertrophic cardiomyopathy [8, 9]. At the neurologic levels, the primary affected sites include proprioceptive neurons of the dorsal root ganglia (DRG), the spinal cord and the dentate nucleus of the cerebellum [10, 11]. The major FA-causing mutation corresponds to a GAA expansion in the first intron of the FXN gene, which leads to the reduced expression of frataxin, a mitochondrial protein involved in iron-sulfur (Fe-S) cluster biosynthesis [12]. Varying from 60 to 1700 repeats, the expansion causes a decreased transcription of the gene, most probably via locus heterochromatinization [13]. The patients express only between 5% and 30% of the normal levels [14].

The events of the physiopathology of FA are well described in heart tissue from patients [15], or cardiomyocytes from cardiac-specific mouse models [16], due to the large size of the cardiac tissue, the high number of affected cell in this tissue, giving a high quantity of material for cellular and biochemical analysis. The difficulty in studying neuronal phenotype at the cellular and molecular level is that affected cells are isolated and diluted in complex tissues comprising several cell types. DRG comprises specialized neuronal subtypes with unique molecular characteristics, including small diameter nociceptive neurons ($TrkA^+$), larger diameter mechanoreceptive neurons ($TrkB^+$ and/or $TrkC^+$) and large proprioceptive neurons ($TrkC^+$). Sensory neurons only represent 15% of the total DRG cells, the other being glial cells [2]. Molecular biology and biochemical approaches such as Western blot, qPCR and enzymatic activity measurements normally used to evaluate Fe-S deficiency, cellular iron dysregulation and mitochondrial activity impairments are not easily applicable in this context, especially due to low material quantity available in DRG neurons [17]. Therefore, data concerning FA neurophysiopathology are limited. Thus, the mechanisms underlying the neurodegeneration and in particular the tissue-specificity in FA are still unknown.

Many efforts have been made in generating partial depletion models with a reduction of frataxin levels closer to what is observed in patients. Several GAA repeat expansion-based mouse models were generated [18, 19], as it is the causative mutation of FA [20]. However, none of them show a robust phenotype, contrarily to the clear, severe and reproducible phenotypes observed in the conditional models (full deletion) [16, 17, 21, 22]. This is mainly due to the fact that GAA repeat expansions are very unstable through cell divisions, and only 200 GAA repeats could be inserted in an attempt to reproduce the transcription decrease seen in FA patients (KIKO model, YG8R and YG22R models [18, 19]).

We have recently established a new neurologic cellular model of Friedreich's ataxia based on mouse primary cultures of DRG sensory neurons from the conditional model that allows the full depletion of frataxin. As the full KO is lethal for any dividing cell, it has to be induced after embryonic development. In this model, frataxin deletion is induced by infecting the cells by AAV9 vectors bearing the Cre recombinase gene, allowing to excise an essential exon from the FXN gene, leading to a total frataxin deficiency (Fig. 1). The following chapter contains our protocol for mouse DRG primary cultures of pure sensory neurons. Although our model consists of full knock out following AAV vectors expression, this protocol can be applied to every mouse model including the GAA repeat expansion-based model.

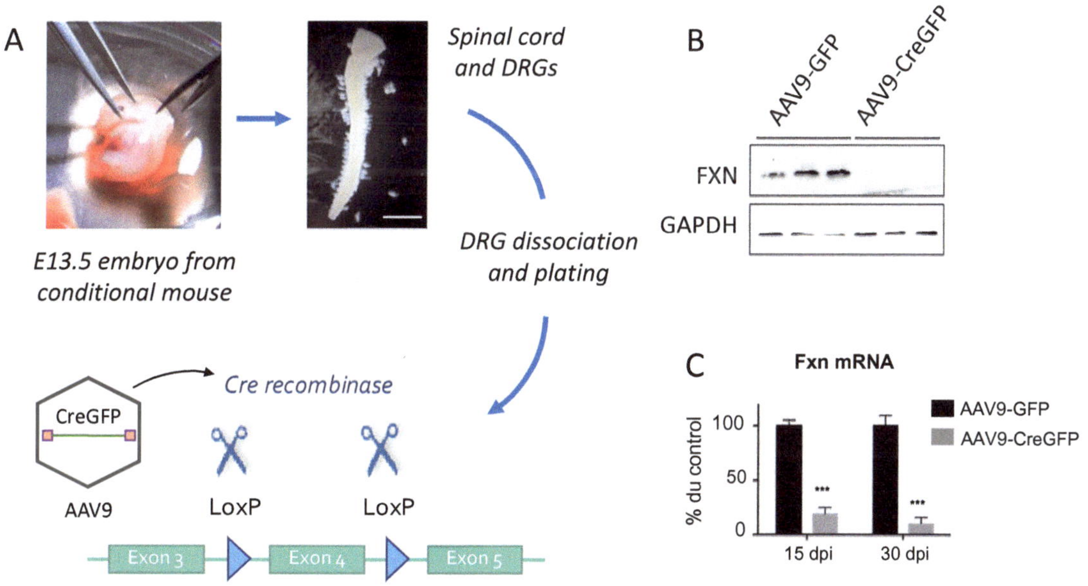

Fig. 1 DRG sensory neuron primary cultures as a model of Friedreich's ataxia. (**a**) Dorsal root ganglia (DRG) are collected on E13.5 mouse embryo, dissociated, and the cell suspension it plated. Following cell attachment to the bottom of the plate, infection with an AAV9 viral vector is performed. Once the viral genome is delivered into the cell, the Cre recombinase is expressed, excising the exon 4 of the gene FXN. Western blot (**b**) and qPCR (**c**) results confirming depletion of frataxin both at the protein and the mRNA levels in cells infected with an AAV9-CreGFP vector. The reminiscent expression corresponds to noninfected cells. The AAV9-GFP infected cells correspond to the wild type (WT). $***p < 0.001$ (student test); scalebar = 200 μm

2 Materials

2.1 Coating of Cell Culture Systems

1. Tissue culture dish 35 × 10 mm style.
2. Multidish PS 4 well nunclon round.
3. Nunclon 4-Well × 1mL MultiDish cell culture dish.
4. 13 mm sterile coverslips.
5. Poly-L-lysine hydrobromide.
   (a) Solution A: 0.1 mg/mL in ultrapure water.
   (b) Solution B: 0.01 mg/mL in ultrapure water.
6. Collagen Type I.
   (a) Solution C: 0.67 mg/mL in ultrapure water with 1/500 acetic acid dilution.
7. Laminin: 3.3 μg/mL in ultrapure water (solution D).
8. Matrigel™ HESC QUALIFIED MATRIX: 1/40 diluted in C-medium (solution E).
9. Glacial acetic acid.
10. Ammonium hydroxide.
11. Sterile gauze compresses.
12. Standard height, nunclon delta treated square BioAssay dish.
13. Parafilm® M.

2.2 Media Preparation

1. Minimum essential medium.
2. Neurobasal™-A medium, no D-glucose, no sodium pyruvate.
3. B-27™ supplement (50×), serum free.
4. Fetal Bovin serum.
5. L-Glutamine 100×.
6. D-Glucose.
7. Nerve growth factor 2.5S.
8. Penicillin/Streptomycin 100×.
9. 5-fluoro-2′-deoxyuridine.
10. Uridine.
11. C-medium: 430 mL MEM, 50 mL FBS, 5 mL P/S (100×), 5 mL L-glutamine (100×), 2 g of D-glucose in 10 mL MEM (4 g/L final), 50 nM NGF.
12. NB medium: 470 mL Neurobasal without Glucose and pyruvate, 5 mL P/S (100×), 5 mL L-glutamine (100×), 2 g of D-glucose in 10 mL MEM (4 g/L final), 50 nM NGF.
13. Antimitotic cocktail 1000×: 5 mL MEM, FUdR 12.3 mg, Uridine 12.2 mg. Dilute it to a 100× solution in MEM (solution F), aliquot and store at −80 °C.

2.3 Dissection

1. Zeiss SEMI 305 stereo microscope.
2. Leibovitz's L-15 medium.
3. Intruments for dissection of mouse embryos:
   (a) Vannas-Tübingen spring scissors.
   (b) Dumont #5S forceps.
   (c) Classical instruments for mouse dissection.
4. Tissue culture dish 35 × 10 mm Style.
5. Tissue culture dish 100 × 20 mm Style.
6. Trypsin (2.5‰), no phenol red: solution G.
7. Agitating block heater.

2.4 AAV Infections

2.4.1 Purified Recombinant AAV9 Viral Vectors

The vectors are produced in the IGBMC in-house viral vector production facility. They are produced following the "helper-free" method, which is based on the adenovirus-free transient cotransfection of all elements that are required for AAV production in host cells such as HEK293 cells: an AAV2 ITR-containing plasmid carrying the gene of interest, a plasmid that carries the AAV2 Rep-Cap and a plasmid that provides the helper genes isolated from adenovirus. Before production, the gene of interest must be inserted into a pAAV vector. Commonly, the vector must bear a fluorescent reporter such as an eGFP in order to identify infected cells. The titer should not be lower than 1×10^{12} GU/mL, as the vectors have to be diluted at 9×10^{9} GU/mL in the culture medium and ideally not less than 100 fold.

3 Methods

3.1 Coating of Cell Culture Dishes

3.1.1 Coating of 35 mm Petri Dishes

1. In 35 × 10 mm petri dishes, dispense 2 mL of poly-L-lysine (solution B).
2. Incubate for 30 min at room temperature (RT).
3. Aspirate the solution and replace by 2 mL of ultrapure water.
4. Subsequently, replace by 2 mL of ultrapure water.
5. Remove completely the water from the petri dish at leave it to dry under the hood, for 1.5 h at RT.
6. Dispense 2 mL of collagen (solution C).
7. Incubate for 15 min at RT.
8. Angle the dish and aspirate the collagen (*see* **Note 1**).
9. Close the dishes and place them in a large square dish.
10. Place a compress in the center of the large plate, dispense 1 mL of ammonium hydroxide on it and close immediately the large dish

11. Incubate for 15 min at RT.
12. Open the dish, discard the compress and open all the 35 mm dishes.
13. Leave to dry overnight (ON) at RT under the working hood.
14. The next morning, close the dishes and keep them sealed with parafilm at 4 °C until use. The coated dishes can be kept up to one month in the fridge.

3.1.2 Coating of 13 mm Coverslips (Must Be Prepared the Day Before the Dissection)

1. Dispense 13 mm cover slides in 4-wells culture plate.
2. Add 350 μL of poly-L-lysine (solution A). Make sure that the solution covers the whole surface of the well.
3. Incubate for 2 h at 37 °C.
4. Wash twice 2 min with 500 μL ultrapure water.
5. Replace by a laminin solution (solution D).
6. Incubate overnight at 37 °C.
7. The next morning, replace by 350 μL of Matrigel (solution E).
8. Incubate for 1 h at RT.
9. Incubate for 1 h at 37 °C.
10. Replace by 350 μL of C-medium until cells are ready to be plated.

3.2 Mouse Dissection and Isolation of Embryonic DRGs

The mice are sacrificed at E13.5 of embryonic development. Each step of the following protocol must be done in a sterile environment: under the hood or next to Bunsen burner.

1. Sacrifice the female.
2. Put the mouse on the back, open the womb on the median line to let appear the organs.
3. Using the forceps, pinch the uterus in the middle, where both sides are joining. Cut and take away both sides of the uterus. Pay attention not to damage the embryos within the uterin horns.
4. Put the uterus in a sterile 10 cm petri dish containing 10 mL of sterile cold L15 medium.
5. Remove the embryos from the uterus by opening it slowly on the median line, always paying attention not to touch the embryos and letting the yolk intact.
6. Isolate every embryo within their placenta, and put each one of them in a 35 mm petri dish containing 1 mL of cold L15 medium. Keep the dishes on ice.

   The following steps have to be repeated for every embryo

7. Take out the embryo from the placenta.

8. Place the embryo on the side. Maintain its position with a forceps in one hand, use iris scissors with the other hand to remove the head, then cut in a vertical line in between the dorsal and the ventral part, in order to remove all the visceral organs, the limb, and the extremity of the tail.
9. Using Dumont #5 forceps in both hands, put the embryo on its dorsal part, and remove the remaining visceral organs, which should allow to expose the vertebrae.
10. Rotate the embryo horizontally, and maintain it with one forceps holding the sides of the embryo. With the other forceps, open slowly the vertebrae being careful not to cut too deep (with the risk of cutting the DRGs). Always maintain the embryo stable with the other hand. When all the vertebrae are incised, you will be able to remove them as a lid and let the spinal cord appear.
11. Rotate the embryo, with the cervical part on top. Put one forceps against the spinal cord, and the other one against the close tissues. This will allow you to stretch the tissue, and start to expose the DRGs.
12. Once you have stretched the tissues all along the spinal cord on both sides, put back the embryo on the horizontal state.
13. Softly pull out the spinal cord, while tightly maintaining the embryo down. If it does not come at once, pull it out in several small steps, in order not to damage the cord. Be careful not to go to fast, which will cause some DRG to stay inside the embryo. It is though still possible to "fish" the remaining DRGs after the spinal cord has been removed.
14. Put the spinal cord with the DRGs in a new 35 mm dish filled with 1 mL cold L15 medium.
15. Carefully detach each DRG from the spinal cords, and get rid of the remaining tissues, keeping only the DRGs in the plate.
16. With a micropipette, transfer the medium containing the DRGs in a 2 mL microtube. Be careful, the DRGs can stick to the sides of the micropipette tips. Try to make 1 tube for 10 embryos. The steps of the dissection are pictured in Fig. 2.

3.3 DRGs Primary Culture Establishment

1. Right after the dissection, centrifuge the tube containing the DRGs at 800 × g for 1 min.
2. Remove the medium and replace it by 1 mL Trypsin (Solution G).
3. Incubate for 35 min at 37 °C under soft agitation (400 rpm on the block heater).
4. Under the hood, transfer the Trypsin solution containing the DRG in a 15 mL Falcon tube containing 1 mL FBS.

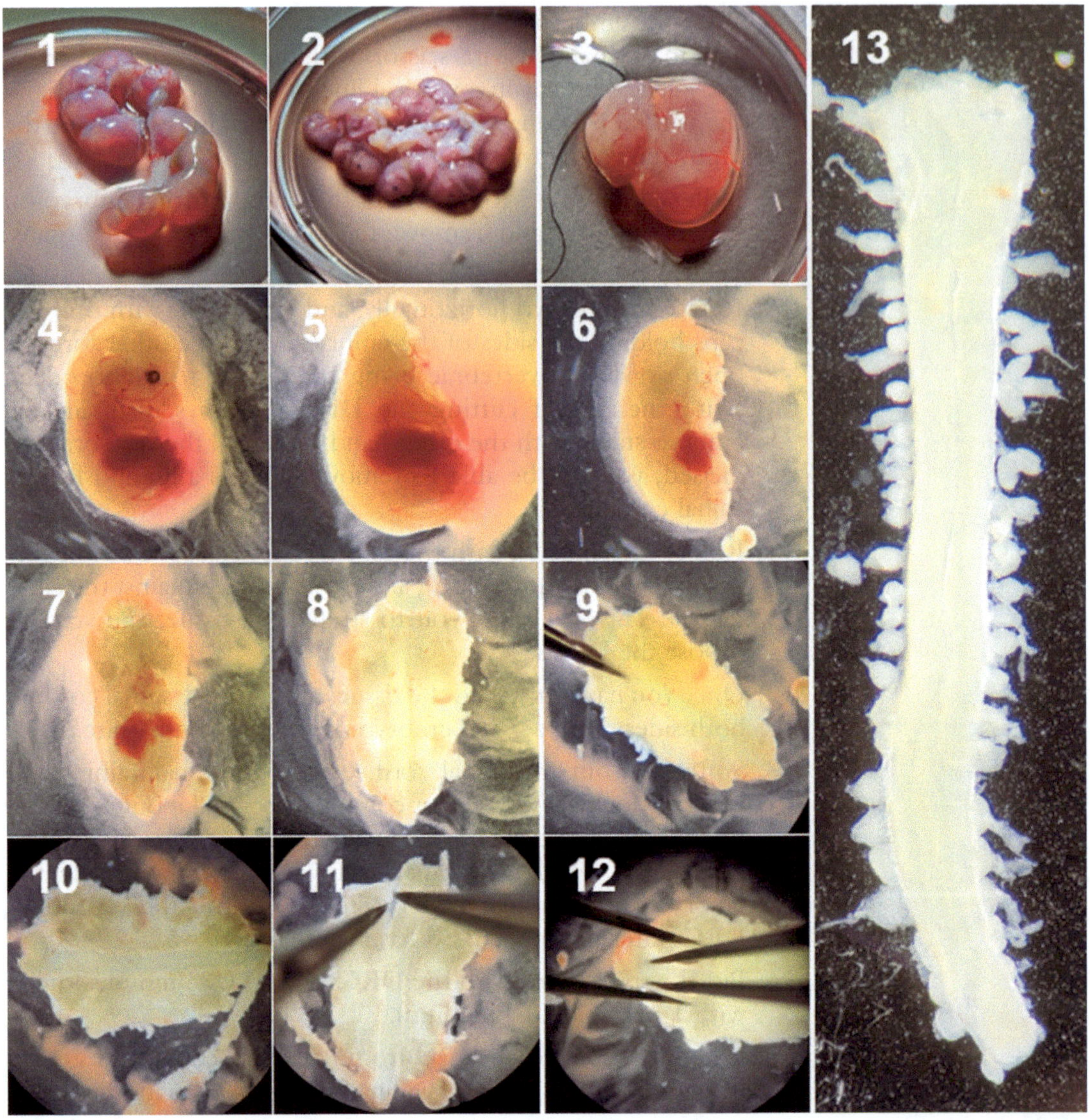

Fig. 2 Pictured steps of mouse E13.5 embryonic dorsal root ganglia dissection. After being removed from the mother, the uterus is placed in a large petri dish containing medium [1]. The uterus is opened, the embryos appear in their placenta [2] and are placed in a small petri dish containing medium [3]. The embryo is removed from its placenta, and placed on its side [4]. The head and visceral organs are successively removed [5, 6]. Embryo back on the dorsal part, the remaining viscera are removed [7]. Vertebrae are incised and removed, letting appear the spinal cord [8–10]. The tissue surrounding DRG localization is stretched, on both sides and all along the spinal cord [11]. The spinal cord is gently pulled out [12] and placed in a small petri dish containing medium [13]. The DRGs are removed from the spinal cord, and the rest of the spinal cord is removed from the dish

5. Wash the trypsin tube with 1 mL of C-medium in order to collect all the DRGs/cells in the 2 mL tube. Put this 1 mL in the 15 mL Falcon tube.
6. Centrifuge at 800 × *g* for 10 min.
7. Remove the supernatant and add 150 μL (volume for 10 embryos) of C-medium.
8. Very gently, triturate the pellet with a 200 μL tip to dissociate the DRG cells.
9. In order to prevent damaging the cells, centrifuge the pellet 500 × *g* for 10 s and transfer the supernatant containing the cells to a 50 mL Falcon tube containing 2 mL C-medium.
10. Add another 150 μL of C-medium and continue the trituration/centrifugation steps until the pellet is dissociated. It is normal that a part of the pellet never dissociates. It contains mainly connective tissues and can be discarded.
11. Count the cells and adjust the concentration to 500,000 cells/mL.

For 35 mm petri dishes

12. With a 10 mL pipette, dispense 1 mL of the cell suspension in the precoated 35 mm petri dish (*see* **Note 2**).
13. Once the suspension is correctly spread in the dish, perform 2 up-and-downs to increase the uniformity of the seeding (*see* **Note 2**).
14. Put the dishes at 37 °C 5% CO_2.
15. After 2 h, angle the dishes to spread the medium on the whole surface of the dish.

For 13 mm coverslips

12. Remove completely the medium from the newly Matrigel-coated coverslips.
13. With the aspirator pipette on, place the coverslips in the center of the well (*see* **Note 3**).
14. Let it to dry for 10 min under the hood.
15. Gently dispense 100 μL of cell suspension on the coverslip, taking care not to spread the medium outside of the slide.
16. Place the cells at 37 °C 5% CO_2.
17. 1 h 30 after, add 250 μL of C-medium in the wells.

3.4 AAV Infections and Culture Protocol

1. On the day of plating (around 4/5 h after plating), transfer the cells in a P2 cell culture laboratory.
2. Dilute the AAV vectors in C-medium to 9 × 10^9 GC/mL.
3. Remove the medium from the dish, and replace it by 1 mL (300 μL for coverslips) of diluted AAV vectors.

4. Incubate at 37 °C 5% CO_2 overnight.
5. The next morning, replace the medium by 1.5 mL (350 μL for coverslips) of C-medium + antimitotic (solution F).
6. Two days after, replace the medium by 1.5 mL (350 μL for coverslips) of NB medium.
7. Replace the medium every 2 or 3 days by 1.5 mL/350 μL NB medium until the culture is ready to be harvested (*see* **Note 4**).

4 Notes

On a general basis, primary neurons are challenging subtypes to culture and maintain *ex vivo*, and DRG sensory neurons are among the most difficult subtypes to handle. In our lab we have developed a reproducible protocol that enables to establish homogenous and healthy DRG sensory cultures (Fig. 3). With the right hints and tips, this protocol allows any researcher to keep DRG sensory neurons in cultures from several weeks to months. Due to their excessively long processes DRG neurons organize in large and complex networks. This specificity leads to a culture structured as one single layer of connected cells. The uniformity of the collagen coating and seeding of cells are key players of the culture quality and survival.

1. Collagen coating: when the collagen is removed after 15 min incubation, the experimenter must make sure that no drop of collagen remains on the bottom of the dish. These drops lead to area of excessive collagen deposition, hence nonuniform attachments of the cells to the plate. To avoid this, the aspira-

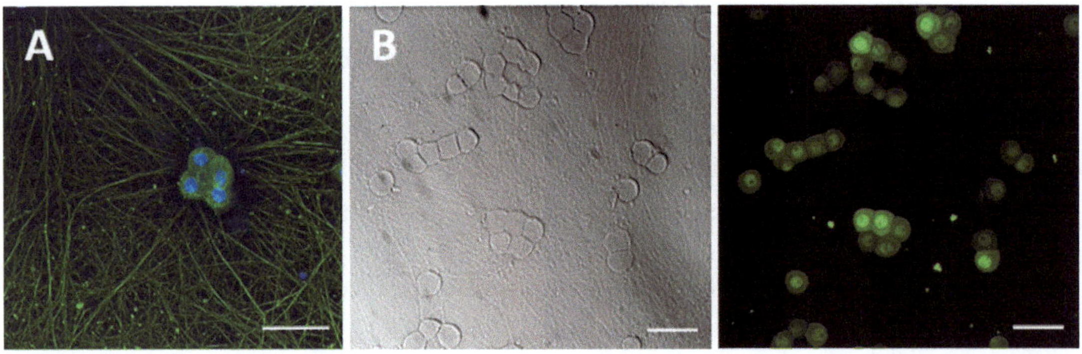

Fig. 3 DRG sensory neuron primary cultures are NF200-positive neuron culture. Primary cultures of mouse DRG sensory neurons were fixed at 15 days, and stained by immunofluorescence with primary antibody against either Neurofilament 200 kDa (NF200; ab4680, Abcam) (**a**) or NeuN (266004, Synaptic Systems) (**b**), and a fluorescent secondary against guinnea pig (A11073, Molecular Probes) or chicken (703-545-155, Jackson ImmunoResearch) IgG. (**c**) Bright field image of culture. Every cell is positive for both NF200 and NeuN, indicating that the culture is purely neuronal, and composed of large sensory neuron cell types (NF200-positive). Scalebars = 50 μm

tion must be kept on for one second after the collagen solution was fully removed. Holding the aspiration for more than one second will make the opposite effect which is that too much collagen is removed, inducing a nonefficient coating and attachment of the cells to the plate.

2. Cell density and seeding homogenization, 35 mm petri dish: the quality of the culture almost essentially depends on the density of the cells and their correct spreading of the dish. As DRG sensory neuron are likely to organize in networks, cell bodies will aggregate in small groups (in general from 2 to 6). The cells attach to the bottom of the dish initially as single cells. After a few hours in culture, they will tend to move from their initial docking point to join surrounding cells. If cells are not evenly spread, some isolated cells will not be able to join a group which will cause them to die. In order to prevent that, the cell suspension density has to be optimized regarding the support. In this protocol we provide optimized densities for 35 mm petri dish and 13 mm coverslips (500,000 cells/mL, 1 mL or 100 μL). In addition, when the suspension is deposited on the petri dish, the medium has to be spread on the maximal area of the dish without touching the edges and the experimenter must perform 2 or 3 up and downs. It is very important that the medium does not touch the sides of the dish. If it is the case, the suspension must be taken back and the petri dish discarded. Moreover, once the cells are spread, the plate must be placed at 37 °C within a few minutes. Hence, keeping the cells at RT for more than 15 min will cause them to aggregate in the center of the plate, which will increase the density at the center.
3. Before going on with the cell deposition, the experimenter must let the coverslip to dry and place it in the center of the well. In order to do that, the medium must be fully removed and the coverslip must be moved to the center with the aspiration pipette. This step will remove the medium from underneath the slide and hence stick it to the bottom. If the well is not completely dried and the cover in the center, the cell suspension will spread outside the coverslip causing the cells to spread on the corners of the well. This time, it is not necessary to perform up-and-downs as only 100 μL of suspension is deposited as one step.
4. In order to keep the culture attached through the multiple medium changes, attention should be taken not to let the culture dry out. In order to prevent that, a bit of medium has to be left in the dish at every change (approximately 200 μL, enough to cover the extremities of the culture). In addition, the medium must be gently and slowly disposed.

Acknowledgments

We thank Aurélie Eisenmann and Alain Martelli for technical assistance. This work was supported by the US Friedreich Ataxia Research Alliance (to H.P.), the Association Française pour l'Ataxie de Friedreich (to H.P.) and the Fondation pour la Recherche Médicale (FRM grant number ECO20160736060 (to O.G.)). This study was supported by the grant ANR-10-LABX-0030-INRT, a French State fund managed by the Agence Nationale de la Recherche under the frame program Investissement d'Avenir ANR-10-IDEX-0002-02.

References

1. Melli G, Höke A (2009) Dorsal root ganglia sensory neuronal cultures: a tool for drug discovery for peripheral neuropathies. Expert Opin Drug Discovery 4:1035–1045
2. Marmigère F, Ernfors P (2007) Specification and connectivity of neuronal subtypes in the sensory lineage. Nat Rev Neurosci 8:114–127
3. Leinninger GM, Edwards JL, Lipshaw MJ, Feldman EL (2006) Mechanisms of disease: mitochondria as new therapeutic targets in diabetic neuropathy. Nat Clin Pract Neurol 2:620–628
4. Estanislao L, Carter K, McArthur J, Olney R, Simpson D, Lidoderm-HIV Neuropathy Group (2004) A randomized controlled trial of 5% lidocaine gel for HIV-associated distal symmetric polyneuropathy. J Acquir Immune Defic Syndr 37:1584–1586
5. Lewis RA (2017) Chronic inflammatory demyelinating polyneuropathy. Curr Opin Neurol 30:508–512
6. McGrath MC (2016) Charcot-Marie-Tooth 1A: a narrative review with clinical and anatomical perspectives. Clin Anat 29:547–554
7. Staff NP, Grisold A, Grisold W, Windebank AJ (2017) Chemotherapy-induced peripheral neuropathy: A current review. Ann Neurol 81:772–781
8. Harding AE (1981) Friedreich's ataxia: a clinical and genetic study of 90 families with an analysis of early diagnostic criteria and intrafamilial clustering of clinical features. Brain 104:589–620
9. Harding AE, Hewer RL (1983) The heart disease of Friedreich's Ataxia: a clinical and electrocardiographic study of 115 patients, with an analysis of serial electrocardiographic changes in 30 cases. QJM 52:489–502
10. Koeppen AH, Mazurkiewicz JE (2013) Friedreich ataxia: neuropathology Revised. J Neuropathol Exp Neurol 72:78–90
11. Koeppen AH (2011) Friedreich's ataxia: Pathology, pathogenesis, and molecular genetics. J Neurol Sci 303:1–12
12. Beilschmidt LK, Puccio HM (2014) Mammalian Fe–S cluster biogenesis and its implication in disease. Biochimie 100:48–60
13. Saveliev A, Everett C, Sharpe T, Webster Z, Festenstein R (2003) DNA triplet repeats mediate heterochromatin-protein-1-sensitive variegated gene silencing. Nature 422:909–913
14. Pandolfo M (2009) Friedreich ataxia: the clinical picture. J Neurol 256:3–8
15. Koeppen AH, Ramirez RL, Becker AB, Bjork ST, Levi S, Santambrogio P, Parsons PJ, Kruger PC, Yang KX, Feustel PJ et al (2015) The pathogenesis of cardiomyopathy in Friedreich Ataxia. PLoS One 10:e0116396
16. Puccio H, Simon D, Cossée M, Criqui-Filipe P, Tiziano F, Melki J, Hindelang C, Matyas R, Rustin P, Koenig M (2001) Mouse models for Friedreich ataxia exhibit cardiomyopathy, sensory nerve defect and Fe-S enzyme deficiency followed by intramitochondrial iron deposits. Nat Genet 27:181–186
17. Piguet F, Montigny C, de Vaucamps N, Reutenauer L, Eisenmann A, Puccio H (2018) Rapid and complete reversal of sensory ataxia by gene therapy in a novel model of Friedreich Ataxia. Mol Ther 26(8):1940–1952
18. Miranda CJ, Santos MM, Ohshima K, Smith J, Li L, Bunting M, Cossée M, Koenig M, Sequeiros J, Kaplan J et al (2002) Frataxin knockin mouse. FEBS Lett 512:291–297
19. Al-Mahdawi S, Pinto RM, Varshney D, Lawrence L, Lowrie MB, Hughes S, Webster Z, Blake J, Cooper JM, King R et al (2006) GAA repeat expansion mutation mouse models of Friedreich ataxia exhibit oxidative stress leading to progressive neuronal and cardiac pathology. Genomics 88:580–590

20. Campuzano V, Montermini L, Moltò MD, Pianese L, Cossée M, Cavalcanti F, Monros E, Rodius F, Duclos F, Monticelli A et al (1996) Friedreich's Ataxia: autosomal recessive disease caused by an Intronic GAA triplet repeat expansion. Science 271:1423–1427
21. Simon D, Seznec H, Gansmuller A, Carelle N, Weber P, Metzger D, Rustin P, Koenig M, Puccio H (2004) Friedreich Ataxia mouse models with progressive cerebellar and sensory ataxia reveal autophagic neurodegeneration in dorsal root ganglia. J Neurosci 24:1987–1995
22. Thierbach R, Schulz TJ, Isken F, Voigt A, Mietzner B, Drewes G, von Kleist-Retzow J-C, Wiesner RJ, Magnuson MA, Puccio H et al (2005) Targeted disruption of hepatic frataxin expression causes impaired mitochondrial function, decreased life span and tumor growth in mice. Hum Mol Genet 14:3857–3864

Chapter 16

GFP Reporters to Monitor Instability and Expression of Expanded CAG/CTG Repeats

Cinzia Cinesi, Bin Yang, and Vincent Dion

Abstract

Expanded CAG/CTG repeats are genetically unstable and, upon expression, cause neurological and neuromuscular diseases. The molecular mechanisms of repeat instability and expression remain poorly understood despite their importance for the pathogenesis of a family of 14 devastating human diseases. This is in part because conventional assays are tedious and time-consuming. Recently, however, GFP-based reporters have been designed to provide a rapid and reliable means of assessing these parameters. Here we provide protocols for quantifying repeat instability and expression using a GFP-based chromosomal reporter and the newly developed ParB/ANCHOR-mediated Inducible Targeting (PInT) and how to validate the results.

Key words Expanded CAG/CTG repeat diseases, GFP reporters, Gene expression, Genome stability, DNA repair

1 Introduction

Huntington disease (HD), myotonic dystrophy (DM1), and several autosomal dominant spinocerebellar ataxias (SCAs) are part of a family of disorders caused by the aberrant expansion of CAG/CTG repeats [1]. The size of the expansion is the primary driver of pathogenesis with longer repeats leading to more severe phenotype [2, 3]. Thus, germline expansion leads to a worsening of the disease phenotypes through generations, a phenomenon known as anticipation. Continual somatic expansions in affected individuals determine, at least in part, how early the symptoms manifest themselves [4]. An attractive hypothesis, therefore, would be to contract the repeat tract to prevent the development of the disease and perhaps slow, stop, or reverse its progression. It is currently unclear how contractions occur even though harnessing this mechanism may have therapeutic implications [5–12]. Thus, measuring and quantifying repeat instability is critical for our understanding of the

Guy-Franck Richard (ed.), *Trinucleotide Repeats: Methods and Protocols*, Methods in Molecular Biology, vol. 2056, https://doi.org/10.1007/978-1-4939-9784-8_16, © Springer Science+Business Media, LLC, part of Springer Nature 2020

molecular mechanisms, diagnostics, and of the design of disease-altering treatments.

The first assay used to detect somatic CAG/CTG repeat instability was Southern blotting, which originally allowed the identification of these dynamic mutations [13–15]. Instability appears as a smear on Southern blots, which is difficult to quantify and requires several micrograms of DNA. In 1995, Monckton et al developed small-pool PCR (SP-PCR) for quantifying repeat instability more precisely and accurately [16]. SP-PCR refers to the use of only a small number, or a small pool, of alleles as templates for PCR amplification. The amplicons are then run on an agarose gel and, because of the low amounts of PCR products, transferred on a membrane. The subsequent Southern blot uses the expected PCR product or an oligonucleotide binding the repeat tract as probes. The results are discrete bands of varying sizes that can be accurately quantified. The approach can detect frequencies of instability down to 10^{-2}. Some recent variations help prevent carry-over contaminations [17], avoiding the use of radioactive probes [18], or making the process significantly faster [19]. This approach remains the gold standard for measuring repeat instability.

One of the most commonly used assays is the GeneScan approach developed in 1996 [20]. In this assay, primers are labeled with a fluorescent dye, the repeat amplified with a PCR using as much as 100 ng of DNA and run into a capillary electrophoresis-based sequencer. This has the advantage of being straightforward, but suffers from a relative lack of sensitivity and potential biases against the amplification of longer alleles compared to small-pool PCR.

In 2001, a plasmid-based assay was developed [21] in which a vector containing a repeat tract is transfected into primate cells, recovered after replication, and transformed into bacteria. The plasmid molecules are then isolated and digested, and the repeat tract is sized on a polyacrylamide gel. This method has been particularly useful to study the effect of *cis*-elements, especially the effect of the position of origins of replication relative to the repeats [21–23]. Similarly, the Lahue lab designed a shuttle plasmid-based assay to detect expansions or contractions [24, 25]. In this assay, plasmids are transfected into human cells and the replicated molecules are recovered and transformed into yeast. The plasmids contain a yeast selectable system that enables quantification of expansions or contractions rates. The advantage is that it eliminates the need for isolating plasmid DNA from *E. coli* and digesting it. The disadvantage is that the assay does not measure both expansions and contractions at the same time and requires two different plasmids to do so. Importantly, this approach has been successful in identifying the role of mismatch repair and histone deacetylases in repeat instability [26–28].

Selectable chromosomal reporters were also designed by the Wilson lab [29, 30]. These assays were based on the use of the *APRT* and *HPRT* genes, whose function can be selected for or against. The insertion of a CAG repeat interferes with the splicing of the reporter. Fortuitously, this works because there was an inefficient branch point cloned in from the DM1 locus [29]. It creates an alternative exon that includes the repeat tract, minus the first CAG. It then brings in 38 bp downstream of the repeat, leading to a frameshift in the mRNA. The strength of the CAG exon inclusion depends on the number of CAG repeats, due to the splicing enhancer nature of CA dinucleotides [31]. The strength of these assays is that they use CAG/CTG repeats that are embedded into the genome and they are easily coupled to siRNA or small molecule treatments. Moreover, they are exquisitely sensitive and can detect as few as one contraction in 10^{-6} cells. Their weakness is that they only assay very specific events: large contractions. Attempts to use the same approach to measure expansions have not been successful to the point of being practical [32]. Nevertheless, these reporters were instrumental in uncovering the role of DNA methylation, R-loop, and transcription-coupled repair in generating contractions [30, 33–37]. An updated version of this assay uses a GFP mini-gene as a read out, making it suitable for higher throughput experiments and allowing to monitor both expansions and contractions at the same time [38, 39]. This comes at the cost of sensitivity, which is only slightly better than SP-PCR [38]. In addition, decreases in repeat instability are more difficult to detect and depend on the background instability present in the sample. This later version is the topic of this review.

In addition to their genetic instability, expanded CAG/CTG repeats accumulate characteristics of heterochromatin at disease loci and, when they reach several hundreds of repeats, are downregulated, but not completely silenced [40]. Conditional transgenic mouse models have shown that sustained expression of the expanded CAG/CTG tract is essential for disease progression [41–43]. The implication is that being able to downregulate the expanded allele, while leaving the expression of the normal allele untouched, would be highly beneficial. There is biochemical [44] and genetic [45, 46] evidence that extra factors required to transcribe through a repeat tract, but the exact mechanism remains an enigma.

Identifying genetic factors that affect the instability and the expression of expanded CAG/CTG repeats is critical, yet it has been slow in part due to the tedious assays available. Here we describe the protocols to be used with our chromosomal GFP-based reporters. The reporter is useful to monitor CAG/CTG repeat instability as well as the effect of expanded CAG/CTG repeats on transcription and splicing.

1.1 A GFP Reporter to Monitor Instability and Gene Expression at Expanded CAG/CTG Repeats

Santillan et al. built a GFP-based reporter that consists of a single copy GFP mini-gene integrated into the genome of HEK293 T-Rex Flp-In cells [39] (Fig. 1). There are two GFP exons interrupted by the intron of the rat *Pem1* gene. The sequences surrounding the CAG repeats are the same as those in the *APRT* and

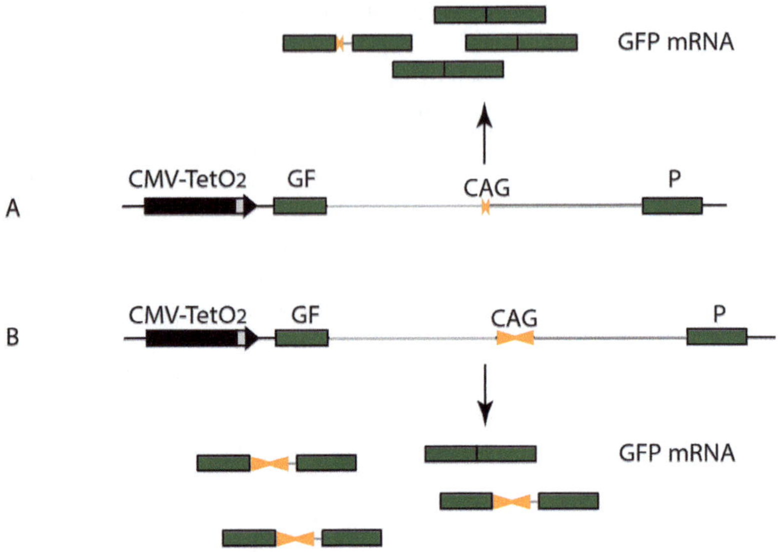

Fig. 1 Schematic of the GFP reporter. GFP reporter consists of an inducible promoter (CMV-TetO_2), an intron (grey line) containing a CAG repeat (orange) and flanked by two GFP exons. Changes in repeat size alter the efficiency of inclusion of the CAG exon, which renders the GFP transcript nonfunctional

HPRT reporters and thus work the same way through influencing splicing. Conveniently, measuring GFP fluorescence by flow cytometry can serve as a proxy for repeat size. Transcription is driven by a doxycycline (dox)-inducible promoter. Consequently, the experimenter has full temporal control of the transcription through the repeat tract. Repeat instability will result in a broadening of the GFP intensity distribution whereas a change in transcription will shift the entire distribution (Fig. 2). Confirmation of repeat size variation can be done in several ways. One straight forward but lengthy method is simply to sort single cells based on their GFP levels, grow the clones, isolate DNA, amplify the repeat tract, and sequence the PCR product using Sanger sequencing. A SP-PCR can also be performed using the sorted or unsorted populations. Changes in GFP expression that occur independently of repeat instability can be confirmed by RT-qPCR, RNA sequencing, and/or Northern blotting.

1.2 ParB/ANCHOR-Mediated Inducible Targeting (PInT)

PInT was designed to address the question of whether a protein of interest (POI) affects gene expression or repeat instability because of a local role or via another function in trans. This problem is a general one. For instance, it is not possible to ascribe a local role to a chromatin modifying enzyme using a loss of function approach, such as knockdown or knockout. The effect observed can also be due to changes in the expression of another, unlinked gene that itself has an effect on the locus of interest. PInT gets around this

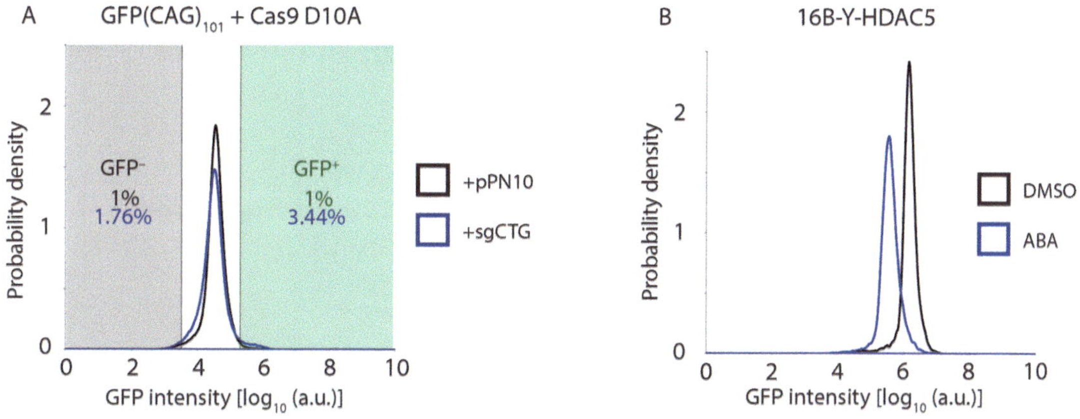

Fig. 2 Example of flow cytometry data. (**a**) The histogram shows variation GFP expression in a population of GFP(CAG)$_{101}$ cells after transfection with vectors expressing the Cas9 nickase and sgCTG. The results were collected 5 days after transfection. In this particular experiment, the treatment induced a 3.44-fold increase in the number of GFP^{+} cells, which indicate the presence of contractions, and 1.76-fold increase in the number of GFP^{-} cells compared to cells transfected with the Cas9 nickase and an empty sgRNA vector. This dataset was published in [38]. The *Y* axis is generated using a kernel density estimation. (**b**) Example flow cytometry data using PInT in a cell line stably expressing PYL-HDAC5 and harboring 16 CAG repeats in the intron of the GFP reporter (16-Y-HDAC5) [47]. The addition of ABA, and presumably targeting of PYL-HDAC5, induces a threefold decrease in the mean GFP expression levels

problem. It is a gain-of-function assay with full spatiotemporal control over the POI.

PInT takes advantage of a site-specific targeting system coupled to a chemical inducer of proximity (CIP—Fig. 3). The site-specific targeting system, ANCHOR, is derived from a bacterial protein, ParB, involved in chromosome partitioning in *B. cenocepacia* [48] and its binding sequence, *parS* (here called INT). INT contains four binding sites for ParB dimers. Once nucleated on these sites, ParB oligomerizes and potentially up to 200 molecules are recruited independently of the flanking sequences [49]. INT also has the advantage of being nonrepetitive, in contrast to other bacterial operator-based targeting methods. The ANCHOR system was first used to visualize DNA resection during double-strand break repair in yeast [49]. More recent uses include the visualization of viral replication as well as gene expression in live mammalian cells [50, 51]. In those cases, INT was introduced into the chromosome or in a viral genome where ParB, fused to a fluorescent protein, could be easily detected by fluorescence microscopy. In PInT, INT is inserted 319 bp from a convenient cloning site within the *Pem1* intron. Here the site contains a CAG/CTG repeat tract of various sizes. To make the targeting inducible, ParB is fused to the plant-derived ABA-insensitive 1 (ABI), which forms a dimer with pyrabactin resistance 1-like (PYL) only in the presence of abscisic acid (ABA)[52]. Hence, fusion of any POI to PYL leads to

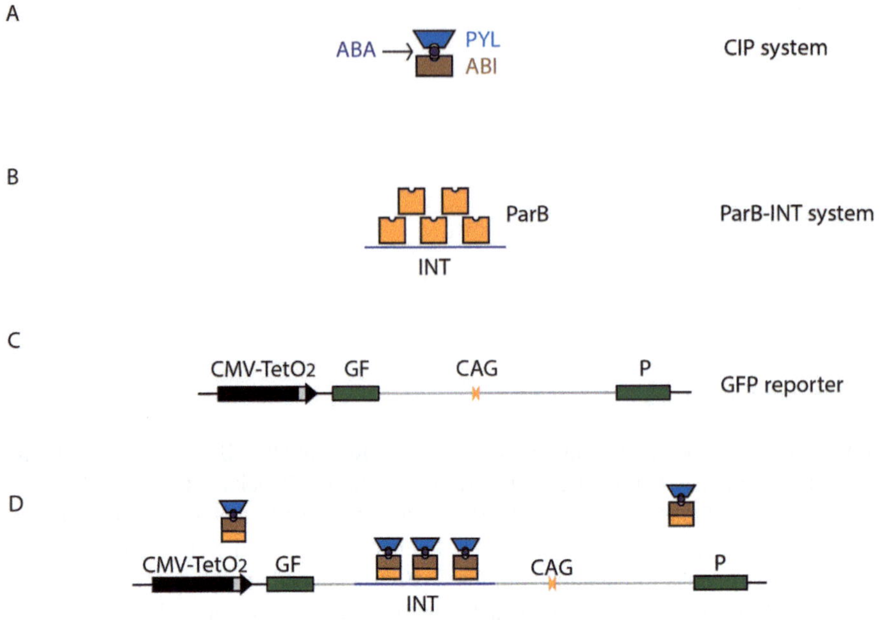

Fig. 3 Schematic of PInT. The system consists of three major parts: a chemical inducer of proximity (CIP) (**a**), the ParB/ANCHOR system (**b**), and the GFP reporter containing the CAG/CTG repeat (**c**). Thus, full spatiotemporal control on the targeting of the POI is achieved and its effect on the GFP reporter can be monitored (**d**)

its inducible and reversible recruitment—merely by washing away ABA from the culture medium.

PInT is highly versatile as it also allows for testing both the effect of a chromatin modifier on gene expression at a sequence of choice as well as the effect of specific intragenic sequences on gene expression. Indeed, several intragenic sequences, including CAG/CTG repeats [40], affect expression in ways that remain poorly understood. Here we provide a protocol for monitoring the effect of a POI on the expression of a GFP reporter containing a repeat tract. In addition, we present a protocol for Chromatin Immunoprecipitation (ChIP) to validate the results.

2 Materials

Prepare all the buffers using Milli-Q water at room temperature.

2.1 Cell Line Maintenance

1. Cell growth medium: DMEM, 10% FBS, 1% of penicillin and streptomycin.
2. Antibiotics: 150 μg/mL hygromycin, 15 μg/mL blasticidin.
3. 12-well plates.

2.2 Cell Line Transfection

1. Poly-D-lysine coated 12-well plates.
2. Lipofectamine 2000 or 3000, Lipofectamine RNAi max.

3. 2 mg/mL Doxycycline dissolved in DMSO.
4. Resuspension buffer: PBS supplemented with 1 mM EDTA.

2.3 PInT System Targeting

1. Cell growth medium: DMEM, 10% FBS, 1% of penicillin and streptomycin.
2. 2 mg/mL Doxycycline dissolved in DMSO.
3. 500 mM ABA dissolved in DMSO.

2.4 Chromatin Immunoprecipitation

1. PBS.
2. Formaldehyde.
3. LB3: 10 mM Tris–HCl pH 8.0, 200 mM NaCl, 1 mM EDTA, 0.5 mM EGTA, 0.1% Na-Deoxycholate (NaDOC), 0.25% Sodium lauroyl sarcosinate (NLS), Protease Inhibitor (Complete Tablets EDTA-free, *EASYpack*, Roche).
4. IP dilution buffer: 1.25% Triton-X, 1 mM EDTA pH 8.0, 0.5 mM EGTA pH 8.0, 16.25 mM Tris–HCl pH 8.0, 137.5 mM NaCl, 1× Complete protease inhibitor (Add fresh).
5. Antibodies: anti-Flag (M2, Sigma), anti-IgG (3E8, Santa Cruz Biotechnology).
6. Protein G Sepharose 4 Fast Flow beads.
7. Wash 1: 0.1% SDS, 1% Triton, 20 mM Tris–HCl pH 8.0, 2 mM EDTA pH 8.0, 300 mM NaCl, filter.
8. Wash 2: 0.1% SDS, 1% Triton, 20 mM Tris–HCl pH 8.0, 2 mM EDTA pH 8.0, 500 mM NaCl, filter.
9. Wash 3: 1% NP-40, 1% Na-deoxycholate, 10 mM Tris–HCl pH 8.0, 1 mM EDTA pH 8.0, 250 mM LiCl, filter.
10. Wash 4: 10 mM Tris–HCl pH 8.0, 1 mM EDTA pH 8.0, filter.
11. 2.5 M Glycine.
12. Crosslink Reversal Buffer: 1% SDS, 0.1 M $NaHCO_3$, 0.5 mM EDTA pH 8.0, 20 mM Tris–HCl pH 8.0, RNase: 100 μg/mL (Add fresh).
13. QIAquick PCR purification kit (Qiagen) or similar columns.
14. Cell sonicator.
15. TPX polymethylpentene tubes (Diagenode).
16. Agarose.
17. TAE electrophoresis buffer.
18. 1.5 mL microtubes.
19. 15 mL tubes.

2.5 Quantitative PCR

1. FastStart Universal SYBR Green Master (Roche).
2. 7900HT Fast Real-Time PCR System or an equivalent qPCR system.

3 Methods

3.1 Cell Line Maintenance

1. Maintain the GFP(CAG)x and PInT cells in DMEM with 10% FBS and 1% of penicillin and streptomycin at 37 °C in the presence of 5% CO_2.
2. Split cell lines (1/5) every 3–4 days with fresh medium in the presence of selection markers (*see* **Note 1**).

3.2 Cell Line Transfection

1. Use poly-D-lysine coated 12-well plates with 600,000 cells per well for all the experiments (*see* **Note 2**).
2. Use Lipofectamine 2000 or 3000 for the transfection of DNA, and Lipofectamine RNAi max to transfect siRNA. Conduct transfections in accordance with the manufacturer's instructions.
3. Six hours after transfection, change the medium to remove the excess of the potentially toxic Lipofectamine reagent. Add doxycycline, dissolved in DMSO, to a final concentration of 2 μg/mL to initiate transcription of the GFP reporter.
4. Change the medium, including the addition of fresh doxycycline, 48 h after transfection. Split the cells if necessary.
5. After another 48 h in culture, gently detach cells using PBS supplemented with 1 mM EDTA (*see* **Note 3**). Use a flow cytometer to measure GFP intensities.

3.3 Flow Cytometry Analysis

1. Collect flow cytometry data using your available flow cytometer. We currently use an Accuri C6 flow cytometer together with the BD Accuri C6 Software (Version 1.0.264.21). We further select the cell populations to be analyzed and quantify the GFP intensities using FlowJo (version 10.5.2). Alternative software may be used.
2. To determine the changes in the number of GFP^+ and GFP^- cells, plot the distribution of GFP intensities as a histogram and draw two gates. One includes the dimmest, the other the brightest 1% of the cells. This is done on the population of cells in the control experiment, for example, transfected with a vector expressing the Cas9 nickase and with an empty sgRNA plasmid. Then ask how much of the test population, here the ones treated with both the nickase and the sgCTG, falls within these gates. Increases suggest that more instability is being generated and vice versa. The 1% cutoff is arbitrary. It represents a compromise between the need for enough events to perform meaningful statistics while making sure that the events that are recorded are indeed expansions and contractions. We propose that users sort cells within their chosen gates and determine repeat sizes by sorting or SP-PCR before assuming that the events they recover are bona fide expansions or contractions. To analyze changes in

gene expression with PInT, we use the mean GFP expression levels and compare multiple independent experiments. We always run a sample treated with DMSO in parallel to one containing ABA. This experimental set up allows direct comparisons between the samples.

3. Export the GFP intensities from FlowJo and use R to plot the results. Our R script includes the geom_density function, which allows smoothing of the curves. The full script is available upon request.

3.4 PInT System Targeting

1. These experiments are conducted as for the GFP(CAG)x cells, without the need for transfection (*see* **Note 4**). Their medium is supplemented with a final concentration of 500 μM ABA or the same volume of DMSO, the vehicle. Add 2 μg/mL doxycycline at the same time to initiate transcription.
2. Split cell 48 h after seeding and add fresh ABA and doxycycline to the growth medium.
3. The flow cytometry step is identical to that of GFP(CAG)x cells.

3.5 Chromatin Immunoprecipitation

To determine whether the targeting indeed is occurring and to quantifying whether the effect seen on gene expression depends on it, we performed a ChIP experiment. We use an antibody against the FLAG-tag found in three copies fused to PYL (*see* **Note 5**). The same protocol can be used to determine the levels of histone acetylation or any other potential protein that might be affected by the targeting.

1. Perform the experiments as indicated above for monitoring GFP expression except that the number of cells needed at the end of the 5 day experiment is 10 million. Therefore, use 10 cm dishes and seed about 4 million cells on the first day.
2. On the fifth day, wash the cells with PBS, incubate with trypsin to detach them for 30 s, replace with 10 mL of growth medium, resuspend, and collect the cells in 15 mL tubes.
3. Take 20 μL cells for counting.
4. Fixation: add formaldehyde to a final concentration of 1%.
5. Shake gently at room temperature for 10 min (*see* **Note 6**).
6. Add Glycine to a final concentration of 0.125 M (from a 2.5 M stock) to quench the formaldehyde. Shake on a wheel for 5 min.
7. Centrifuge the samples at 100×*g* for 5 min, discard supernatant.
8. Add PBS to the cell pellet to obtain 10 million cells/mL, then distribute cells to 1.5 mL microcentrifuge tubes to have 10 million cells per tube (*see* **Note 7**).

9. Centrifuge the samples for 3 min at 100 × *g*, discard the supernatant.
10. The pellets can be frozen at −80 °C at this step for later use.
11. Resuspend the cell pellet in 1 mL of cold LB3 buffer containing freshly added proteinase inhibitors. Keep on ice and transfer in TPX polymethylpentene tubes (*see* **Note 8**).
12. Sonicate the samples with a Diagenode Bioruptor Standard Sonicator at the high power setting, with cycles of 30 s on and 30 s off, for 25–30 min (*see* **Note 9**).
13. Centrifuge 15 min at 4 °C at maximum speed.
14. Collect supernatant of each sample. Keep 20 μL to assess the sonication pattern.
15. Store sonicated cell extracts at −80 °C.
16. Add 80 μL of crosslink reversal buffer to the 20 μL of samples.
17. Incubate from 6 h to overnight at 65 °C.
18. Purify the samples with a Qiagen QIAquick PCR Purification Kit, and elute into 20 μL of water. Load samples on a 1% TAE agarose gel and run for 45 min at 80 V. An optimal sonication pattern will show a DNA smear around 300–500 bp.
19. Resuspend thoroughly the protein G Sepharose 4 Fast Flow beads by gently turning the tubes over several times. Pipet out 70 μL of slurry into a 1.5 mL microtube.
20. Centrifuge the beads at 800 rpm for 2 min at 4 °C to remove the storage buffer and wash twice with ice-cold PBS and then once with ice-cold IP dilution buffer (*see* **Note 10**).
21. Add a final concentration of 1 mg/mL BSA and 0.3 mg/mL salmon sperm DNA. The salmon sperm DNA needs to be denatured at 95 °C for 5 min and then immediately incubate on ice prior to addition to the IP dilution buffer. Add 35 μL of this buffer to the beads and block by shaking on a wheel for 1 h at 4 °C.
22. Once the sonication pattern has been deemed acceptable, keep 20 μL as IP input. Dilute the cell extract 1/5 with IP dilution buffer. Each IP sample needs 200 μL of extract (2 million cells) and 800 μL of IP dilution buffer.
23. Preclean each extract for 30 min to 1 h at 4 °C on a wheel by adding 20 μL of the blocked protein G bead slurry for every 1 mL of diluted sample.
24. Spin the samples for 2 min at 800 rpm, and transfer supernatant into a new tube.

25. Add 50 μL of blocked G beads and 3 μg of the antibody to the sample and incubate overnight on a wheel at 4 °C.
26. Spin IPs for 2 min at 800 rpm at 4 °C.
27. Discard supernatant and wash sequentially with wash buffer 1, 2, and 3. Then twice with wash buffer 4. Every wash consists of 5 min on the wheel at 4 °C, followed by centrifugation for 2 min at 800 rpm at 4 °C.
28. At the end of the last wash, discard buffer.
29. Add 100 μL of crosslink reversal buffer to the beads. In the meantime, thaw the input sample and add 80 μL of the crosslink reversal buffer.
30. Incubate overnight at 65 °C.
31. Purify the samples with the Qiagen QIAquick PCR Purification Kit, and elute with 50 μL of water.

3.6 Quantitative PCR

1. We perform the qPCR with the FastStart Universal SYBR Green Master using a 7900HT Fast Real-Time PCR System in a 384-Well Block Module. Alternative equivalent set ups may also be used.
2. Dilute DNA samples 25 times to obtain *Ct* values between 20 and 30. Primers used to detect enrichment at the INT sequence and *ACTA1* gene were published in [47] and are listed in Table 1.
3. Include three technical replicates for each sample.
4. Analyze the qPCR curves with the SDS Software v2.4 to obtain Ct values for each sample.
5. Plot the data as a function of the percentage of the input. To do so, use the following equation: %Input = $2^{\Delta Ct} * 100\%$, where ΔCt is the Ct difference between the input and the immunoprecipitated samples for a given locus. Be sure to adjust the values for differential dilutions of the input and immunoprecipitated samples.

Table 1
Primers for qPCR of the INT and *ACTA1* loci

Primer name	Target sequence	Primer sequence
oVIN-0969	INT forward	5′ TGAATACCATGCGCTCTA
oVIN-0970	INT reverse	5′ GCCGTTCGTGGCAGAGAT
oVIN-1075	*ACTA1* forward	5′ AGCGCGGCTACAGCTTCAC
oVIN-1076	*ACTA1* reverse	5′ CAGCCGTGGCCATCTCTT

4 Notes

1. In our HEK293-derived cells, hygromycin and blasticidin are used at concentrations of 150 μg/mL and 15 μg/mL, respectively.
2. During the experiments, use dialyzed calf serum and do not include the selection markers or the antibiotics.
3. Do not use Trypsin–EDTA to detach cell from plate here, the cells will aggregate over time and clog the flow cytometer.
4. We found that the best results are obtained by stably integrating the components of the CIP first and then use the Flp recombinase to insert the GFP reporter at a predetermined site in HEK293 T-Rex Flp-In cells (D) [47].
5. We obtained best results using the M2 mouse antibody against FLAG coupled to Protein G beads. The protocol can be adapted to pull down other substrates, but the antibodies and beads must be adjusted accordingly.
6. The exact time of fixation is essential to achieve the perfect sonication pattern.
7. The cell number is critical for proper shearing.
8. These tubes are important to improve sonication and shearing efficiency.
9. Note that some optimization may be necessary.
10. Centrifuging faster will damage the beads.

Acknowledgments

We thank members of Joachim Lingner's lab for help setting up the ChIP protocol and Dinis Barros for help with the figures. This work is supported by Swiss National Foundation professorships (#172936) to V.D. and by the UK Dementia Research Institute, which receives its funding from DRI Ltd, funded by the UK Medical Research Council, Alzheimer's Society and Alzheimer's Research UK.

References

1. Orr HT, Zoghbi HY (2007) Trinucleotide repeat disorders. Annu Rev Neurosci 30:575–621
2. Holmans PA, Massey TH, Jones L (2017) Genetic modifiers of Mendelian disease: Huntington's disease and the trinucleotide repeat disorders. Hum Mol Genet 26:R83–R90
3. Tezenas S, Durr A, Rakowicz M et al (2014) Prediction of the age at onset in spinocerebellar ataxia type 1, 2, 3 and 6. J Med Genet 51:479–486
4. Lòpez-Castel A, Cleary JD, Pearson CE (2010) Repeat instability as the basis for human diseases and as a potential target for therapy. Nat Rev Mol Cell Biol 11:165–170
5. Usdin K, NCM H, Freudenreich CH (2015) Repeat instability during DNA repair: Insights

from model systems. Crit Rev Biochem Mol Biol 50:142–167

6. Schmidt MHM, Pearson CE (2016) Disease-associated repeat instability and mismatch repair. DNA Repair 38:117–126
7. Mcginty RJ, Mirkin SM (2018) Cis- and trans-modifiers of repeat expansions: blending model systems with human genetics. Trends Genet 34:448–465
8. Polyzos AA, Mcmurray CT (2017) Close encounters: moving along bumps, breaks, and bubbles on expanded trinucleotide tracts. DNA Repair 56:144–155
9. Polleys EJ, NCM H, Freudenreich CH (2017) Role of recombination and replication fork restart in repeat instability. DNA Repair 56:156–165
10. Freudenreich CH (2018) R-loops: targets for nuclease cleavage and repeat instability. Curr Genet 64(4):789–794
11. Dion V (2014) Tissue specificity in DNA repair: Lessons from trinucleotide repeat instability. Trends Genet 30:220–229
12. Massey TH, Jones L (2018) The central role of DNA damage and repair in CAG repeat diseases. Dis Model Mech 11(1):pii: dmm031930.
13. Harley HG, Brook JD, Rundle SA et al (1992) Expansions of an unstable DNA phenotypic region and in myotonic dystrophy. Nature 355:545–546
14. Aslanidis C, Jansen G, Amemiya C et al (1992) Cloning of the essential myotonic dystrophy region and mapping of the putative defect. Nature 355:548–551
15. Buxton J, Shelbourne P, Davies J et al (1992) Detection of a unstable fragment of DNA specific to individuals with myotonic dystrophy. Nature 355:547–548
16. Monckton DG, Wong LJ, Ashizawa T, Caskey CT (1995) Somatic mosaicism, germline expansions, germline reversions and intergenerational reductions in myotonic dystrophy males: small pool PCR analyses. Hum Mol Genet 4:1–8
17. Aeschbach L, Dion V (2017) Minimizing carry-over PCR contamination in expanded CAG/CTG repeat instability applications. Sci Rep 7(1):18026
18. Tomé S, Nicole A, Gomes-Pereira M, Gourdon G (2014) Non-Radioactive Detection of Trinucleotide Repeat Size Variability. PLOS Currents Muscular Dystrophy. 2014 Mar 6. Edition 1. https://doi.org/10.1371/currents.md.ad50113b899fa1352ce70c087eead706
19. Dandelot E, Gourdon G (2018) The flash-small-pool PCR: how to transform blotting and numerous hybridization steps into a simple denatured PCR. Biotechniques 64:262–265
20. Mangiarini L, Sathasivam K, Seller M et al (1996) Exon 1 of the HD gene with an expanded CAG repeat Is sufficient to cause a progressive neurological phenotype in transgenic mice. Cell 87:493–506
21. Cleary JD, Nichol K, Wang YH, Pearson CE (2002) Evidence of cis-acting factors in replication-mediated trinucleotide repeat instability. Nat Genet 31:37–46
22. Panigrahi GB, Cleary JD, Pearson CE (2002) In vitro (CTG)*(CAG) expansions and deletions by human cell extracts. J Biol Chem 277:13926–13934
23. Panigrahi GB, Lo A, Foiry L, Pearson CE, Melton DW (2011) Maternal germline-specific effect of DNA ligase I on CTG/CAG instability. Hum Mol Genet 20(11):2131–2143. https://doi.org/10.1093/hmg/ddr099
24. Claassen DA, Lahue RS (2007) Expansions of CAG. CTG repeats in immortalized human astrocytes. Hum Mol Genet 16:3088–3096
25. Farrell BT, Lahue RS (2006) CAG CTG repeat instability in cultured human astrocytes. Nucleic Acids Res 34:4495–4505
26. Keogh N, Chan KY, Li G, Lahue RS (2017) MutSbeta abundance and Msh3 ATP hydrolysis activity are important drivers of CTG • CAG repeat expansions. Nucleic Acids Res 45:10068–10078
27. Gannon AM, Frizzell A, Healy E, Lahue RS (2012) MutS b and histone deacetylase complexes promote expansions of trinucleotide repeats in human cells. Nucleic Acids Res 40:10324–10333
28. Debacker K, Frizzell A, Gleeson O, Kirkham-mccarthy L, Mertz T, Lahue RS (2012) Histone deacetylase complexes promote trinucleotide repeat expansions. PLoS Biol 10(2): e1001257
29. Gorbunova V, Seluanov A, Dion V, Sandor Z, Meservy JL, Wilson JH (2003) Selectable system for monitoring the instability of CTG/CAG triplet repeats in Mammalian cells. Mol Cell Biol 23:4485–4493
30. Lin Y, Dion V, Wilson JH (2006) Transcription promotes contraction of CAG repeat tracts in human cells. Nat Struct Mol Biol 13:179–180
31. Gersappe A, Pintel DJ (1999) CA- and purine-rich elements form a novel bipartite exon enhancer which governs inclusion of the minute virus of mice NS2-specific exon in both singly and doubly spliced mRNAs. Mol Cell Biol 19:364–375
32. Lin Y, Dion V, Wilson JH (2005) A novel selectable system for detecting expansion of CAG CTG repeats in mammalian cells. Mutat Res 572:123–131

33. Dion V, Lin Y, Jr LH, Waterland RA, Wilson JH (2008) Dnmt1 deficiency promotes CAG repeat expansion in the mouse germline. Hum Mol Genet 17:1306–1317
34. Hubert L, Lin Y, Dion V, Wilson JH (2011) Topoisomerase 1 and single-strand break repair modulate transcription-induced CAG repeat contraction in human cells. Mol Cell Biol 31:3105–3112
35. Lin Y, Leng M, Wan M, Wilson JH (2010) Convergent transcription through a long CAG tract destabilizes repeats and induces apoptosis. Mol Cell Biol 30:4435–4451
36. Lin Y, Dent SYR, Wilson JH, Wells RD, Napierala M (2010) R loops stimulate genetic instability of CTG CAG repeats. PNAS 107:692–697
37. Gorbunova V, Seluanov A, Mittelman D, Wilson JH (2004) Genome-wide demethylation destabilizes CTG. CAG trinucleotide repeats in mammalian cells. Hum Mol Genet 13:2979–2989
38. Cinesi C, Aeschbach L, Yang B, Dion V (2016) Contracting CAG/CTG repeats using the CRISPR-Cas9 nickase. Nat Commun 7:13272
39. Santillan BA, Moye C, Mittelman D, Wilson JH (2014) GFP-based fluorescence assay for CAG repeat instability in cultured human cells. PLoS One 9(11):e113952
40. Dion V, Wilson JH (2009) Instability and chromatin structure of expanded trinucleotide repeats. Trends Genet 25:288–297
41. Yamamoto A, Lucas J (2000) Reversal of neuropathology and motor dysfunction in a conditional model of Huntington' s disease. Cell 101:57–66
42. Mahadevan MS, Yadava RS, Yu Q, Balijepalli S, Frenzel-McCardell CD, Bourne TD, Phillips LH (2006) Reversible model of RNA toxicity and cardiac conduction defects in myotonic dystrophy. Nat Genet 38:1066–1070
43. Zu T, LA D, Kaytor MD, Berlinger MS, Zoghbi HY, Clark HB, Orr HT (2004) Recovery from polyglutamine-induced neurodegeneration in conditional SCA1 transgenic mice. J Neurosci 24:8853–8861
44. Parsons MA, Sinden RR, Izban MG (1998) Transcriptional properties of RNA polymerase II within triplet repeat-containing DNA from the human myotonic dystrophy and Fragile X Loci. J Biol Chem 273:26998–27008
45. Cheng H, Chern Y, Chen I, Liu C, Li S, Yan Y, Cohen SN, Cheng T (2015) Effects on murine behavior and lifespan of selectively decreasing expression of mutant huntingtin allele by Supt4h knockdown. PLoS Genet 11(3):e1005043
46. Liu C, Chang C, Chern Y et al (2012) Spt4 Is selectively required for transcription of extended trinucleotide repeats. Cell 148:690–701
47. Yang B, Borgeaud A, Aeschbach L, Dion V (2018) Uncovering the interplay between Epigenome editing efficiency and sequence context using a novel inducible targeting system. bioRxiv. https://doi.org/10.1101/368480
48. Dubarry N, Pasta F, Lane D (2006) ParABS systems of the four replicons of Burkholderia cenocepacia: new chromosome centromeres confer partition specificity. J Bacteriol 188:1489–1496
49. Saad H, Gallardo F, Dalvai M, Tanguy-le-gac N, Lane D, Bystricky K (2014) DNA dynamics during early double-strand break processing revealed by non-intrusive imaging of living. PLoS Genet 10(3):e1004187
50. Germier T, Kocanova S, Walther N, Bancaud A, Shaban HA, Sellou H, Politi AZ, Ellenberg J, Gallardo F, Bystricky K (2017) Real-time imaging of a single gene reveals transcription-initiated local confinement. Biophys J 113:1383–1394
51. Mariamé B, Kappler-Gratias S, Kappler M, Balor S, Gallardo F, Bystricky K (2018) Real-time visualization and quantification of human cytomegalovirus replication in living cells using the ANCHOR DNA labeling technology. J Virol 92:1–22
52. Liang F, Ho WQ, Crabtree GR (2011) Engineering the ABA plant stress pathway for regulation of induced proximity. Sci Signal 4:1–10

Chapter 17

Gene Therapy for Huntington's Disease Using Targeted Endonucleases

Magdalena Dabrowska and Marta Olejniczak

Abstract

Huntington's disease (HD) is a hereditary neurological disorder caused by expansion of the CAG repeat tract in the huntingtin gene (*HTT*). The mutant protein with a long polyglutamine tract is toxic to cells, especially neurons, leading to their progressive degeneration. Similar to many other monogenic diseases, HD is a good target for gene therapy approaches, including the use of programmable endonucleases. Here, we describe a protocol for *HTT* gene knock out using a modified Cas9 protein (nickase, Cas9n) and a pair of sgRNAs flanking the repeats. Recently, we showed that excision of the CAG repeat tract resulted in a frameshift mutation and premature translation termination. As a model, we used HD patient-derived fibroblasts electroporated with a pair of plasmid vectors expressing CRISPR-Cas9n tools. Efficient *HTT* inactivation independent of the CAG tract length was confirmed by Western blotting. A modified version of this protocol involving precise excision of the CAG repeats and insertion of a new DNA sequence by homology directed repair may also be used for the generation of new isogenic cellular models of HD.

Key words Gene therapy, Polyglutamine diseases, CRISPR, Cas9, CAG repeats, HDR

1 Introduction

Huntington's disease (HD) is a hereditary neurological disorder that is caused by a mutation in the first exon of the *HTT* gene. HD patients contain abnormally expanded CAG repeats that translate into a polyglutamine (polyQ) tract in one allele of the *HTT* gene. The accumulation of polyQ-rich huntingtin protein induces a toxic gain-of-function property and affects various cellular activities. It is also postulated that long CAG repeats in transcripts may form a hairpin structure that is responsible for RNA toxicity. HD symptoms involve the loss of neurons in the striatum and cortex accompanied by reactive gliosis and astrocytosis, which lead to progressive movement abnormalities and dementia [1].

Despite many years of research searching for the best therapeutic strategy and considerable progress in the development of antisense and RNA interference (RNAi) technologies, HD is still

Guy-Franck Richard (ed.), *Trinucleotide Repeats: Methods and Protocols*, Methods in Molecular Biology, vol. 2056, https://doi.org/10.1007/978-1-4939-9784-8_17, © Springer Science+Business Media, LLC, part of Springer Nature 2020

incurable [2]. Programmable nucleases, such as CRISPR-Cas9, are currently the most promising tools for targeted genome modifications in a variety of cell types and organisms. RNA-guided Cas9 endonucleases generate double-strand breaks (DSBs), which are repaired by two major mechanisms: nonhomologous end joining (NHEJ) and homology-directed repair (HDR) [3]. NHEJ is prone to errors resulting in indel (*in*sertion/*del*etion) mutations in target sites that may cause frameshifts and/or premature STOP codon generation. Therefore, this method can be used to knock out the expression of protein-coding genes. The more accurate but less frequently used HDR enables precise DNA modifications. In this strategy, exogenously delivered oligodeoxynucleotide (ODN) or plasmid DNA containing homology arms serves as a template for DNA synthesis and faithful repair. To increase the specificity of genome editing, one of two cleavage domains of Cas9 is mutated to form a nickase (Cas9n) that cuts only one DNA strand. DSBs are induced by using a pair of single-guide RNA (sgRNA)-Cas9n complexes targeting opposite DNA strands. This modification reduces off-target activity up to 1500-fold [4, 5] and increases the number of HDR events compared to those of wild-type Cas9 (wtCas9) [6, 7].

Several genome-editing approaches have been applied in experimental therapy for HD [8]. In an allele-selective strategy, single-nucleotide polymorphisms (SNPs) were used as a target for CRISPR-Cas9 to cut and inactivate only the mutant allele [9, 10]. In another nonallele selective strategy, *HTT* inactivation was achieved by excision of a DNA fragment containing CAG repeats by a pair of sgRNAs and wtCas9 [11].

Recently, we developed a similar strategy for *HTT* knock out by CAG repeat excision [12]. In contrast to the previous study, we use Cas9 nickase, which is more precise than wtCas9. Here, we describe a protocol for *HTT* gene knock out with this strategy. A pair of sgRNAs (sgRNA1 and sgRNA4) is designed to target sequences upstream and downstream of the CAG repeats and induce double cuts on the opposite DNA strands (Fig. 1a). Plasmid-encoded sgRNAs coexpressed with Cas9n and a GFP marker are electroporated into HD patient-derived fibroblasts containing different numbers of CAG repeat tracts (Fig. 1b). GFP-positive cells are sorted by FACS prior to DNA, RNA and protein

Fig. 1 (continued) performed in the fibroblasts (**b**) and HEK293T cells (**c**). Both cell lines were electroporated with plasmids encoding the Cas9n protein, sgRNA1 and sgRNA4 pair. Additionally, HEK293T cells were electroporated with a 179 nt ssODN as the HDR template. Two days after electroporation, fibroblast cells were sorted by FACS based on GFP expression and cultured until they reached 80% confluence. DNA, RNA and proteins were isolated and used for PCR, Sanger sequencing, qRT-PCR and Western blot analyses, respectively. After electroporation, the HEK293T cells were plated in a 150 mm cell dish and cultured until single cells formed colonies. The colonies were separated into a 48 well plate using cloning rings. When the cells reached 80% confluence, DNA was isolated from each single-cell-derived clone. The product size and sequence was confirmed by PCR and Sanger sequencing

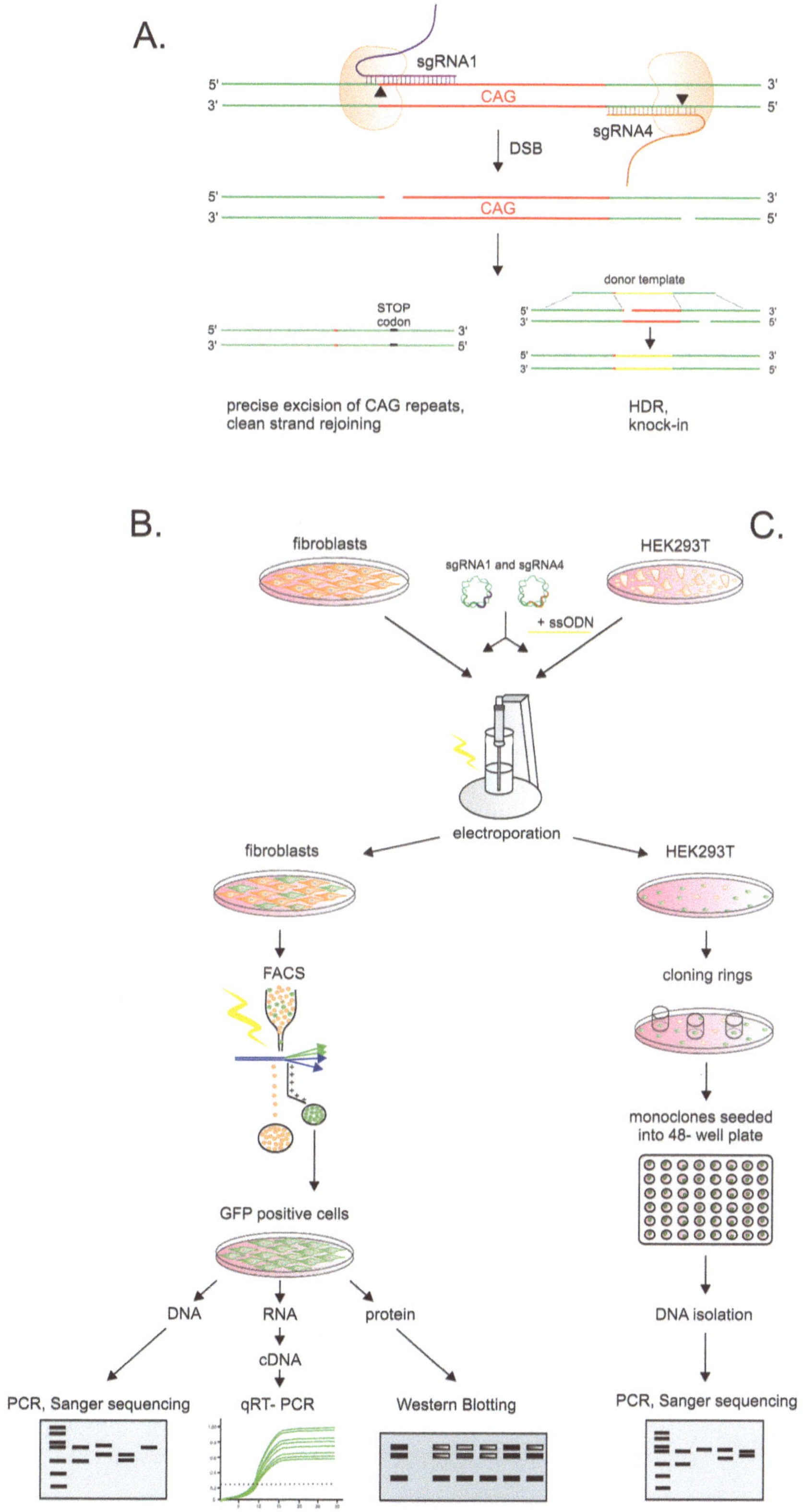

Fig. 1 A strategy utilizing a pair of sgRNAs and the Cas9n protein for precise excision of the CAG repeat tract (knock-out) or insertion of a new sequence by HDR (knockin), respectively (**a**). Schematic representation of procedures

isolation. Precise excision of CAG repeats and premature stop codon generation in the DNA and mRNA are confirmed by PCR and Sanger sequencing. The HTT protein level should be efficiently reduced by ~70% and confirmed by Western blotting.

The above strategy may also be useful for the generation of new isogenic models of HD. Therefore, in a modified version of the protocol, HEK293T cells are transfected with a pair of plasmids encoding Cas9n, sgRNA1 and sgRNA4 together with the donor template (e.g., ssODN) (Fig. 1c). The presence of a new sequence in the *HTT locus* resulting from HDR is confirmed by PCR and Sanger sequencing analysis of single-cell-derived clones.

2 Materials

2.1 Cloning

1. Plasmid: pSpCas9n(BB)-2A-GFP (D10A nickase mutant; Addgene, Cambridge, MA, USA, ID: PX461).
2. DNA oligonucleotides for sgRNA construction.
3. U6-Fwd primer (Table 1).
4. Restriction enzyme: FastDigest BpiI.
5. T4 DNA ligase, 20 U/μL.
6. 10× T4 DNA ligase buffer.
7. DNase- and RNase-free water.
8. Ampicillin.
9. LB medium.

Table 1
List of primers used

Name	Sequence
U6-Fwd	GAGGGCCTATTTCCCATGATTCC
HD1F	CCGCTCAGGTTCTGCTTTTA
HD1R	GGCTGAGGCAGCAGCGGCTG
HD_F	CGACAGCGAGTCAGTGATTG
HD_R	ACCACTCTGGCTTCACAAGG
GAPDH_F	GAAGGTGAAGGTCGGAGTC
GAPDH_R	GAAGATGGTGATGGGATTTC
sgRNA1s	CACCGCTGCTGCTGCTGCTGCTGGA
sgRNA1a	AAACTCCAGCAGCAGCAGCAGCAGC
sgRNA4s	CACCGGCTTCCTCAGCCGCCGCCGC
sgRNA4a	AAACGCGGCGGCGGCTGAGGAAGCC

10. LB agar medium.
11. ChemiComp GT116 *E. coli* (InvivoGen, San Diego, CA, USA).
12. Gene JET Plasmid Miniprep Kit (Thermo Fisher Scientific).
13. GenElute HP Endotoxin-Free Plasmid Maxiprep Kit.
14. Petri dishes, 100 mm.
15. PCR tubes.
16. Ice.
17. Fridge.
18. Thermocycler.
19. Microbiological incubator at 37 °C.
20. Bacterial incubator shaker at 37 °C.

2.2 Cell Culture

1. Patient-derived fibroblasts: GMO4208, 21/44 CAG in the *HTT* gene; GMO4281, 17/68 CAG in the *HTT* gene; and GMO9197, 21/151 CAG in the *HTT* gene (Coriell Cell Repositories, Camden, NJ, USA).
2. HEK293T cells (ATCC).
3. Minimal essential medium (MEM).
4. Dulbecco's modified Eagle's medium (DMEM) supplemented with 10% FBS, L-glutamine, and antibiotics.
5. Phosphate-buffered saline (PBS).
6. 10× trypsin–EDTA solution.
7. 0.4% Trypan blue solution.
8. TC20 automated cell counter and counting slides (Bio-Rad).
9. Tissue culture plates, pipettes, microtubes, 50 mL and 5 mL polypropylene tubes.
10. 5% CO_2 humidified incubator.
11. Water bath.
12. Microscope.
13. Centrifuge.

2.3 Electroporation

1. SpCas9n(BB)-2A-GFP (D10A nickase mutant) plasmid with cloned oligos corresponding to sgRNA1 and sgRNA4.
2. Single-stranded oligodeoxynucleotide (ssODN) as a donor template for HDR.
3. Neon transfection system: E and E2 buffers, R buffer, and 100 μL and 10 μL tips (Invitrogen).
4. 50 mg/mL Normocin.
5. 60-mm and 150-mm cell culture dishes.

2.4 Cell Sorting (Fibroblasts)

1. BD FACSAria III sorter (BD Biosciences).
2. FACSDIVA software (BD Biosciences).
3. Cell culture medium with 50% FBS.
4. FACS polystyrene tubes, 5 mL.

2.5 Single-Cell-Derived Clones (HEK293T)

1. Sterile cloning rings.
2. Cell culture plates, 48 wells.
3. Silicone grease and tweezers.

2.6 Genomic DNA Extraction

1. DNA isolation kit (Norgen, Thorold, ON, Canada).
2. 0.5× Direct-Lyse buffer: 10 mM Tris pH 8.0, 2.5 mM EDTA, 0.2 M NaCl, 0.15% SDS, and 0.3% Tween-20 [13].
3. Spectrophotometer DS-11 (DeNovix).

2.7 Polymerase Chain Reaction (PCR)

1. Phusion High-Fidelity PCR Master Mix (Thermo Fisher Scientific).
2. Target-specific primers: HD1F and HD1R (Table 1).
3. DNase- and RNase-free water.
4. Any kit for purification of PCR products.
5. Thermal cycler.
6. PCR tubes.
7. Ice.

2.8 Gel Electrophoresis and Gel Extraction

1. Agarose powder.
2. TBE electrophoresis buffer.
3. Ethidium bromide.
4. Gel cast, combs, and gel electrophoresis tanks.
5. Gel imaging system, G:BOX (Syngene).
6. UV transilluminator.
7. Scalpel.
8. Gel extraction kit (Thermo Fisher Scientific or equivalent provider).

2.9 RNA Isolation

1. Total RNA isolation kit, Direct-zol RNA MiniPrep (Zymo Research, Irvine, CA, USA).

2.10 cDNA Synthesis

1. Superscript III Reverse Transcriptase (Life Technologies).
2. Random hexamer primers.
3. dNTPs.
4. Ribonuclease inhibitor, RNaseOUT (Invitrogen).
5. DNase- and RNase-free water.

6. Thermal cycler.
7. PCR tubes.
8. Ice.

2.11 Quantitative Real-Time PCR

1. SsoAdvanced™ Universal SYBR® Green Supermix (Bio-Rad).
2. DNase- and RNase-free water.
3. Target-specific primers: HD_F, HD_R, GAPDH_F and GAPDH_R (Table 1).
4. 96-well plates.
5. CFX Connect™ Real-Time PCR Detection System (Bio-Rad).
6. CFX Manager software (Bio-Rad).

2.12 Protein Isolation

1. PB buffer: 60 mM Tris base, 2% SDS, 10% sucrose, and 2 mM PMSF.
2. PCR tubes.
3. Thermocycler.
4. Spectrophotometer.

2.13 Western Blot Analysis

1. Tris–acetate SDS-polyacrylamide gel (3–8%, NuPAGE™, Invitrogen).
2. Tris–acetate SDS running buffer (Novex, Carlsbad, CA, USA).
3. Milk (nonfat dry milk).
4. 10× PBS: 1 tablet in 100 mL (BioShop, Burlington, ON, CA).
5. PBST: PBS, 0.1% Tween 20.
6. Transfer buffer: 25 mM Tris–HCl pH 8.3, 192 mM glycine, 20% methanol, and 0.1% SDS.
7. Primary antibodies: anti-plectin, 1:1000, ab83497 (Abcam, Cambridge, UK) and anti-huntingtin, 1:1000, MAB2166 (Millipore, Burlington, MA, USA).
8. Secondary antibodies: anti-mouse HRP conjugate, 1:2000, A9917 (Sigma-Aldrich) and anti-rabbit HRP conjugate, 1:2000, 711-035-152 (Jackson ImmunoResearch, West Grove, PA, USA).
9. Western blotting device.
10. Western blotting detection solution (WesternBright™ Quantum Kit).
11. Gel imaging system (G:BOX).
12. Gel-Pro Analyzer (Media Cybernetics).

3 Methods

3.1 Cloning a sgRNA into the pSpCas9n(BB)-2A-GFP Vector for Coexpression with Cas9n

1. Digest the pSpCas9n(BB)-2A-GFP plasmid with BpiI enzyme according to the manufacturer's instructions (*see* **Notes 1** and **2**).
2. Run the digested products in a 1% agarose gel, and extract the linearized plasmid using a gel extraction kit (*see* **Note 3**).
3. Measure the DNA concentration using a spectrophotometer.
4. Construct complementary sense (s) and antisense (a) oligonucleotides that correspond to the desired sgRNAs (*see* **Notes 4** and **5**): sgRNA1s, sgRNA1a, sgRNA4s and sgRNA4a (Table 1).
5. Prepare a 100 μM solution of each oligo. Anneal the two complementary oligonucleotides. Assemble the annealing mixture as follows: 1 μL of sense oligo, 1 μL of antisense oligo and 8 μL of 1× DNA annealing buffer. Heat the mixture at 95 °C for 5 min, and then anneal at room temperature for 1 h. Dilute the annealed duplexes 1:100 in RNase- and DNase-free water.
6. Ligate the sgRNA duplex into the linearized pSpCas9n(BB)-2A-GFP plasmid. Set up a ligation reaction as follows: 50 ng of linearized plasmid, 2.5 μL of diluted oligonucleotides, 1 μL of 10× T4 ligase buffer, 0.5 μL of T4 DNA Ligase, and up to 10 μL of H_2O. Incubate the reaction at 4 °C overnight (*see* **Note 6**).

3.2 Bacterial Transformation

1. Thaw ChemiComp GT116 competent cells on ice, and incubate for 5 min on ice.
2. Pipet 45 μL of competent cells into prechilled 1.5-mL tubes, and return the tubes to the ice.
3. Add 5 μL of the ligation reaction mixture to the cells.
4. Incubate the tube on ice for 30 min.
5. Incubate the tube in a 42 °C water bath for 30 s.
6. Place the tube on ice for 2 min.
7. Add 350 μL of room temperature LB medium.
8. Incubate the tubes at 37 °C for 1 h with shaking at 300 rpm.
9. Spread 200–400 μL of the above mixture onto LB agar plates containing 100 μg/mL ampicillin.
10. Incubate the plates at 37 °C overnight.

3.3 Identification of Bacterial Colonies

1. After overnight incubation, pick approximately two colonies, and inoculate them into 3 mL of LB medium with ampicillin (100 μg/mL) in round-bottom tubes. Incubate the growth culture in a bacterial shaker with shaking at 180 rpm overnight at 37 °C.

2. Isolate the plasmid DNA using a miniprep kit (*see* **Note 7**).
3. Inoculate ~0.5 mL of the overnight culture from point 1 into 150 mL of LB medium and 100 μg/mL ampicillin in a bacterial shaker with shaking at 180 rpm overnight at 37 °C.
4. After overnight incubation, isolate the plasmid DNA using an Endotoxin-free Maxiprep Kit according to the manufacturer's instructions.
5. Measure the concentration of the isolated plasmid by using a spectrophotometer.
6. Store the DNA at −20 °C or use immediately.

3.4 Fibroblast and HEK293 Cell Cultures

1. Grow the fibroblasts in MEM supplemented with 10% FBS, L-glutamine (2 mM) and antibiotic (100 U penicillin, 10 mg streptomycin, and 25 μg amphotericin) in a 10 cm culture plate in a 5% CO_2 incubator at 37 °C.
2. Grow the HEK293T cells in DMEM supplemented with 10% FBS, L-glutamine and antibiotics in a 10 cm dish in an incubator supplied with 5% CO_2.
3. Change the medium every 2 days, and harvest the cells when they exceed 80% confluence.
4. Wash the cells with 10 mL of PBS.
5. Harvest the cells using a 1× trypsin–EDTA solution, and the incubate the cells at 37 °C for 3–5 min in an incubator supplied with 5% CO_2.
6. Examine the cells under a microscope to ensure that they have completely detached from the plates, and add 5 mL of complete medium to neutralize the trypsin.
7. Add 7 μL of cells suspended in medium to 7 μL of trypan blue, and then count the cells using a cell counter.

3.5 Electroporation

1. Electroporate the cells with the Neon™ Transfection System (*see* **Note 8**). Harvest 1×10^6 to 5×10^5 fibroblast cells, resuspend the cells in PBS, and electroporate the cells with 10 μg of plasmid DNA (5 μg of each plasmid containing sgRNA1 and sgRNA4) (*see* **Note 9**) in 100 μL tips according to the manufacturer's instructions. Use the following parameters: 1350 V, 30 ms, and 1 pulse.
2. Electroporate 5×10^4 HEK293T cells suspended in R buffer with 125 ng of plasmid (62.5 ng of each plasmid containing sgRNA1 and sgRNA4) and 0.5 μL of 10 μM ssODN in 10 μL tips using the following parameters: 1150 V, 20 ms, and 2 pulses (*see* **Note 10**).

3. Seed the fibroblasts after electroporation into a 60 mm cell culture plate with MEM supplemented with 10% FBS and L-glutamine without antibiotics.
4. Plate the HEK293T cells in a 150 mm plate (~1000 cells per plate), and grow the cells until they form single cell clones.
5. Four hours after electroporation, add 100 μg/mL Normocin to the medium.
6. Check the transfection efficiency 24 h after electroporation. The percentage of fluorescent cells (GFP expression) can by estimated by using a fluorescence microscope (*see* **Note 11**).

3.6 Fluorescence-Activated Cell Sorting (FACS) (See Note 12*)*

1. Sort the cells 48 h post-electroporation.
2. Wash the cells with PBS, harvest them using 1× trypsin–EDTA solution, add complete medium and centrifuge.
3. Suspend the cell pellet in 1 mL of PBS. Set the configuration of the flow cytometer as follows: a 100-m nozzle and 20 psi (0.138 MPa) of sheath fluid pressure.
4. Collect the sorted cells into tubes containing 2.5 mL of medium supplemented with 50% FBS.
5. Analyze the data with FACSDIVA software.
6. Seed the cells into a 6-well plate, add 100 μg/mL Normocin to the medium and maintain them until they reach confluence. Then, collect the cells for genomic DNA extraction (fibroblasts), or seed them into a 150-mm plate (HEK293T cells).

3.7 Single-Cell-Derived Clones from HEK293T Cells

1. Gently wash cells seeded into a 150 mm plate with 10 mL of PBS.
2. Mark individual colonies.
3. Using sterile curved forceps, center the cloning ring over a cell colony (*see* **Note 13**).
4. Add 20 μL of trypsin–EDTA solution directly into the cylinder, and incubate at 37 °C for 2 min in a 5% CO_2 incubator. Monitor the colony under a microscope.
5. Neutralize the trypsin by adding 80 μL of DMEM.
6. Transfer the detached cells from a single colony to a 48-well plate.
7. Grow the cells in a 48-well plate until they reach 60%–80% confluence (*see* **Note 14**).

3.8 DNA Extraction

1. Extract DNA from the fibroblasts using a Cell and Tissue DNA Isolation Kit according to the manufacturer's instructions. Measure the DNA concentration using a spectrophotometer.
2. Isolate DNA from individual HEK293T colonies using 0.5× Direct-Lyse buffer as described by Ramlee et al. [13].

3.9 PCR and Gel Electrophoresis

1. Mix 5 μL of 2× Phusion Master Mix, 1 μL of primers (10 μM mixture of the forward and reverse primers), 100 ng of DNA template and H_2O to a final volume of 10 μL (*see* **Note 15**). Incubate the mixture in a thermal cycler at 98 °C for 3 min, followed by 12 cycles at 98 °C for 15 s and 60 °C for 15 s, an additional 21 cycles at 98 °C for 15 s and 62 °C for 15 s, and a final incubation at 72 °C for 5 min.
2. Run the PCR products with gel loading dye on a 1.3% agarose gel. Use an appropriate DNA ladder. Visualize the products using a gel imaging system.
3. Purify the PCR products.
4. Confirm the sequence of the purified PCR products using Sanger sequencing with the forward primer HD1F (Table 1) (*see* **Note 16** and **17**).

3.10 RNA Isolation and cDNA Synthesis

1. Remove the medium from the cell culture plate, and wash the cells once with PBS.
2. Add an appropriate amount of TRIzol reagent directly into a cell culture dish, and isolate the RNA using a Direct-zol RNA MiniPrep kit according to the manufacturer's instructions. Use the DNase treatment step.
3. To elute the RNA, add DNase- and RNase-free water or TE buffer, and measure the RNA concentration using a spectrophotometer.
4. To perform cDNA synthesis, mix 0.5–1 μg of RNA, 1 μL of 10 μM dNTPs, and 0.25 μL of random primers (500 μg/mL).
5. Incubate the samples at 65 °C for 5 min, and then place them on ice for 1 min. Perform a quick spin, and prepare a new mixture containing 4 μL of 5× First Strand Buffer, 1 μL of 0.1 M DTT, 1 μL of RNase OUT and 1 μL of Superscript III RT.
6. Mix by pipetting, and incubate at 25 °C for 5 min, 55 °C for 60 min and 70 °C for 15 min. Store the cDNA at −20 °C.

3.11 Quantitative Real-Time PCR Analysis

1. Use 700 ng of complementary cDNA for quantitative polymerase chain reaction (qPCR) using SsoAdvanced™ Universal SYBR® Green Supermix (Bio-Rad). Prepare three replicates of each sample with HTT and GAPDH primers.
2. Mix 5 μL of SsoAdvanced™ Universal SYBR® Green Supermix with 1 μL of 10 μM primers (HTT or GAPDH), 3 μL of H_2O and 1 μL of cDNA (*see* **Note 18**).
3. Incubate the samples in the CFX Connect™ Real-Time PCR Detection System under the following conditions: incubation at 95 °C for 30 s, followed by 40 cycles at 95 °C for 15 s and 60 °C for 30 s, and then incubation at 65 °C–95 °C (delta 0.5 °C per 5 s).
4. Analyze the data by using CFX Manager software.

3.12 Protein Isolation

1. Remove the medium from the cells described above, and wash the cells with PBS.
2. Use trypsin–EDTA solution to detach the cells from the dish.
3. Neutralize the trypsin–EDTA solution by using MEM containing 10% FBS.
4. Centrifuge the cells for 5 min at 268 × *g*. Remove the supernatant from the cell pellet.
5. Use PB buffer to isolate total proteins. Add approximately 30 μL of PB buffer to the cell pellet, and denature the proteins in a thermal cycler for 5–10 min at 90 °C.
6. Measure the protein concentration by using a spectrophotometer.
7. Store the isolated proteins at −20 °C, or use immediately for Western blot analysis.

3.13 Western Blotting

1. Mix 30 μg of protein with a sample loading buffer containing 2-mercaptoethanol, and boil for 5 min at 95 °C.
2. Load 12 μL of HiMark™ Prestained Protein Standard and ~15 μL of each sample onto a Tris–acetate SDS-polyacrylamide gel (3–8%), and run the electrophoresis in Tris–acetate SDS running buffer at 170 V and 4 °C.
3. After electrophoresis, equilibrate the SDS-PAGE gels in transfer buffer for 15 min at room temperature.
4. Cut the membrane roughly to the size of the SDS-PAGE gel. Remember the approximate size of the huntingtin (350 kDa) and plectin (500 kDa) proteins. Place the nitrocellulose membrane immediately in transfer buffer.
5. Cut eight pieces of Whatman 3-mm chromatography paper (four pieces per site) to the size of the gel, and wet each piece in transfer buffer.
6. Make a gel sandwich in the following order: (top) one sponge, four wet pieces of Whatman paper, one wet layer of 3-mm nitrocellulose membrane, SDS gel, four wet pieces of Whatman paper and one sponge (bottom). Take care to remove air bubbles by rolling each layer with a clean roller.
7. Electrophoretically transfer the proteins to the membrane at 30 V overnight.
8. Check the transfer efficiency by Ponceau staining. Wash the membrane with PBST. During this step, the membrane may be cut into two pieces containing the huntingtin or plectin protein bands.
9. Place the membrane into a petri dish, and block nonspecific binding using 5% milk dissolved in PBST for 1 h.

10. Prepare the primary and secondary antibody solutions in milk (*see* **Note 19**).
11. Decant the milk, add the primary antibody solution to the membrane in a clean Petri dish, and incubate for 2 h at room temperature in a 3D blot mixer. The membrane should be completely covered by the primary antibody solution. If 10 mL is not sufficient to completely cover the membrane, larger volumes may be used.
12. Decant the primary antibody solution, and wash the membrane three times for 5–20 min with 50 mL of PBST at room temperature in a 3D blot mixer.
13. Add the secondary antibody solution, and incubate the membrane for 1 h at room temperature in a 3D blot mixer.
14. Remove the antibody solution, and wash the membrane three times for 5–20 min with 50 mL of PBST at room temperature in a 3D blot mixer.
15. Prepare the Western blotting detection solution according to the manufacturer's instructions, and add it to the membrane, ensuring that the entire membrane is covered with a thin layer of liquid. Incubate for 5 min in the dark.
16. Put the membrane in a Petri dish cover to dry, and place directly into the G-BOX.
17. Perform several exposures of the membrane such that each band of interest and the marker have the maximum signal. Typically, reference proteins such as plectin give a strong signal and require separation from the huntingtin band.
18. Perform quantified analysis of the bands using Gel-Pro Analyzer

4 Notes

1. The pSpCas9n(BB)-2A-GFP plasmid also expresses the GFP protein, which reveals the transfection efficiency.
2. The Cas9n protein and target-specific sgRNA are encoded in the same vector. For double nicking application, use a 1:1 ratio of plasmids expressing sgRNA1 and sgRNA4.
3. After digestion of the plasmid, ensure that the digestion was completed properly. Check the sample after digestion and without digestion on a 1% agarose gel with a 1 kb DNA ladder.
4. To design other sgRNAs, use CRISPOR (http://crispor.tefor.net/) [14] or other software as described in Cui et al. [15]. This tool identifies suitable target sites and predicts potential

off-targets for each intended part of the genome. Order the necessary oligos as specified by the online tool.

5. An extra "G" has to be added at the 5′ end of the sgRNA when the guide sequence does not begin with "G". The U6 RNA polymerase III promoter that expresses the sgRNA prefers a guanine nucleotide as the first base of its transcript. This trick facilitates sgRNA expression.
6. To properly conduct ligation, purify the digested plasmid, and if necessary, dephosphorylate the cut ends. The digested bands can be isolated from the agarose gel and dephosphorylated using a commercial kit. This step may be necessary to avoid self-ligation and circularization of the plasmid DNA.
7. Verify that the sgRNA oligos were cloned into the plasmid by sequencing from the U6 promoter using the U6-Fwd primer or performing a PCR with correctly designed primers. The primers should be located near an appropriate restriction site in the plasmid sequence.
8. For transfection of HEK293T and fibroblast cells, we recommend nucleofection (Neon transfection system). The Neon™ website contains many protocols and conditions suitable for various cell lines.
9. Vectors delivered into cells via electroporation have to be highly concentrated (concentration between 1 and 5 μg/μL) and free of bacterial toxins. The DNA amount should not exceed 10% of the total reaction volume because this amount influences the transfection efficiency and cell viability after nucleofection.
10. The donor template can be a ssODN, plasmid or PCR product that contains the sequence necessary for strand synthesis during HDR. The ssODN is comprised of two homology arms and the desired sequence. The homology arms need to be complementary to the sequences around the DSB, and their lengths depend on the size of the inserted sequence (usually approximately 30–70 nt). In our experiments, a 179 nt ssODN was used that consisted of two 60 nt homology arms and the 59 nt GFP sequence.
11. The electroporation efficiency depends on the vector size. If the plasmids are more than 8 kb, the transfection efficiency tends to be lower [16].
12. Sort the cells into collection tubes with appropriate medium and a high concentration of FBS. Cells are weak after sorting and need more supplements for recovery.
13. Methods used to generate a monoclonal cell line include serial dilutions or single-cell sorting (one cell per well) into a 96-well plate by using a FACS device. Cells can also be seeded into a

150 mm dish and detached after they reach the appropriate confluency by using cloning rings. Colonies have to be separated from each other to avoid cross-contamination.

14. One or two weeks may be required to form colonies from a single cell. Change the medium supplemented with FBS and antibiotics every 2 days. For better cell growth, make conditioned medium (1:1 ratio of filtered medium from HEK293T cells and new complete DMEM).
15. Using high-fidelity polymerases is important to minimize errors during PCR amplification. Design PCR primers outside the sequence complementary to the homology arms to avoid detection of residual donor template.
16. Modified DNA (after excision of the CAG repeats from the *HTT* gene) is clearly visible on a gel as a shorter PCR product. The products can by purified by using any gel extraction kit. Only purified PCR products can be used for Sanger sequencing.
17. Generally, indel mutations can be detected by mismatch cleavage assays, such as T7E1, a Surveyor assay or other methods, such as ddPCR (droplet digital PCR), IDAA (indel detection by amplicon analysis), deep sequencing, or qEva-CRISPR [17]. However, PCR amplification of the *HTT* gene region, including polymorphic CAG repeats, and the subsequent T7E1 analysis result in the generation of multiple bands in both the treated and untreated control cells. Therefore, a determination of the exact indel frequency in this polymorphic, highly repetitive gene region is difficult using methods based on heteroduplex recognition. We suggest using the qEva-CRISPR assay, which allows for successful analysis of targets located in "difficult" genomic regions [17].
18. Prepare and aliquot the real-time PCR reaction mixture in the dark. Light as well as repeated cycles of thawing and freezing inactivate fluorescent dyes.
19. Dilute the primary antibodies (anti-huntingtin and anti-plectin) and secondary antibodies (anti-mouse HRP conjugate and anti-rabbit HRP conjugate) in PBS/0.1% Tween-20 buffer containing 2.5% nonfat milk to final dilutions of 1:1000 and 1:2000, respectively.

Acknowledgments

This work was supported by a grant from the National Science Center (2015/18/E/NZ2/00678) and from the quality-promoting subsidy under the Leading National Research Center (KNOW) program for 2014–2018.

References

1. Bates GP, Dorsey R, Gusella JF et al (2015) Huntington disease. Nat Rev Dis Primers 1:15005. https://doi.org/10.1038/nrdp.2015.5
2. Wild EJ, Tabrizi SJ (2017) Therapies targeting DNA and RNA in Huntington's disease. Lancet Neurol 16:837–847. https://doi.org/10.1016/S1474-4422(17)30280-6
3. Shibata A, Steinlage M, Barton O et al (2017) DNA double-strand break resection occurs during non-homologous end joining in G1 but is distinct from resection during homologous recombination. Mol Cell 65:671–684.e5. https://doi.org/10.1016/j.molcel.2016.12.016
4. Cho SW, Kim S, Kim Y et al (2014) Analysis of off-target effects of CRISPR/Cas-derived RNA-guided endonucleases and nickases. Genome Res 24:132–141. https://doi.org/10.1101/gr.162339.113
5. Ran FA, Hsu PD, Lin CY et al (2013) Double nicking by RNA-guided CRISPR cas9 for enhanced genome editing specificity. Cell 154:1380–1389. https://doi.org/10.1016/j.cell.2013.08.021
6. Kocher T, Peking P, Klausegger A et al (2017) Cut and paste: efficient homology-directed repair of a dominant negative KRT14 Mutation via CRISPR/Cas9 nickases. Mol Ther 25:2585–2598. https://doi.org/10.1016/j.ymthe.2017.08.015
7. Eggenschwiler R, Moslem M, Fráguas MS et al (2016) Improved bi-allelic modification of a transcriptionally silent locus in patient-derived iPSC by Cas9 nickase. Nat Publ Gr:1–14. https://doi.org/10.1038/srep38198
8. Mosbach V, Poggi L, Richard G-F (2019) Trinucleotide repeat instability during double-strand break repair: from mechanisms to gene therapy. Curr Genet 65:17–28. https://doi.org/10.1007/s00294-018-0865-1
9. Shin JW, Kim K-H, Chao MJ et al (2016) Permanent inactivation of Huntington's disease mutation by personalized allele-specific CRISPR/Cas9. Hum Mol Genet 25(20):4566–4576. https://doi.org/10.1093/hmg/ddw286
10. Monteys AM, Ebanks SA, Keiser MS, Davidson BL (2017) CRISPR/Cas9 editing of the mutant Huntingtin Allele in vitro and in vivo. Mol Ther 25:12–23. https://doi.org/10.1016/j.ymthe.2016.11.010
11. Yang S, Chang R, Yang H et al (2017) CRISPR/Cas9-mediated gene editing ameliorates neurotoxicity in mouse model of Huntington's disease. J Clin Invest 127:2719–2724. https://doi.org/10.1172/JCI92087
12. Dabrowska M, Juzwa W, Krzyzosiak WJ, Olejniczak M (2018) Precise excision of the CAG tract from the Huntingtin gene by Cas9 nickases. Front Neurosci 12:75. https://doi.org/10.3389/FNINS.2018.00075
13. Ramlee MK, Yan T, Cheung AMS et al (2015) High-throughput genotyping of CRISPR/Cas9-mediated mutants using fluorescent PCR-capillary gel electrophoresis. Sci Rep 5:15587. https://doi.org/10.1038/srep15587
14. Haeussler M, Schönig K, Eckert H et al (2016) Evaluation of off-target and on-target scoring algorithms and integration into the guide RNA selection tool CRISPOR. Genome Biol 17:148. https://doi.org/10.1186/s13059-016-1012-2
15. Cui Y, Xu J, Cheng M et al (2018) Review of CRISPR/Cas9 sgRNA design tools. Interdiscip Sci Comput Life Sci 10:455–465. https://doi.org/10.1007/s12539-018-0298-z
16. Yumlu S, Stumm J, Bashir S et al (2017) Gene editing and clonal isolation of human induced pluripotent stem cells using CRISPR/Cas9. Methods 121–122:29–44. https://doi.org/10.1016/j.ymeth.2017.05.009
17. Dabrowska M, Czubak K, Juzwa W et al (2018) qEva-CRISPR: a method for quantitative evaluation of CRISPR/Cas-mediated genome editing in target and off-target sites. Nucleic Acids Res 46:e101. https://doi.org/10.1093/nar/gky505

Index

Guy-Franck Richard (ed.), *Trinucleotide Repeats: Methods and Protocols*, Methods in Molecular Biology, vol. 2056, https://doi.org/10.1007/978-1-4939-9784-8, © Springer Science+Business Media, LLC, part of Springer Nature 2020

P

R

S

T

Y

FSC
www.fsc.org
MIX
Papier aus verantwortungsvollen Quellen
Paper from responsible sources
FSC® C105338

If you have any concerns about our products,
you can contact us on
ProductSafety@springernature.com

In case Publisher is established outside the EU,
the EU authorized representative is:
Springer Nature Customer Service Center GmbH
Europaplatz 3, 69115 Heidelberg, Germany

Printed by Libri Plureos GmbH
in Hamburg, Germany